Caralluma (*Sensu lato*)
Antiobesity Plants

The Authors

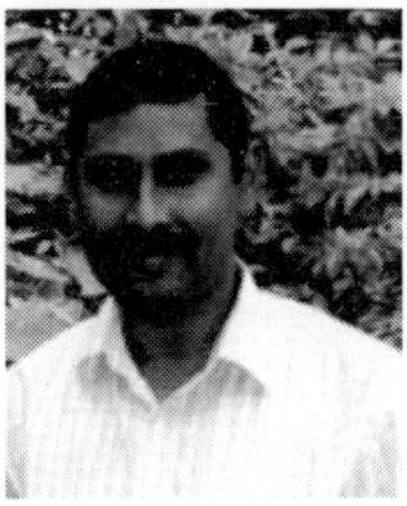

Dr. S. Karuppusamy obtained his M.Sc. (1996) degree from Madurai Kamaraj University and Ph.D (2002) from Gandhigram University, Tamil Nadu. He was a Post Doctoral Fellow at Sri Krishndevaraya University (2000 – 2004), Anantapur. At present he is working as Assistant Professor, Department of Botany, The Madura College, Madurai since 2004. He has published 75 scientific papers in nationally and internationally reputed journals. He is the co-author of Flora of Andhra Pradesh (Vol. 5) and Flora of Eastern Ghats (Vol. 3 & 4). He is the recipient of Young Botanist Award 2006 from Indian Botanical Society. He is the Principal Investigator of two major research projects from UGC, New Delhi and NIF, Ahmedabad. He is life member of many scientific societies in India.

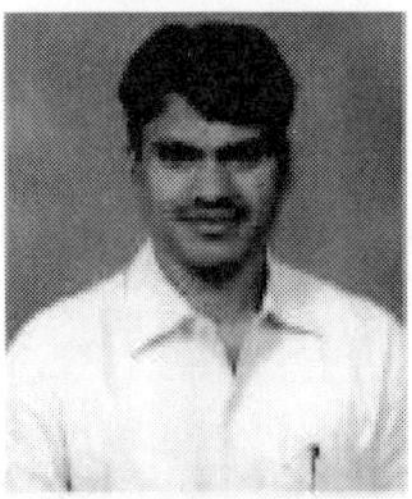

Dr. A. Ugraiah, has completed his Master and doctoral degree from Sri Krishnadevaraya University, Anantapur, A.P. Dr. Ugraiah has been working as a Research Associate since 2011 in Dept. of Crop Physiology, University of Agricultural Science, GKVK, Bangalore. So far he has published eight research papers in national and international journals. He got "BEST PAPER PRESENTATION AWARD" and selected for "YOUNG BOTANIST AWARD" during his doctoral degree. He has attended several national and internal seminars.

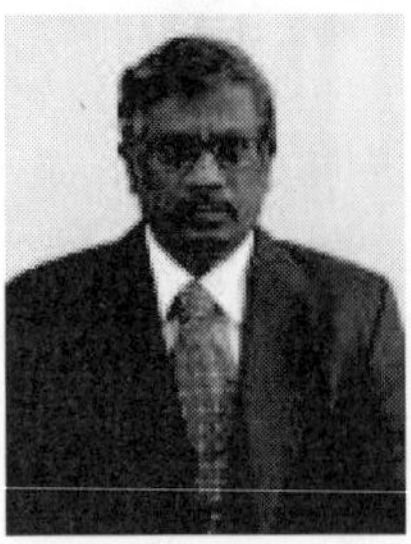

Prof. T. Pullaiah obtained his M.Sc. (1973) and Ph.D. degrees in Botany from Andhra University. He was a Post Doctoral Fellow at Moscow University, Russia, during 1976-78. He traveled widely in Europe and visited Universities and Botanical Gardens in about 16 countries. Professor Pullaiah joined Sri Krishnadevaraya University as Lecturer in 1979 and became Professor in 1993. He held several positions in the University, which include Dean, Faculty of Life Sciences, Head of the Department of Botany, Chairman, BOS in Botany, Head of the Department of Sericulture, Co-ordinator and Chairman, BOS in Biotechnology, Principal, S.K.University College and Warden S.K.U.Hostels. Prof. Pullaiah has published 44 books, 245 research papers and 35 popular articles. He is Principal Investigator of 20 major Research Projects totaling more than a Crore of Rupees funded by DBT, DST, CSIR, UGC, BSI, WWF, GCC, BRNS etc. Under his guidance 50 students obtained their Ph.D. degrees and 34 students their M.Phil. degrees. He is recipient of Best Teacher Award from Government of Andhra Pradesh, Prof. P. Maheshwari Gold Medal of Indian Botanical Society, Prof. Y.D.Tyagi Gold medal of Indian Association for Angiosperm Taxonomy and Scientist of the Year Award from National Environmental Science Academy. He was Vice President of Indian Botanical Society and presently Councilor of the same. He was a member of Species Survival Commission of IUCN.

Caralluma (*Sensu lato*)
Antiobesity Plants

S. Karuppusamy
Department of Botany
The Madura College
Madurai – 625 011
Tamil Nadu

&

A. Ugraiah
T. Pullaiah
Department of Botany
Sri Krishnadevaraya University
Anantapur – 515 003
Andhra Pradesh

2013
Regency Publications
A Division of
Astral International Pvt. Ltd.
New Delhi – 110 002

ISBN 978-81-89233-80-8

Published by : **REGENCY PUBLICATIONS**
A Division of
Astral International Pvt. Ltd.
81, Darya Ganj, Near Hindi Park,
Delhi Medical Association Road,
New Delhi - 110 002
Phone: 011-4354 9197, 2327 8134
Fax: +91-11-2324 3060
E-mail: info@astralint.com
Website: www.astralint.com

Laser Typesetting : **Classic Computer Services**
Delhi - 110 035

Printed at : **Salasar Imaging Systems**
Delhi - 110 035

PRINTED IN INDIA

Preface

Stapeliads are the most attractive group of succulent Asclepiads giving an aesthetic view to the dry areas of India with its assorted and beautifully ornamented flowers. Although the differently coloured flowers with cacti like habits, the determination of scientific names to certainty is often found to be difficult since in the available taxonomic works on Indian plants, these species are described vaguely and collectively incorporating a number of colour variants under each name. Moreover, presently since the rockery or rock gardening is getting wide popularity in the country, there is a trend of introducing exotic cacti in gardens and nurseries, thus leading to great complications in its taxonomic evaluation. This led us to undertake detailed systematic account on the group with the three year project "Taxonomic revision of genus *Caralluma* in India" funded by DST, New Delhi.

The work was initiated by examining the specimens in all the major Indian herbaria. We visited all over India for collection of fresh specimens, our close observation revealed a lot of intraspecific morphological variations, even in the specimens collected from the same locality. This necessitated observation of the plants under cultivation. Accordingly live specimens have been brought from different parts of the country and introduced in the botanical garden at Sri Krishnadevaraya University, Anantapur, Andhra Pradesh state. Most of the specimens from the country easily acclimatized to the local conditions because driest climatic condition prevails throughout the year in Anantapur. We continued our studies with live specimens collected from the field and also some specimens we could not collect in flowering condition. We did not observe complete flower of *Boucerosia procumbens* (Gravely et Mayuranathan) Plowes even after bimonthly visit to the natural habitat from the year 2006. All other plants were collected from the original habitat with flowering and fruiting conditions. Thus, the present book is the result of our continued observation of the plants in natural habitat and under cultivation and also evaluation of their characters for about eight years.

The taxonomic monograph of the 16 Indian species and 10 varieties of the genus *Caralluma* R.Br. and its allies is presented here. Many of the binomials established by earlier workers have been reduced to synonyms after going back to the original publications. One new name *Caralluma adscendens* var. *bicolor* is proposed to replace the earlier taxonomic concept. One species name retained its position *Boucerosia lasiantha* Wight due its original long lasting characters found in live specimens. Both the native and cultivated plants occurring in the country as on date are included. Moreover we included the medicinal importance of the Indian stapeliads, phytochemistry and pharmacology of each species pointed out elaborately. For the conservation purpose we did microporpagation work for almost all Indian *Caralluma* species and established microshoots in garden pots. Necessary information was given on micropropagation techniques of Indian stapeliad succulents. In the last section of the book an illustrative chapter on pioneer workers in Stapeliad taxonomy is added which gives chronological evolution about Stapeliad taxonomy for the young taxonomists.

It is hoped that the book, complete in decription, illustrations, photographs, molecular taxonomy, phytochemistry, pharmacology and notes on cultivation may be helpful to the researchers for undertaking further studies with confidence, as well as to the gardeners, nursery men and plant lovers.

We thank authorities of Botanical Survey of India for permitting us to consult the Herbaria and Libraries. We are also thankful to authorities of Royal Botanical Gardens, Kew for the images of Type specimens. Soumen Aditya spared the photographs of *Caralluma moorei* and *Caralluma sarkariae* var. *longipedicellata*, and we gratefully acknowledge the same.

S. Karuppusamy

A. Ugraiah

T. Pullaiah

Contents

List of Abbreviations

BLAT:	Blatter Herbarium, St. Xavier College, Mumbai
CAL:	Central National Herbarium, Howrah,
Cm:	Centimeter
DD:	Forest Research Institute, Dehra Dun
et al.,:	*et alia* (and others, of people)
FBI:	Hooker's Flora of British India
Fl.:	Flowering season
Fr.:	Fruiting season
Gamble:	Gamble and Fischer's Flora of the Presidency of Madras
m:	metre(s)
MH:	Madras Herbarium, BSI, Southern circle, TNAU campus, Coimbatore
mm:	millimeter(s)
Ori.:	Oriya
p.p.:	*pro parte,* in part
sq. Km.:	Square kilo-metre(s)
ssp.:	subspecies
Tel:	Telugu
Tam.:	Tamil
var.:	Varieties (variety)
Vern.:	Vernacular name(s)

Chapter 1
Introduction

India with its vast geographical area of about 329 m ha, ranks seventh largest country in the world. The diverse physical features and tropical monsoon climate supports rich biological diversity in different ecological habitats. India represents one of the 12 mega diversity centres in the world. The main natural habitats in India are mountains, forests, grasslands, plains, rivers, wetlands, coastal and marsh areas and islands.

India is having 2.4 per cent of global area and exhibits 10 per cent of floral diversity and 6.67 per cent of faunal diversity. India has about 48,000 species of plants representing about 10 per cent of the world's flora (Hajra and Mudgal, 1997), which include ca. 17,500 (Pullaiah, 2008) species of vascular plants with 33.7 per cent of endemism.

India with its highly diverse geology, topography and climate is endowed with a very rich heritage of biological diversity. India is a mega biodiversity country with a high level of endemism of its flora and fauna. The endemic plants and animals by virtue of being restricted only to a particular ecological niche, habitat, biogeographic regions or a country, are comparatively more vulnerable, and therefore merit special consideration in the conservation. In India, a lot of work needs to be done on identification, mapping and biogeography of endemic and endangered plants, for developing strategies for their conservation. About 5725 species of plants are endemic to India distributed in 25 endemic centres, which represents more than one-third of the total recorded species of flowering plants (Nayar, 1996).

According to APG I, II and III, the Asclepiadaceae is a former plant family now treated as a sub family (sub family Asclepiadoideae) under the family Apocynaceae (Angiosperm Phylogeny Group, 2009). They form a group of perennial herbs, twining shrubs, lianas or rarely trees but notably also contain a significant number of leafless stem succulents, belonging to the order Gentianales. The name comes from the type genus *Asclepias* (milkweeds).

World wide the sub family is represented by 348 genera and 2,900 species. They are mainly located in the tropics to subtropics, especially in Africa and South America. The florally advanced tribe Stapeliae within this family contains the relatively familiar stem succulent genera such as *Huernia, Stapelia, Hoodia* and *Caralluma*. They are remarkable for the complex mechanisms they have developed for pollination, which independently parallel the unrelated Orchidaceae, especially in the grouping of their pollen into pollinia. The fragrance from the flowers, often called "carrion", attracts flies, the flies pollinate the flowers. In India, Asclepiadoideae is represented by 43 genera with 243 species, of which five genera are endemic to India (Jagatap and Singh, 1999).

Succulent Asclepiads have a global distribution and are represented in nearly all types of habitats. They are often bizarre growth-forms and attractive flowers have long attracted the attention of botanists, both amateur and professional, and horticultural enthusiasts. Despite the widespread intrest in Stapeliad succulents, and their ecological and economic importance, relatively little attention has been paid to their conservation needs.

Economically the subfamily is of little value. Some genera are of horticultural interest; *Asclepias, Hoya* and related species are grown as outdoor or pot plants, *Dischidia, Stapelia, Caralluma* and *Ceropegia* species can be found all over the world in special hobbyist collections.

Stapeliads

The genera of plants within the subtribe Stapeliae are all to varying degrees stem succulents. Many of the species resemble cacti, though are not closely related, as an example of convergent evolution. The stems are often angular, mostly four-angled in cross-section, but in some species there are six or more, with some species of *Hoodia* having more than thirty angles. The leaves, in most species, are reduced to rudiments, sometimes hardened and thorn-like, arranged on bumps or tubercles on the angles. Some species, however, still have recognisable leaves, most notably the Indian species *Frerea indica*, and some members of *Tridentea*. Stapelias are most abundant in warm, dry climates. In Africa, there are two separate regions where Stapeliads have most diversified: northeast Africa, and Southern Africa. Several species are endemic to the small island of Socotra off the Horn of Africa. The Arabian Peninsula, and most specifically the country of Yemen, contains another concentration of species. Several more are found in the drier parts of Pakistan, Afghanistan, India, Nepal, and Myanmar. A single species, *Caralluma europaea* is found in Europe, in the very southern part of the Iberian peninsula. Stapeliads are often regarded as a climax group within the family because of their often structurally complex flowers. Certain aspects of these reproductive parts mirror the pollination systems in the Orchid family and represent a case of parallel evolution though both groups are quite unrelated and have developed similar, though not identical means to achieve the ultimate goal of pollination and therefore reproduction. Most stapeliads use flies as pollinators, that are attracted to odours resembling dung or rotting meat, emanating from the flowers. Many of the flowers also bear some physical resemblance to rotting animal carcasses, leading to their popular name of 'carrion flowers'. However, not all stapeliads smell bad, or attract flies. Some species use beetles, bees, wasps, butterflies or moths as pollinators. Stapeliad flowers range in size from mere millimetres in species of *Echidnopsis* and *Pseudolithos* to those of *Stapelia gigantea* that can reach 40 cm in diameter, and are some the largest of flowers to be found on any species of succulent.

Stapeliads have represented approximately 30 accepted genera with 400 species. All species are of palaeotropical origin, and many have evolved life-forms with fleshy subterranean parts or stem succulents. The tribe Stapeliae includes the genus *Caralluma, Ceropegia* and of 30 other genera which are collectively known as stapeliads. As stem succulents, with often large and attractive flowers, they are very well known to hobbyist growers and can be found in collections all over the world. In the wild, most of the species are confined to the more arid parts of Africa, but there are also several species occurring in Arabia, India, and Myanmar. Two European species are closely related to those of North Africa. The species mainly form small, widely scattered or sometimes solitary populations. It is becoming increasingly apparent that stapeliads are a comparatively old plant group, in which plate tectonics and changes of climate have led to several migratory processes. This perspective allows for the introduction of a relatively large number of genera in the stapeliads, a view supported by most of the recent studies. Research work so far, however, has mainly been limited to morphological characters and unfortunately has led to divergent concepts of species and even genera.

Northeast Africa is assumed to be the centre of evolution for the stapeliads, but most of the species occur in southern Africa today. This secondary centre (Albers 1983) has evolved its own genera: *Hoodia, Huerniopsis, Lavrania, Notechidnopsis, Ophionella, Orbeanthus, Orbeopsis, Pectinaria, Quaqua, Stapelia, Stapeliopsis, Tavaresia, Trichocaulon, Tridentea,* and *Tromotriche.* The genus *Stapelianthus* is endemic to Madagascar. Only a few genera, like *Huernia* and *Duvalia,* are known on both sides of the equator, the vast majority of the North African species belongs to the genus *Caralluma.* The species from India and Myanmar are included here. Despite intensive research which has been done by Gilbert (1990) the genus still needs attention. With the aid of modern methods it seems to be possible to elucidate this complex. Most of the other large genera of the stapeliads have been revised recently or revisions are in preparation (*Duvalia, 14* spp., Meve, in press; *Echidnopsis,* 31 spp., Bruyns 1988; *Hoodia, 13* spp., Bruyns 1993; *Huernia, 69* spp., Leach 1988; *Lavrania, 5* spp., Bruyns 1993; *Orbea, 21* spp., Leach 1978; *Orbeopsis,* 11 spp., Leach 1978; *Pachycymbium sensu* Gilbert, 31 spp., Gilbert 1990; *Piaranthus* 7 spp., Meve 1994; *Quaqua 24* ssp., Bruyns 1983; *Stapelia, 45* spp., Leach 1985; *Tridentea, 20* ssp., Leach 1980). Valuable information on the distribution and ecology of the species is included in most of the revisions. The *Hoodia/Trichocaulon* complex, which has also been studied by Plowes (1992) still needs a satisfactory nomenclature. Lavranos has contributed to the knowledge of most of the taxa in a valuable way by describing new species and introducing new genera which he had found and collected on field trips in Africa and Arabia. Little is known about the population behaviour of the stapeliads. Observations on *Hoodia* spp. in Namibia indicated that some specimens have a lifespan of approximately 60 years. Albers and Meve (1991) demonstrated, in contrast, that some karroid species with creeping life form behave like ephemerals, *e.g.* within nine years a large *Duvalia caespitosa* population was substituted by a *Stapelia pillansii* population. Further long-term studies of enormous importance for studying conservation status, are needed for other taxa. The myiophilous pollination syndrome of the stapeliads is now being investigated more carefully (Meve and Liede 1994). The knowledge of pollinators of the other taxa is still very poor (Meve and Liede 1994). Species of the stapeliads can be quite readily propagated by seed, but most of the specimens which are cultivated by specialists are of wild origin or from material exchanged among colleagues. Many of the species are not easy to grow on their own roots, so grafting seems to be a very successful way to keep them alive and make them bloom sooner.

Systematic Treatment of Stapeliads

Brummit (1992) compiled 315 genera in the family Asclepiadaceae which include stapeliads. Today the number of species is estimated in this family at more than 2000. In an intensive study of the family, Liede and Albers (1994) determined that about 500 correctly described genera exist. These are arranged in taxonomic order into three sub-families (Periplocoideae, Gonolobeae, Asclepiadoideae), the Asclepiadoideae comprise four tribes (Marsdeniae, Asclepiadeae, Gonolobeae, Stapeliae) according to Bruyns and Forster (1991). After tribe Fockeae is added to this subfamily by Kunze, Meve and Liede (1994). But recent taxonomists placed the Asclepiads as a subfamily Asclepiadoideae under the family Apocynaceae (Endress, 2004). The Asclepiadoideae, as traditionally defined, have repeatedly been shown to be an apomorphic derivative of the Apocynaceae. It has often been recommended that the Asciepiadaceae be subsumed within the Apocynaceae in order to make the latter monophyletic. APG III provided a unified classification for the Apocynaceae, which consists of 424 genera distributed among five subfamilies: Rauvolfioideae, Apocynoideae, Periplocoideae, Secamonoideae, and Asclepiadoideae. In APG III classification (Chase and James, 2009), Stapeliads have been classified under subfamily Asclepiadoideae, tribe Ceropegiae, subtribe Stapeliinae. This tribe comprises about 46 genera include; *Anisotoma, Anomalluma, Apteranthes, Australluma, Baynesia, Boucerosia, Brachystelma, Caralluma, Caudanthera, Ceropegia, Conomitra, Cosmostigma, Duvalia, Duvaliandra, Echidnopsis, Edithcolea, Heterostemma, Hoodia, Huernia, Larryleachia, Lavrania, Leptadenia, Neoschumannia, Notechidnopsis, Ophionella, Orbea, Orbeanthus, Orbeopsis, Orthanthera, Pectinaria, Piaranthus, Pseudolithos, Quaqua, Rhytidocaulon, Richtersveldia, Riocreuxia, Sisyranthus, Socotrella, Stapelia, Stapelianthus, Stapeliopsis, Stephanotis, Tavaresia, Tridentea, Tromotriche, White-sloanea*

Genus *Caralluma*

The genus *Caralluma* was first named by R. Brown (1810) to describe an Indian species with very characteristic elongated flowering succulent stem. Wight and Arnott (1834) have split the genus and described two new genera *Boucerosia* and *Hutchinia*. Genus *Boucerosia* was characterized to include species with flowers in terminal umbels, from India, Arabia and the Mediterranean area of the world. *Hutchinia* was erected for Indian species with a few flowers in terminal umbles and creeping underground succulent stems. In 1892, N.E. Brown compiled all the genera under the genus

Caralluma. After the number of similar succulent species described under the genus from South Africa, it was making more controversy in taxonomy of this succulent group. Schumann (1895) has tried to divide the genus into three sections – *Eucaralluma* (= *Caralluma*), *Lalacruma* and *Boucerosia*. Since the Schumann's work, many number of species dumped in these groups were all succulents called as stapeliads. It was remained for a century till White and Sloane published their monumental work *The Stapeliae*. They also followed N.E. Brown's classification in their Stapeliae and again all the succulent stapeliae named under single genus *Caralluma*.

In 1990, Gilbert tried to classify the genus *Caralluma* in his 'A review of *Caralluma* R.Br. and its segregates'. He has segregated the genus two most important characters such as morphology of stem and structure of pollinaria. He retained the genus *Frerea* as a monotypic genus in India, *Caralluma* got divided into 4 subgenera – *Boucerosia* (27 sp.), *Desmidorchis* (5 sp.), *Caralluma* (2 sp.) and *Urmalcala* (3 sp.). Of these *Desmidorchis* is not represented in India. Plowes (1995) believed that taxonomy of the genus *Caralluma* had full of species in dust-bin and it could not be fitted into other existing genera. He has segregated execratively the genus *Caralluma* into 17 different genera. He proposed 11 new genera in addition with resurrecting 6 older names. According to Plowes (1995), Indian species fall into 4 categories – *Caraluma* R. Brown, *Cryptolluma* Plowes (= *Caralluma edulis*), *Boucerosia* Wight and *Borealluma* Plowes (*Caralluma tuberculata*). Meve and Liede (2002) tried to solve the taxonomic problem of the tribe Ceropegiae using modern tools of molecular phylogeny. They have suggested clearly the Indian genus *Caralluma* segregated into 4 groups – *Boucerosia* Wight, *Caralluma* R. Brown, *Caudanthera* Meve et Liede (*Caralluma edulis*) and *Apteranthes* Meve et Liede (*Caralluma tuberculata*).

Caralluma R.Br. (*sensu lato*) has been usually accepted to include about 120 taxa, with a wide African, Asian, South African and Southeast European distribution (Mabberley, 1993). It belongs to subtribe Stapeliinae (tribe Ceropegiae, sub family Asclepiadoideae and family Apocynaceae), which has its centre of origin in East Africa (Meve and Liede, 2004). The genus possesses xerophytic succulent herbs, represented by 16 species and 8 varieties in India. Of these 5 species and 5 varieties are endemic to Peninsular India (Jagtap and Singh, 1999). They are growing in arid, rocky regions in the foothills of Western Ghats and Eastern Ghats. Out of 16 species, 14 species of *Caralluma* are distributed in Deccan Peninsula. Gravely and Mayuranathan (1931), while reviewing the Indian genus *Caralluma* (Asclepiadaceae), described 2 new species and 3 new varieties from Peninsular India. Many species are narrow endemics, confined only small areas of distribution.

In *Caralluma* like other members of the Asclepiadoideae, require the agency of insects to bring about pollination and fertilization; and two species growing within a moderate distance of each other would become very liable to be cross-fertilized with each other's pollen. These hybrids would not necessarily be found in the neighborhood of their parents, as the seeds being provided with a large tuft of long fine hairs, would be liable to be carried to a considerable distance by the wind. The new hybrid established in another place, in turn, in course of time, might give rise to other hybrids (Gravely and Mayuranathan, 1931).

The genus *Caralluma* R. Brown is now segregated into 17 genera by Plowes (1995) of which 4 genera *i.e., Caralluma, Boucerosia, Apteranthus* and *Caudanthera* can be encountered in India. *Caralluma sensu str.*, and *Boucerosia* can easily be distinguished, at least so far as Indian forms are concerned, by the arrangement of the flowers and by the nature of the stems. In *Caralluma sensu str.*, the flowers arise in the axils of the rudimentary and evanescent leaves all along the distal portion of the stem whereas in *Boucerosia* the flowers are terminal (usually in compact umbels though sometimes solitary); *Apteranthus* with the single species known from Sunderbani (Jammu) flowers in compact umbels arising at sub-apical portion of stem but not in series, always isolated, while in *Caudanthera* flowers glabrous, single or paired; arising in axils of leaves. *Caralluma sensu str.*, the stems are almost always more or less distinctly tapered distally, usually very markedly so, at least fully matured where as in *Boucerosia* the stems are of approximately uniform thickness throughout. Karthikeyan *et al*. (2009) included all the Indian *Caralluma* under only one genus *Caralluma*.

Much of the nomenclatural turmoil in the stapeliads in recent years is because leading specialists have had varying interpretations about the meaning and use of the terms 'monophyly' and 'paraphyly' (see Podani, 2010). This has led to there being different ideas as to what genera should be accepted, and what criteria and techniques should be used to define those genera. Some workers prefer to use "broad concept" and to lump together all those species that share few basic features but this approach may consequently result in plants that lack a similarity in other features being put together within the same genus. On the other hand, other workers aim for homogenous genera whose included species share as many morphological characters as possible, and to exclude those species that are too dissimilar: this therefore makes it easy to place any individual plant into an appropriate genus and it helps to ensure that all the species within such clear-cut genera are likely to be closely related. This is the approach Plowes (2011) adopted. It is useful too because morphologically or geographically anomalous taxa are not overlooked due to having been buried in a non-critical broadly based name that covers up such confounding but important details. The adoption of taxon names that are narrowly and precisely delimited is also useful for ecological and environmental studies as they help to define and delimit different ecological biomes where biogeographical isolation has led to the evolution of new taxa, and they thereby focus attention on the existence of such biomes and on the flora and fauna that occur in them.

Floral colour differences are usually a poor criterion for separating species, but pattern differences have better diagnositic value. As pointed in revisions of the species that remained in *Caralluma* (Plowes 1995, 1996, 2010) there are a number of morphological features that can and should be used as diagnostic tools for determining relationships among species and genera but some of these had hitherto (and even since then) not been utilised by certain other workers. At the species level these diagnostic characters include colour patterns and the textures and shapes of corollas and coronas. At the generic level useful characters include the location of floral placement sites on the stem, stem morphology, manner of branching, and the nature of the vestigial remnants of rudimentary leaves and leaf organs. The shapes and structure of the gynostegium and of the pollinaria are of particular importance for the correct grouping of taxa and their placement into homogenous genera of related species.

Many workers tried to solve the intricate problem of classifying various taxa of Indian *Caralluma* but still more ambiguity persisted, which made the identity of this genus a subject of controversy. Out of 16 species of *Caralluma*, 13 species are solely endemic to South India. Many of them are rare and endangered specifically *Boucerosia truncato-coronata*, *Caralluma bhupinderiana*, *Caralluma sarkarieae* and *Boucerosia procumbens* (Nayar, 1996). Many species are not collected after the type collections even from the type localities.

Identification of some of the species in the genus is problematic due to their morphological plasticity. Usually all these species are distributed in narrow endemic areas and it is essential to identify the locality to conserve the population of this rare plant group.

Chapter 2
Medicinal Uses

Almost all the plants in Asclepiadoideae of Apocynaceae are of medicinal value. Asklepios means the God of Medicine in Greek Mythology mentioned by Linnaeus in his *Species Plantarum*. Generally Asclepiadoideae plants are the sources of cytotoxic and cardiac glycosides and contain high potentiality products for curing many diseases of animals and human beings. The plants are also abundant in esterified polyoxy pregnane glycosides, which therefore promise a source of antitumour and anticancer agents (Hayashi *et al.*, 1988; Luo *et al.*, 1993).

The species *Caralluma* found in India are edible and form a part of the traditional medicine system of the country. The medicinal properties of *Caralluma* include carminative, febrifugal, anthelmintic, antirheumatic, antidiabetic and antihyperglycemic, anti-pyretic, anti-inflammatory, antinociceptive and antioxidant effects (Table 2.1). *Caralluma* extracts have also been found to be appetite-suppressants. Plants belonging to the genus *Caralluma* are rich in esterified polyhydroxy pregnane glycosides (Table 2.2), some of which showed antitumour activity and others were postulated as precursors of cardenolides (Deepak *et al.*, 1989, 1997). Rizwani *et al.* (1990) and Ramesh *et al.* (1999b) reported the presence of flavone glycosides. Several members of the genus *Caralluma* have found medicinal uses in the treatment of rheumatism, diabetes, and leprosy and as antiseptics and disinfectants (Neuwinger, 1994).

Previous studies on the plants of the genus *Caralluma* have reported the isolation of several pregnane glycosides or their esters (Ahmed *et al.* 1988; Tanaka *et al.* 1990; Lin *et al.* 1994; Qiu *et al.* 1999), with antitumor activity (Deepak *et al.* 1989, 1997) and recently showed antitrypanosomal activity (Abdel-Sattar *et al.* 2008).

The compounds, which are present in *Caralluma*, are ingredients in the preparation of drugs. In Table 2.1 biological activities of the genus *Caralluma* are given while Table 2.2 gives the chemical compounds reported in *Caralluma*.

Table 2.1: A List of Biological Activities of the Genus *Caralluma*

Biological Activity	*Plant Name*	*Reference*
Analgesic activity	*Caralluma adscendens*	Tambe *et al.* (2010)
Anthelmintic activity	*Caralluma edulis*	Chopra *et al.* (1956)
Antiarthritic activity	*Caralluma stalagmifera*	Reddy *et al.* (1996)
Antigastric ulcer activity	*Caralluma arabica*	Zakaria *et al.* (2002)
Antihyperglycemic activity	*Caralluma arabica*	Radhakrishnan *et al.* (1999)
	Caralluma attenuata	Venkatesh *et al.* (2003)
Antiinflammatory activity	*Caralluma arabica*	Zakaria *et al.* (2001)
	Caralluma attenuata	Ramesh *et al.* (1998)
	Caralluma umbellata	Ramesh *et al.* (1999a)
	Caralluma stalagmifera	Reddy *et al.* (1996)
	Caralluma tuberculata	Ahmad *et al.* (1983)
	Caralluma adscendens	Naik and Jadge (2009), Jadge *et al.* (2009)
	Caralluma adscendens var. *attenuata*	Madhuri *et al.* (2010)
Antinociceptive activity	*Caralluma arabica*	Zakaria *et al.* (1999, 2001)
	Caralluma attenuata	Ramesh *et al.* (1998)
	Caralluma umbellata	Ramesh *et al.* (1999a)
Antirheumatic activity	*Caralluma edulis*	The Wealth of India (1992)
Antitumor activity	*Caralluma tuberculata*	The Wealth of India (1992)
Appetite suppressant	*Caralluma fimbriata*	Mary Shomon (2006)
Carminative	*Caralluma edulis*	The Wealth of India (1992)
Cytoprotective	*Caralluma arabica*	Zakaria *et al.* (2002)
Febrifugal	*Caralluma edulis*	The Wealth of India (1992)
Hypoglycemic activity	*Caralluma tuberculata*	Ahmed and Shaikh (1989)
	Caralluma attenuata	Jayakar *et al.* (2004)
Immunostimulating activity	*Caralluma adscendens*, *Caralluma stalagmifera*, *Boucerosia lasiantha*	Madhuri *et al.* (2010)
Antioxidant activity	*Caralluma edulis*, *Caralluma adscendens*, *Caralluma adscendens* var. *attenuata*, *Caralluma flava*, *Caralluma stalagmifera*, *Boucerosia lasiantha*	Ansari *et al.* (2005), Tatiya *et al.* (2010), Madhuri *et al.* (2010) Marwah *et al.* (2007), Madhuri *et al.* (2010) Madhuri *et al.* (2010)
Antiobesogenic and anti-atherosclerotic activity	*Caralluma adscendens* var. *fimbriata*	Radhakrishnan *et al.* (1999); Kamalakkannan *et al.* (2010)
Antitrypanosomal activity	*Caralluma* sp.	Abdel Sattar *et al.* (2009)

Table 2.2: A List of Phytochemical Compounds Isolated from Genus *Caralluma*

Plant Name	*Compounds*	*Reference*
Caralluma arabica	Flavone glycoside, Luteolin-4'-O-neohesperidoside	Kamil *et al.* (1999)
Caralluma burchardii	Squalene, sitosterol acetate, lupeol acetate, guimanenol, 3,4-seco-triterpene	Castro *et al.* (1980)
Caralluma attenuata	Flavonoid glycoside, Luteolin-4'-O-neohesperidoside	Ramesh *et al.* (1998)
	Flavone glycoside, Luteolin-4'-O-neohesperidoside	Ramesh *et al.* (1999b)
Caralluma dalzielli	Pregnane glycosides	Leo *et al.* (2005)
Caralluma edulis	Hexocosanediol, boucerosin, saponin, glycosides	Wealth of India (1992)
Caralluma lasiantha	Bisdesmosidic C-21 steroidal pregnane glycosides	Qiu *et al.* (1999)
	Flavone glycoside, Luteolin-4'-O-neohesperidoside	Ramesh *et al.* (1999b)
Caralluma negevensis	Pregnane glycosides	Braca *et al.* (2002)
	Two Megastigmane glycosides, two flavone glycosides	Bader *et al.* (2003)
Caralluma penicillata	Penicillosides A-C, C-15 oxypregnane glycosides	Abdel-Sattar *et al.* (2001)
	oxypregnane glycosides	Abdel-Sattar *et al.* (2002)
Caralluma retrospiciens	Two pregnane ester aglycones	Khalil (1995)
	Pregnane glycosides	Halim and Khalil (1996)
	Six polyoxypregnane glycosides	Halaweish *et al.* (2004)
Caralluma russeliana	Pregnane glycosides	Al-Yahya *et al.* (2000)
Caralluma tuberculata	Boucerin	Von Eum and Reichstein (1948)
	Dihydroboucerin	Nikaido *et al.* (1967)
	Flavone glycosides, Luteolin-4'-O-neohesperidoside	Rizwani *et al.* (1990)
	Two Pregnane glycosides, Caratubersides A and B	Ahmad *et al.* (1988)
	Four pregnane glycosides, Boucerosides AI, AII, BI and BII	Hayashi *et al.* (1988)
	Ten pregnane glycosides	Tanaka *et al.* (1990)
Caralluma umbellata	Flavone glycoside, Luteolin-4'-O-neohesperidoside	Ramesh *et al.* (1999b)
	Pregnane glycoside, Carumbelloside I and II	Lin *et al.* (1994)
	C-21 steroidal glycosides, Carumbelloside III, IV and V	Qiu *et al.* (1997)

Contd...

Table 2.2–*Contd...*

Plant Name	*Compounds*	*Reference*
Caralluma adscendens var. *fimbriata*	Pregnane Glycosides	Kunert *et al.* (2008)
Caralluma stalagmifera	Steroidalglycosides, stalagmosides I–V (**1–5**)	Kunert *et al.* (2006)
Caralluma indica	Indicosides I and II (**7** and **8**),	
Caralluma umbellata	Pregnane steroid	Suresh Babu *et al.* (2008)
	Steroidal glycosides	Kunert *et al.* (2009)

Caralluma adscendens (Roxb.) R. Brown

Tatiya *et al.* (2007) have reported antibacterial activity of various extracts of stem of *Caralluma adscendens* against *Bacillus pumilus, Escherechia coli,* and *Staphylococcus aureus*. Jadge *et al.* (2009) have reported anti-inflammatory activity of aqueous and ethanolic extracts of whole plant of *Caralluma adscendens* in rats. The anti-inflammatory activity was evaluated by using Digital Plethysmometer. The study was carried out by using dose of 250 mg/kg of ethanolic and aqueous extract orally. All extracts showed significant activity for all dose as compared to diclofenac sodium. Mali *et al.* (2009) have observed hypoglycemic effect of *Caralluma adscendens* in alloxan induced experimental rats.

Antioxidant and hypolipidemic effects of *Caralluma adscendens* were evaluated by Tatiya *et al.* (2010) using DPPH *in vtro* lipid peroxidation and reductive ability methods. The treatment showed significant decrease in total cholesterol, LDL, triglyceride and TC/HDL and an increase in HDL in the treated diabetic animal group. *In vitro* antioxidant activity showed that the butanolic extract exhibited potent free radical scavenging effects (Tatiya *et al.*, 2010).

Petroleum ether, ethyl acetate and methanolic extracts of *Caralluma adscendens* aerial parts at the doses of 100 and 200 mg/kg was evaluated by Tambe *et al.* (2010a) for the analgesic activity using the hot plate and acetic acid induced abdominal constrictions in mice. *Caralluma adscendens* aerial parts extract showed significant analgesic properties in all the models studied.

Caralluma adscendens (Roxb.) R. Brown var. *attenuata* (Wight) Grav. et Mayur. (Syn.: *Caralluma attenuata* Wight; *Stapelia adscendens* Roxb.)

Extracts showed antihyperglycemic activity (Venkatesh *et al.*, 2003).

Luteolin-4′-O-neohesperidoside, *i.e.*, luteolin-4′-O-[α-(L-rhamnopyranosyl-(1→2)-β-D-glucopyranoside)] isolated from *Caralluma adscendens* var. *attanuata* has significant anti-inflammatory action (Ramesh *et al.*, 1998). Its antinoceceptive activity is less pronounced when compared with its anti-inflammatory activity.

Madhuri *et al.* (2010) reported antioxidant, anti-inflammatory, antiobesity and antimicrobial activity of *Caralluma adscendens* var. *attenuata*.

Caralluma adscendens (Roxb.) R. Brown var. *fimbriata* (Wall.) Gravely et Mayuranathan. (Syn.: *Caralluma fimbriata* Wall.)

Tribes in India use *Caralluma adscendens* var. *fimbriata* to suppress hunger and enhance endurance. In 2006, the division of Nutrition at St. John's National Academy of Health Sciences in Bangalore, India, assessed the effect of using 1 g of *Caralluma adscendens* var. *fimbriata* extract in 50 overweight adults against a placebo group for 60 days. Waist circumference and hunger levels showed a significant decline in the experimental group compared to the placebo group. There was no significant difference between groups with regard to weight, body mass index, hip circumference, body fat and energy intake. This study provided support for the use of *Caralluma* extract as an appetite suppressant but found that the supplement did not have a significant impact on weight loss.

The Indian tribes have consumed *Caralluma* for centuries as a vegetable. People use it during famines to decrease appetite and as a thirst quencher. The Indian Health Ministry has included *Caralluma adscendens* var. *fimbriata* on a list of medicinal plants as a vegetable eaten raw or used in pickles and curries. There are no adverse side effects or toxicity levels.

Rebecca *et al.* (2007) have observed the effect of *Caralluma fimbriata* extract on appetite, food intake and anthropometry in adult Indian men and women. Waist circumference and hunger levels over the observation period showed a significant decline in the experimental group when compared to the placebo group. While there was a trend towards a greater decrease in body weight, body mass index, hip circumference, body fat and energy intake between assessment time points in the experimental group, these were not significantly different between experimental and placebo groups.

Radhakrishnan *et al.* (1999) have observed *Caralluma* for weight loss. Indian Cactus is promising appetite suppressant and diet aid. *Caralluma fimbriata* is a succulent plant, that has been used as a natural appetite suppressant in India for centuries. It's another new arrival in the family of various cactii that are being used for their appetite suppressant, blood sugar lowering, and weight loss properties, much like the increasingly popular *Hoodia gordonii* from the Kalahari Desert in Africa.

Kumar *et al.* (2008) reported antifungal and anthelmintic of *Cralluma adscendens* var. *fimbriata*.

Caralluma arabica N.E.Br. (Syn.: *Caralluma aucheri* (Decne) N.E.Br.)

The plant is widespread in the tropics; in Arabia and Middle East. *Caralluma arabica* is a species found in the wild in United Arab Emirates. In 2001, a group from the Ministry of Health in Abu Dhabi evaluated both oral and topical application of extract from *Caralluma arabica* at doses of 200 and 400 mg/kg for anti-inflammatory properties in rats. Results found the extracts in all models studied showed significant anti-inflammatory properties, supporting its traditional use in treating painful and inflammatory conditions.

Plant collected in spring and sold in the market, to be eaten with cooked food "saloonah" as a nutritice and tonic. The plant is emollient, diuretic, it treats liver diseases, diabetes, hypertension, Flowers replenish from thirsty, externally for wounds and cuts. Juice of stem is used to curdle milk and given to sick to speed convalescence, burns, itchy skin and sunburns. *Caralluma arabica* is commonly used in traditional medicine as decoction in the United Arab Emirates (UAE) for the treatment of many disease conditions. Certain species of *Caralluma* are used in folk medicine as antipyretic, antirheumatic and reported to possess significant anti-inflammatory activity (Ahmad *et al.*, 1983).

Zakaria *et al.* (2001) investigated anti-nociceptive and anti-inflammatory properties of *Caralluma arabica*. *Caralluma arabica* extract significantly reduced the increase in hind paw volume induced by carrageenan injection when used orally or topically (Zakaria *et al.*, 2001). Methanolic extract showed anti-nociceptive and anti-inflammatory properties (Zakaria *et al.*, 2001). Zakaria *et al.* (2002) reported that the *C. arabica* extract protects gastric mucosal cells against experimental gastric mucosal damage. This effect confirms results of other studies on *Caralluma* species and seems to be mediated by multi-mechanisms including increased gastric production of prostaglandins and mucin and reduced gastric acidity.

Antinociceptice activity – Hot plate - Zakaria *et al.* (1999, 2001)

Antinociceptice activity – Tail flick - Zakaria *et al.* (1999, 2001)

Antinociceptice activity – Writhing - Zakaria *et al.* (1999, 2001)

Anti-inflammatory activity was evaluated using cotton pellet granuloma method (Zakaria *et al.*, 2001). Results of this study confirm the use of *Caralluma arabica* traditionally for the treatment of painful and inflammatory conditions and indicate transdermal absorption of the plant extract.

Zakaria *et al.* (2002) evaluated the antigastric ulcer activity of 10 per cent ethanolic extract of *Caralluma arabica*, at the doses of 200 and 400 mg/kg, using experimental gastric ulcer models induced by phenylbutazone or indomethacin and 80 per cent ethanol or 0.2N NaOH, and cold restraint stress. Some experiments were carried out to study the effects of *C. arabica* extract on gastric acid secretion in pyloric ligation induced ulcer and gastric wall mucin production. The 10 per cent ethanolic extract of *C. arabica* produced a dose-dependent reduction in all experimentally induced gastric lesions used in the present study. The cytoprotective activity of *C. arabica* in ethanol-induced ulcer was completely abolished by pretreatment with indomethacin. Induction of gastric ulcer reduced gastric wall production of mucin to 50.8 per cent of its initial value. This reduction was completely prevented by pretreatment with *C. arabica* extract. *C. arabica* extract significantly reduced total gastric acidity (from 22.4 to 9.2 mEq/L) and volume of gastric secretions (from 9.98 to 2.03 ml). Results of this study revealed that the *C. arabica* extract protects gastric mucosal cells against experimental gastric mucosal damage. This effect confirms results of other studies on *Caralluma* species and seems to be mediated by multi-mechanisms including increased gastric production of prostaglandins and mucin and reduced gastric acidity.

Chemistry: Flavonoids *e.g.*, Luteolin-6-O-β-D-glucopyranoside 3-O-α-L-rhamnopyranoside and Kaempferol-3-O- β-D-glucopyranoside-4- O-α-L-rhamnopyranoside have been isolated (Kamil *et al.*, 2002).

Caralluma dalzielli N.E.Br.

It is used in folk medicine as antiplasmodic and analgesic remedy. In Bandigara region of Mali the plant is applied on suppurating wounds, while the stems are grounded and eaten raw as tonic remedy for bodily exhaustion and cardiac problems (NeuWinger, 2000; Iwu, 1993). The stems are reported crushed and eaten raw as a tonic and stimulant for faintness due to fasting, pain in the chest and epigastreum, etc. A decoction is used in the Tenkodogo area of Upper Volta as an antemetic. Moorish people in the Western Sahara extract a strong poison by maceration in sheep's urine.

Chemistry: Twenty-seven new pregnane glycosides were isolated from the whole plant of *Caralluma dalzielii,* and their structures elucidated from extensive 2D NMR analysis as well as ESI-MS experiments. All isolated compounds were tested for their antiproliferative activity on J774.A1, HEK-293, and WEHI-164 cell lines. Moderate to high potency of cytotoxicities were found in almost all tested compounds, confirming the significant cytotoxic activity of pregnane glycosides (De Leo *et al.*, 2005).

Caralluma edulis Benth. et Hook.f.

The fleshy herb is eaten as a vegetable. The juicy stem is reported to possess carminative, febrifugal, anthelmintic and anti-rheumatic properties. Stem, dried and powdered, is taken as a stimulant. It is also useful in leprosy and diseases of blood.

Ansari *et al.* (2005) evaluated the antioxidant activity of five vegetables traditionally consumed by South-Asian migrants in Bradford, Yorkshire, UK in the DPPH scavenging assay. And *in vitro* non-enzymatic inhibition of bovine brain lipid peroxidation. In both antioxidant assays a strong activity was shown by extracts derived from *Caralluma edulis.*

Caralluma edulis did not show any hypoglycemic effect in normal as well as in diabetic rabbits (Wadood *et al.*, 1989).

Chemistry: The aerial parts contain 1, 26-hexacosanediol, boucerosin, a saponin and a mixture of glycosides, which on hydrolysis yields boucerin, dihydroboucerin, cymarose, sarmentose, oleandrose and digitoxose. The plant also contains tomentogenin and sitosterol is also reported from the plant (Heneidak, 2001).

Eighteen fatty acids, four hydrocarbons and sterol have been isolated from the ethyl acetate fraction of the vegetative part of the medicinal herb *Caralluma edulis* (Rizwani *et al.*, 1993).

Caralluma europaea (Guss.) N.E.Br.

The essential oil of the stems and fruits of *Caralluma europaea* from Lampedusa Island has been obtained by hydrodistillation and its composition analyzed (Pietro *et al.* 2010). It contains 74 volatile compounds, of which 16 were aromatic and 58 non-aromatic. Stems and fruits contained 1.4 per cent and 2.7 per cent of aromatic compounds respectively, while non-aromatic were 88.3 per cent and 88.8 per cent. Non-aromatic hydrocarbons were the most abundant compounds in both organs, followed by fatty acids. In stems accounted for 38 compounds while fruits for 53. Carmen *et al.* (2009) have analysed the floral headspace compounds by the GC-MS method. The main components were, among the monoterpenoids, terpinolene (23.3 per cent), α-terpinene (19.1 per cent) and linalool (18.4 per cent), whereas, among the carbonylic compounds the major constituents were heptanal (2.0 per cent), octanoic acid (2.4 per cent) and hexanoic acid (1.7 per cent). Heneidak (2001) have investigated on the extracts of *Caralluma europaea*, it contains varieties of glycoside flavonoids namely luteolin-3-O-glucoside, chrysoeriol-4-O-neohersperidoside, quercetin-O-pentosyl-hexoside, apigenn-4-O-neohesperidoside, and quercetin-3-O-rutinoside.

Apteranthes europaea (Guss.) Plowes (=*Caralluma europaea*) was found to be rich in rather uncommon flavone glycosides. Of these, luteolin 42-neohesperidoside represents the major flavonoid of all samples; luteolin-32-*O*-(62-*O*-sinapoylglucoside)-42-*O*-neohesperidoside and luteolin-32-*O*-(62-*O*-feruloylglucoside)-42-*O*-neohesperidoside are reported here for the first time. Flavonol glycosides also occur, but in much smaller quantities (Meve and Heneidak, 2005).

Caralluma flava N.E.Br.

Marwah *et al.* (2007) reported that *Caralluma flava* is edible. Marwah *et al.* (2007) investigated the antioxidant activity of wound-healing herbs using *in vitro* DPPH and phosphomolybdenum assay methods. Out of the 19 plants screened, the aqueous ethanol extract of *Caralluma flava* showed the best DPPH scavenging activities with per cent IP value 31.5 per cent, after 15 min of incubation at an effective test concentration of 50μg/ml. Although *Caralluma flava* showed less antioxidant activity in the DPPH assay, very strong antioxidant activity had been demonstrated in the phosphomolybdenum assay. The Total Antioxidant Capacity as gallic acid equivalent of 335mg/g of ethanol extract was obtained in the phosphomolybdenum assay. Total phenolic content was 23.6 mg GAE/g of ethanol extract.

Chemistry: *Caralluma flava* possesses pregnane glycosides and triterpenes.

Caralluma negevensis Zohary

The plant is used by Bedouins to treat chronic lung diseases, such as tuberculosis and cancer (Bader *et al.*, 2003).

Chemistry: Megastigmane glycosides and two flavonol glycosides reported such as luteolin-3,4-di-O-beta-d-glucopyranoside and leuteolin3-O-beta-d-glucopyranoside-4-O-alpha-l-rhamnopyranosyl-beta-d-glucopyranoside (Bader *et al.* 2003).

Caralluma penicillata (Defl.) N.E.Br.

World Distribution: Saudi Arabia, Yemen.

Used in Saudi traditional medicine for the treatment of snake bite and scorpion stings (Al-Yahya *et al.*, 1983).

Chemistry: The chloroform fraction of the defatted ethanol extract from aerial parts of *Caralluma penicillata* yielded three C-15 oxypregnane glycosides, penicillosides A-C (Abdel Sattar *et al.*, 2001). The ether fraction of defatted ethanol extract of the aerial parts of *C. penicillata* yielded four new oxypregnane glycosides penicillosides D-G (Abdel Sattar *et al.*, 2002).

Pregnane glycosides previously isolated from genus *Caralluma penicillata* were tested by Abdel-Sattar *et al.* (2009) for their antitrypanosomal activity. Penicilloside E showed the highest antitrypanosomal activity ([IC_{50}] 1-01 μg/ml) followed by caratuberside C ([IC_{50}] 1.85 μg/ml), which exhibited the highest selectivity index (SI 12.04). It was noticed that acylation is required for the antitrypanosomal activity while glycosylation at C-20 has no significant effect on the activity.

Caralluma quadrangula (Forssk.) N.E.Br.

Marwah *et al.* (2007) reported that the entire plant of *Caralluma quadrangula* plant is edible; in some communities, the juice expressed from its stem is added to fresh milk as a general tonic.

Marwah *et al.* (2007) investigated the antioxidant activity of wound-healing herbs using *in vitro* DPPH and phosphomolybdenum assay methods. Out of the 19 plants screened, the aqueous ethanol extract of *Caralluma quadrangula* showed very low DPPH scavenging activities with per cent IP value 14.5 per cent, after 15 min of incubation at an effective test concentration of 50μg/ml. Some what surprising was that *C. quadrangula*, a member of succulent asclepiads, lacks antioxidant activity in the DPPH assay but demonstrated very strong antioxidant activity in the phorsphomolybdenum assay. The Total Antioxidant capacity as gallic acid equivalent of 893mg/g of ethanol extract was obtained in the phosphomolybdenum assay. Total phenolic content was 18.7 mg GAE/g of ethanol extract.

Chemistry: *Caralluma quadrangula* possesses pregnane glycosides and triterpenes.

Caralluma retrospeciens (Ehrenb.) N.E.Br.

Chemistry: Two pregnane ester glycosides were isolated from *Caralluma retrospeciens* (Halim and Khalil, 1996). These are beta-benzoxyloxy-20-isovaleroxyloxy-8-beta, 14-beta-dihydroxy-pregnane-3-O-[beta-D-glucopyranosyl-(1→6)-beta-D-glycopyranosyl-(1-→4)-beta-D-(3-O-methyl-6-doxy)-galactopyranosde] (caretroside A) and the bioside 12 beta-benzoyloxy-8-beta, 14-beta-dihydroxypregn-20-one-3-O-[beta-D-oleandropyranosyl -(1→4)-beta-D-cymaropyranoside] (Halim and Khalil, 1996).

Six related polyoxypregnane glycosides were isolated and characterized from *Caralluma retrospeciens* leaves (Halaweish *et al.*, 2004). The compounds were identified as 12 beta-benzoyloxy-8beta, 14 beta-dihydroxypregn-20-one-3-O-[3-O-methyl-6-deoxy-beta-D-allopyranosyl-(1→4)- beta-D-cymaropyranosyl-(1→4) –beta-D-cymaropyranoside], 12 beta-benzoyloxy-8beta, 14 beta-dihydroxypregn-20-one-3-O-[beta-D-glucopyranosyl-(1→4)-3-O-methyl-6-deoxy-beta-D-allopyranosyl-(1→4)-beta-D- cymaropyranoside, 12 beta-benzoyloxy-8-beta, 14 beta-dihydroxypregn-20-one-3-O-[beta-D-glucopyrnosyl-(1→4)-3-O-methyl-6-deoxy-beta-D-galactopyranosyl-

(1→6)-beta-D-glucopyranoside], 12beta- benzoyloxy-8beta, 14 beta- dihydroxypregn-20-one-3-O-[beta-D-glucopyranosyl-(1→6)beta-D-glucopyranosyl -(1→4)- 3-O-methyl-6-deoxy- beta-D-galactopyranosyl-(1→4)-3-O-methyl-6-deoxy-beta-D-galactopyranoside], 12 beta-benzoyloxy- 11 alpha-isovaleroyloxy -8 beta, 14 beta-dihydroxypregn-20-one-3-O-[beta-D-glucopyranosyl -(1→4)-3-O-methyl-6-deoxy-beta-D-galactopyranosyl-(1→4) -3-O-methyl-6-deoxy-beta-D-galactopyranoside], and 12 beta-benzoyloxy—11 alpha-isovaleroyloxy-8 beta, 14 beta-dihydroxypregn-20-one-3-O-[beta- D-glucopyrnosyl-(1→4)-3-O-methyl-6-deoxy-beta-D-allopyranosyl-(1→4)-beta-D-cymaropyranosyl-(1→4) –beta-D-cymaropyranoside. The compounds showed cytotoxic activities towards brine shrimp having IC_{50} values of 1.19x 10(-4), 8.83 x 10(-5), 2.64 x 10(-4), 2.26 x 10(-4), 2.39 x 10(-4), and 1.7 x 10(-4) M, respectively.

Caraluma russeliana (Brongn.) Cufod

Chemistry: The aerial parts of *Caralluma russeliana* yielded four new pregnane glycosides, russeliosides A-D (1-4), in addition to a known flavone glycoside, luteolin 4'-O-beta-D-neohesperidoside (Al-Yahya *et al.*, 2000). The structures of compounds 1-4 were elucidated using a combination of spectroscopic methods.

The aerial parts of *Caralluma russeliana* yielded new pregnane glycosides Russeliosides A-D, in addition to a known flavone glycoside, luteolin 4'-O-beta-D-neohesperidoside (Abdul-Aziz *et al.*, 2000). The chloroform extract of aerial parts of *Caralluma russeliana* yielded four acylated pregnane glycosides namely russeliosides E-H, three were found new (Abdel-Sattar *et al.*, 2007).

Pregnane glycosides previously isolated from genus *Caralluma russelliana* were tested by Abdel-Sattar *et al.* (2009) for their antitrypanosomal activity. Penicilloside E showed the highest antitrypanosomal activity ([IC_{50}] 1-01 μg/ml) followed by caratuberside C ([IC_{50}] 1.85 μg/ml), which exhibited the highest selectivity index (SI 12.04). It was noticed that acylation is required for the antitrypanosomal activity while glycosylation at C-20 has no significant effect on the activity.

Caralluma sinaica (Decne) A.Berger (Syn: *Boucerosia sinaica* Decne)

People of Asir region of Saudi Arabia chew *Caralluma sinaica* to lower glucose level. It was observed that administration of *C. sinaica* in different doses to healthy animals can cause significant decrease in glucose level (Habibuddin *et al.*, 2008).

Chemistry: Heneidak (2001) has reported the presence of luteolin-3-4-O-diglucoside, luteoline-3-O-(6-O-sinapolyglucoside)-4-O-glucoside, vincenin-2, and quercetin-O-ramnosyl-pentosyl-hexoside in the extracts.

Caralluma stalagmifera C.E.C. Fisch.

The aqueous and butanol extracts of the whole plant was tested on carragenin-induced rat paw-edema and kaolin-induced arthritis in rats. Both the extracts have shown significant anti-inflammatory and antiarthritic activities (Reddy *et al.*, 1996).

Madhuri *et al.* (2010) reported antioxidant, anti-inflammatory, antiobesity and antimicrobial activity of *Caralluma stalagmifera*.

Chemistry: New steroidal glycosides, stalagmosides I–V (*1–5*), together with the known compounds carumbelloside III, lasianthosideA, and lasianthosideB, were isolated by Kunert *et al.* (2006) from whole plants of *Caralluma stalagmifera*. Their structures were elucidated by extensive NMR spectroscopic studies.

Caralluma tuberculata N.E.Br.

The plant is useful in tonic properties. Either eaten raw or cooked as vegetable and is also reputed to be a cure for diabetes, rheumatism and diseases of blood (Ali, 1986; Hoope, 1975). The alcoholic extract of *Caralluma tuberculata* was shown to possess hypoglycemic activity (Ahmed *et al.*, 1993). The fresh juice of *C. tuberculata* was shown to possess hypoglycemic activity (Ahmed and Moin-Uddin-Shaik, 1989).

The juicy stem of *Caralluma tuberculata* is bitter tonic, febrifuge, stomachic and carminative useful in rheutmatism and consumed as vegetable, especially when cooked with minced meat (Shinwari *et al.*, 2006).

Caralluma tuberculata showed protection against mucosal damage caused by indomethacin (Al-Harbi *et al.*, 1994). Al-Harbi *et al.* (1994) was of the opinion that the protective effects of *Caralluma tuberculata* in addition to its effects on mucus production and on protein sulfhydryl concentration may be mediated through its free radical and prostaglandin inducing properties.

Pretreatment with *Caralluma tuberculata* extract significantly reduced the clastrogenicity in mice (Al Bekairi *et al.*, 1992). These results indicated the involvement of different phytoconstituents acting by different routes (Al-Bekari *et al.*, 1992).

Chemistry: Five pregnane glycosides were isolated by Abdel-Sattar *et al.* (2008) from *Caralluma tuberculata* (1-5), in addition to a known one (russelioside E, 6). The structures of the isolated compounds were elucidated by the analysis of NMR data and FAB-MS experiments. All the isolated compounds were tested for their antimalarial and antitrypanosomal activities as well as their cytotoxicity against human diploid embryonic cell line (MRC5).

Luteolin-4′-O-β-D-glucopyranosyl (2→1)-α-rhamnopyranoside was isolated from *Carallulma tuberculata* (Rizwani *et al.*, 1990).

Pregnane glycosides are potent cytotoxic agents which may represent new leads in the development of anti-tumour drugs, particularly in the treatment of breast cancer, because of the structural similarity to estrogenic agonists. *Caralluma* species are natural sources of a wide variety of pregnane glycosides. Waheed *et al.* (2011) isolated, using an activity-guided fractionation approach, novel pregnane glycosides for testing on breast cancer and other tumour lines. The effect of crude extracts, specific organic fractions and isolated compounds from *Caralluma tuberculata* was tested by Waheed *et al.* (2011) on the growth and viability of MCF-7 estrogen-dependent, and MDA-MB-468 estrogen-independent breast cancer cells, Caco-2 human colonic cells, HUVECs and U937 cells. Neutral red uptake and MTT assays were used. Apoptosis was detected by Western blot of poly-(ADP ribose) polymerase (PARP) as were other markers of nuclear fragmentation (DNA ladder assay, staining of cells with nuclear dye DAPI). The involvement of caspases was investigated using the pan-caspase inhibitor Z-VAD-FMK. The ethyl acetate fraction of *Caralluma tuberculata* was found to be the most potent anti-proliferative fraction against all three cancer cell lines. Two novel steroidal glycosides were isolated from the active fraction after a series of chromatographic experiments. The structure of the isolated compounds was elucidated solely based on 2D-NMR (HMBC, HETCOR, DQF-COSY) and MS spectral analysis as compound 1: 12-O-benzoyl-20-O-acetyl-3β,12β,14β,20β-tetrahydroxy-pregnan-3-ylO-β-D-glucopyranosyl-(1→4)-β-d-glucopyranosyl-(1→4)-3-methoxy-β-d-ribopyranoside, and as compound 2: 7-O-acetyl-12-O-benzoyl-3β,7β,12β,14β-tetrahydroxy-17β-(3-methylbutyl-O-acetyl-1-yl)-androstan-3-ylO-β-d-glucopyranosyl-(1→4)-6-deoxy-β-d-allopyranosyl-(1→4)-β-d-cymaropyranosyl-(1→4)-β-d-cymapyranosyl-(1→4)-β-d-cymaropyranoside. Compound 1 (pregnane glycoside) and compound 2 (androstan glycoside) induced apoptosis at <25μM after 48h as assessed by cell shrinkage, PARP cleavage, DNA fragmentation, and reversal with the caspase inhibitor. This study showed that two novel steroid glycosides, isolated from *Caralluma tuberculata*, possess moderate, micromolar cytotoxic activity on breast cancer and other cells *in vitro*, which may indicate a source of activity *in vivo* of interest to future drug design.

Pregnane glycosides previously isolated from genus *Caralluma tuberculata* were tested by Abdel-Sattar *et al.* (2009) for their antitrypanosomal activity. Penicilloside E showed the highest antitrypanosomal activity ([IC_{50}] 1-01 μg/ml) followed by caratuberoside C ([IC_{50}] 1.85 μg/ml), which exhibited the highest selectivity index (SI 12.04). It was noticed that acylation is required for the antitrypanosomal activity while glycosylation at C-20 has no significant effect on the activity.

The antihyperglycaemic and hypolipidaemic effects of the methanolic extract of *Caralluma tuberculata* were investigated by Abdel-Sattar *et al.* (2011) in streptozotocin (STZ)-induced diabetic rats. The antihyperglycaemic activity was assessed by the reduction in fasting blood glucose (54 per cent at 4th week) and the peak of blood glucose at 120min of an oral glucose tolerance test in diabetic rats. Further, the tested extract also increased plasma insulin by 206.8 per cent. The hypolipidaemic action of the extract was evident by the significant decrease in the levels of total cholesterol, triglycerides and LDL-cholesterol by 41.5 per cent, 36.7 per cent and 49.1 per cent,

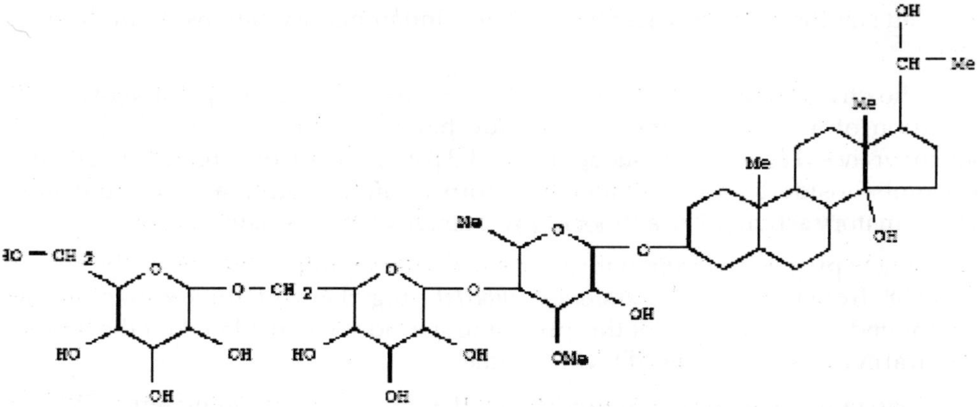

Caratuberoside D

respectively, compared to diabetic rat values. Interestingly, the extract increased the cardio-protective lipid HDL-cholesterol by 147.97 per cent as compared to diabetic rat value. This data suggests that the methanolic extract of *C. tuberculata* has both antihyperglycaemic and hypolipidaemic effects in STZ-induced diabetic rats that may need further studies to be used in the management of diabetes and associated hyperlipedaemia.

Chemistry: Pregnane glycosides, Caratuberosides A-D were isolated from *Caralluma tuberculata.*

Boucerosia indica (Wight et Arn.) Plowes (Syn.: *Caralluma indica* (Wight et Arn.) N.E.Br.)

New steroidal glycosides, indicosides I and II, together with the known compounds carumbelloside III, lasianthosideA, and lasianthosideB, were isolated by Kunert *et al.* (2006) from whole plants of *Boucerosia indica*. Their structures were elucidated by extensive NMR spectroscopic studies.

Boucerosia lasiantha Wight (Syn.: *Caralluma lasiantha* Wight)

Chemistry: From the whole plant of *Boucerosia lasiantha*, two new bisdesmosidic C-21 steroidal (pregnane) glycosides, named as lasianthoside-A and -B, were isolated by Qiu *et al.* (1999) and their structures elucidated solely based on extensive 2D-NMR and MS/MS spectral analysis as caralasigenin 3-*O*-β-D-glucopyranosyl(1→4)-β-D-digitalopyranoside-20-*O*-α-L-rhamnosyl(1→6)-β-D-glucopyranoside and caralumagenin 3-*O*-β-D-glucopyranosyl(1→4)-β-D-digitalopyranoside-20-*O*-α-L-rhamnosyl(1→6)-β-D-glucopyranoside. In addition, a known flavonoid glycoside, luteolin neohesperidoside, was also isolated

Madhuri *et al.* (2010) reported antioxidant, anti-inflammatory, antiobesity and antimicrobial activity of *Boucerosia lasiantha*.

Boucerosia umbellata (Haw.) Wight et Arn. (Syn.: *Caralluma umbellata* Haw.)

Stems are used in stomach disorders and abdominal pains. *Caralluma umbellata* showed significant antinociceptive and anti-inflammatory actions (Ramesh *et al.*, 1999).

The phytochemical study using *Caralluma umbellata* whole plant allowed the isolation of a novel pregnane glycoside named Carumbelloside I (3-O-β-D-glucopyranosyl (1→6)-β-D-glucopyranosyl-3 β-14 β-dihydroxypregn-5-en-20-one). Carumbelloside-I was evaluated for both antinociceptive activity and anti-inflammatory activity. The antinociceptive activity was evaluated in mice

A new pregnane steroid with an unusual formyl group was isolated by Babu *et al.* (2008) from the stems of *Caralluma umbellata*, together with three known steroid compounds. The structure of this pregnane steroid was elucidated on the basis of spectral evidence including 2D NMR studies.

Two new pregnane compounds named as 3b-hydroxy-pregn-5-ene (CRUR I) and 3b,14 b-dihydroxy pregn-5-ene (CRUR II) were isolated from *Caralluma umbellata* roots and their structures elucidated by extensive spectroscopic studies like IR, H^1, C_{13}- NMR, and MS (Kishore *et al.*, 2010).

Orbea decaisneana (Lem.) Bruyns (=*Caralluma decaisneana* (Lem.) N.E.Br.

In Senegal an extract of the aerial parts enters in a treatment for mental problems and epilepsy. Plant sap is applied to teeth with caries. Plant sap is considered very toxic and milk is taken as an antidote to poisoning. In Mali dried powdered stems are thrown in the water as fish poison; it is considered slow-acting. In Niger the stems are macerated in water and the extract used as bait for guinea fowl. In Algeria nomads put the plant sap or pulped plants on bait to poison jackal. It is sometimes used as criminal poison.

Antiobesity Properties of *Caralluma*

Caralluma adscendens var. *fimbriata*

Caralluma adscendens var. *fimbriata* is regarded amongst the foremost new fad things in weight loss medicine. The extract of the plant has been gradually increasing its acceptance within USA and Europe as words of its capability is spreading to those areas. *Caralluma adscendens* var. *fimbriata* is amongst India's best kept secrets and currently it's advancing to recommend for weight loss, settle for added activity and become healthier, and have additional energy. The plant is clump forming succulents. It is often found growing wild in urban centers of India and it's additionally found to be offered and seen planted at around a boundary marker in gardens and as a roadside shrub.

Methods of Utilization of *Caralluma*

The *Caralluma* is found in India and Africa. It acts as appetite suppressant. It enhances energy. It helps regulate blood glucose levels. It quenches thirst which may be employed by folks whereas partaking in work all day long and in want of energy. The historical usage is that *Caralluma* is employed as a daily vegetable in India, significantly tribal India. It is often eaten in many forms: cooked with salt and spices as an everyday vegetable, utilized in preserves like pickles and chutneys and eaten raw. Indian tribals suppress hunger and enhance endurance whereas on a day's hunt by chewing chunks of *Caralluma*. It is utilized in India as a medicinal plant, now it is available easily in form of *Caralluma* actives. *Caralluma* additionally works in ways in that which is believed that pregnane glycosides play an area in why *Caralluma* is in a position to stop fat accumulation by blocking citrate lyase. It's hydroxycitrate (HCA) that has been proven to contribute to weight loss in humans while not stimulating the central nervous system. The parts that *Caralluma* have an effect are on the appetite management center of the brain. *Caralluma* is believed to possess an inhibitory result on the sensory mechanism of the hypothalamus.

Caralluma actives is created from plant extracts that has been utilized by Indians for thousands of years. Explorers who required travelling an awfully long term on expeditions used *Caralluma* actives. The intake of *Caralluma* actives created a potential for the explorers to travel on with their expeditions for long periods of their time while not eating as a result of the plant suppressing their hunger. Except for this, *Caralluma* actives boosted their overall endurance, which allowed them to become additionally productive in their tasks. This can be the explanation why lots of makers ensure that their merchandise contain this natural herb. However, it should be made sure that a product contains the important *Caralluma* actives, or if they use the proper quantity of it to administer positive results which is why it should be verified on who is exactly selling it.

Caralluma Suppress Hunger

Caralluma product is currently used as appetite suppressant diet pills. *Caralluma* believed to be an efficient part that may stop activities of some enzymes. This may then cause minimal formation of fats and in flip forcing the fat reserves to be burned. Except for that, it's conjointly known to be effective in lowering the blood sugar. *Caralluma* is currently growing popularity for its fitness and health advantages. Thus it is for those that are searching for an effective mechanism to lose weight or management weight gain. It is not rare for a few those who are currently at their ideal body weight to seek additional weight loss in order to improve their performances in sports, or meet needed weight classification for participation in an event which requires low body weight. However, others are also driven by achieving a more engaging body image. The golden rule in weight loss is to avoid foods that are high in sugars that contribute to increased body mass and are detrimental to the general health. Further, weight gain has been associated with excessive alcohol consumption.

Functioning of *Caralluma* for Weight Loss

Caralluma despite the reduction of consumption of food, the consumer doesn't feel the shortage of energy that commonly happens to some those that are on a strict diet. This was also proven safe since it's been cooked as a vegetable and used to preserve chutneys and pickles. In fact, some additionally take them raw.

The key phytochemical constituents of the herb *Caralluma* are pregnane glycosides, flavone glycosides, megastigmane glycosides, and saponins. *Caralluma fimbriata* is thought to help weight loss by blocking the activity of several enzymes, which then blocks the formation of fat, forcing fat reserves to be burned; and it has an effect on the appetite control centre of the brain, which results in the suppression of appetite while still enhancing stamina and endurance.

In a Clinical Study which included 22 people (7 in control group taking Placebo and 15 taking *Caralluma* extract), the *Caralluma* group lost between 1 and 9 pounds. Additionally, those taking *Caralluma* lost 1 to 3 inches around the waist, and an average of 1.82 inches off the hips. There was no significant weight loss for the people taking a placebo, and some actually gained weight. The study found the supplement to be safe (Source: Annual World Conference on Anti-Aging Better Nutrition. Atlanta. Mar. 2008. Vol. 70(3): 1-30).

Mechanism of Action

It is postulated that the pregnane glycosides and perhaps constituents in standardized extract of *Caralluma* principles prevent fat accumulation via blocking

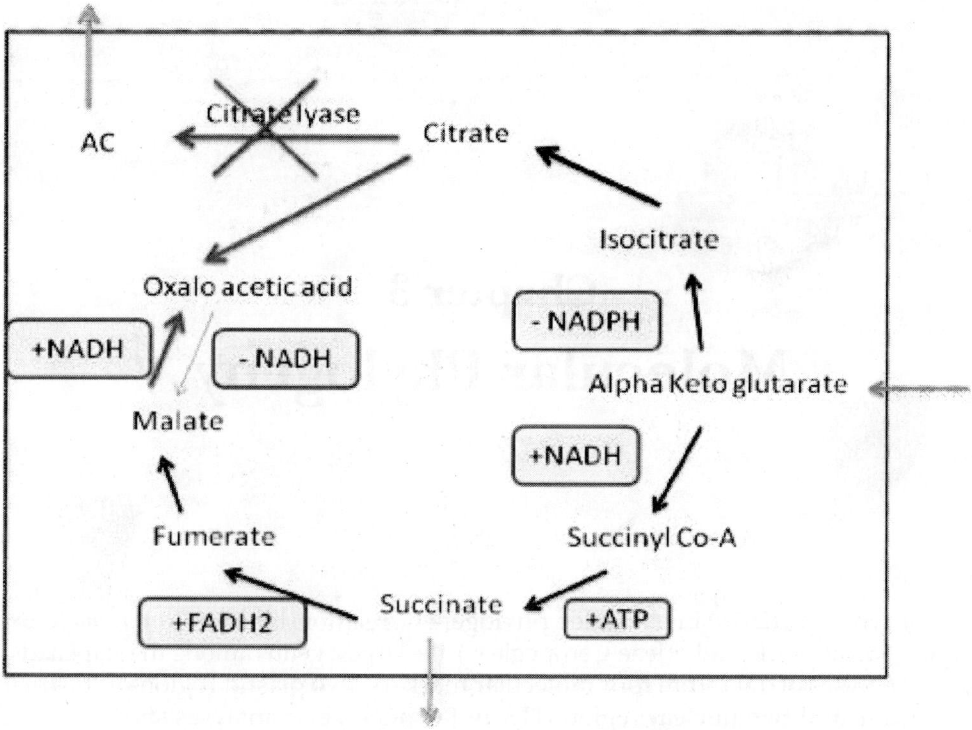

Figure 2.1: Mechanism of Action of *Caralluma* Extract

citrate lyase enzyme system (Preuss *et al.*, 2004). Because standardized extract of *Caralluma* is a competitive inhibitor of ATP-citrate lyase, an extra mitochondrial enzyme involved in the initial 25 steps of de novo lipogenesis. *Caralluma* also has hydroxycitrate (HCA) as active component. HCA has been reported to cause weight loss in humans without stimulating the central nervous system (Jena *et al.*, 2002; Soni *et al.*, 2004). Consequently, HCA reduces the transformation of citrate into acetyl coenzyme-A, a step necessary for the formation of fatty acids in the liver. In addition to its effect on citrate lyase, the postulated blocking of malonyl coenzyme-A by Standardized extract of *Caralluma* could further lead to a decrease in fat formation in the metabolic pathway (Ohia *et al.*, 2001). New fat cells are formed as preadipocytes. Standardized extract of *Caralluma* inhibit new fat cell formation by acting on malonyl coenzyme. It also inhibits this hunger sensory mechanism of the hypothalamus. The pregnane glycosides contained in standardized extract of *Caralluma* interfere with the signaling mechanism and create a signal on its own, seeming to fool the brain into thinking that the stomach is full, even when the person has not eaten much. More specifically, it is believed that the pregnane glycosides in standardized extract of *Caralluma* inhibit the hunger sensory mechanisms of the hypothalamus. It could be assumed that the appetite-suppressing activity of *Caralluma* is attributed to the presence of the aforementioned pregnane glycosides.

Chapter 3
Molecular Phylogeny

Bruyns *et al.* (2010) investigated phylogenetic relationships for *Caralluma* R. Br. (Apocynaceae-Asclepiadoideae-Ceropegieae), the largest genus among the stapeliads, using analyses of data from four molecular markers: two plastid regions *psbA-trnH* and *trnT-F* and two nuclear regions ITS and ncpGS. Their analyses show that the stapeliads consist of two lineages, with *Caralluma* dominating one of these lineages. Within this lineage, *Caralluma* is not monophyletic, with its species distributed among two major clades. One of these clades contains species of *Caralluma* and representatives of *Anomalluma* Plowes, *Echidnopsis* Hook. f. and *Rhytidocaulon* P.R.O. Bally, while in the other clade the small genera *Edithcolea* N.E. Br., *Frerea* Dalz. and *Pseudolithos* P.R.O. Bally are embedded among species of *Caralluma*. They discussed morphological features that characterize some of the clades. *Caralluma* is mainly paleotropical in its distribution and is the most widely distributed group among the stapeliads, from the Canary Islands in Macaronesia to the Indian subcontinent. They showed that the Indian subcontinent has been invaded four times by species of *Caralluma*, while its greatest diversity is found in North-East Africa and southern Arabia.

Mahmood *et al.* (2010) investigated genetic variations within and between two species of *Caralluma viz.*, *Caralluma tuberculata* and *Caralluma edulis* collected from different locations in Pakistan. Random primers OPC series was used for genetic characterization. Ten RAPD markers were used and only 6 of them gave reproducible results with all the primers showing polymorphism (79 per cent) among the samples of both the species. The primer OPC5 showed highest number of bands (89). UPGMA cluster analysis of molecular data showed mixed grouping of samples of both the species and failed to differentiate the species at molecular level. Morphological data of both the species was also recorded for comparison with the molecular data. Based on morphological data the two species of *Caralluma* were clustered into two groups, *viz.*, *C. tuberculata* and the *C. edulis*, while molecular data showed a high level of genetic diversity as both species have shown mixed patterns.

Madhuri *et al.* (2011) investigated genetic variations among six species of *Caralluma viz., Caralluma adscendens* var. *fimbriata, Caralluma stalagmifera, Caralluma adscendens* var. *attenuata, Caralluma longipetala, Boucerosea lasiantha, Boucerosea umbellata* distributed in peninsular India. Accurate authentication to prevent adulteration of target plant with other species is one of the great challenges to plant systematics. Random Amplified Polymorphic DNA fingerprints (RAPD) were used to estimate genetic diversity/similarity among six species of *Caralluma*. Random primers OPA, OPB, OPD and OPN series were used for amplification of DNA segments distributed randomly throughout the genome. Molecular data showed a high level of genetic diversity even at variety level of *Caralluma* species using OPB6, OPB7, OPB8, OPB9, OPB10, and OPB11. Two major groups were identified by NTSY pc-program 2.01 version with 22 per cent similarity.

Molecular Phylogeny of *Caralluma* (*Sensu lato*) Species Occurring in India

S. Siddharthan*

School of Biological Sciences, The University of Hong Kong, Pokfulam Road, Hong Kong

The generic names of *Caralluma* (*sensu lato*) are still a confusion among botanists. Therefore in the present study we used molecular systematics, to study the major phylogenetic groupings among 13 species and 4 varieties (total of 17 taxa) and to provide taxonomic revisions for the Carallumas occurring in India. Nuclear ITS, chloroplast *trnL* intron and *trnLF* intergenic spacers were used for the study. For combined analysis some published sequences (Meve and Liede, 2002) of the *Caralluma* allies were used.

Experimental

Plant Material

Seventeen taxa (13 species and 4 varieties) of *Caralluma s.l.* which occur in India were collected from the original localities. The voucher specimens are available in the herbarium of Sri Krishnadevaraya University, Anantapur, India. The names of plants used in this study, their location, voucher information and Genbank accession numbers are listed in Table 3.1. The names of taxa from Genbank along with their accession numbers are listed in Table 3.2. The stem succulent *Ceropegia dichotoma* was used as outgroup.

DNA Extraction, PCR Amplification and Sequencing

DNA extraction was extracted by the CTAB method (Doyle and Doyle, 1987). About 20 - 50 mg of silica gel dried or fresh leaf material was ground using a glass pestle in an eppendorf tube along with 600 µl of 2× cetyl trimethyl ammonium bromide (CTAB) buffer (50 mM Tris-HCl, pH 8.0, 10 mM EDTA, 2 per cent CTAB, 1.4 M NaCl

* *Present Address*: Post Doctoral Fellow, Department of molecular systematics, Indian Institute of Science, Bangalore).

Table 3.1: *Caralluma s.l.* Species Used in the Study, their Location, Voucher Specimen and Genbank Accession Numbers of ITS, *trnL* and *trnLF* Regions

Sl.No.	Species/Vareity	Location	Voucher	ITS	trnL	trnLF
1	*Apteranthes tuberculata* (N.E.Br.) Meve et Liede	Lalda plain hills, Sunderbehni, Jammu district, Jammu	SKU 31763	HM366926	HM366931	HM366937
2	*Boucerosia lasiantha* (Wight) N.E.Br.	Gooty hills, Anantapur district, Andhra Pradesh	SKU 27970	EU267902	EU267100	EU267090
3	*B. nilagiriana* Subba Rao et Kumari	Madhukarai, Kudrimalai, Tamil Nadu	SKU 28512	HM366922	HM366927	HM366933
4	*B. pauciflora* (Wight) N.E.Br.	Vallanadu forest, Palayamkottai, Tamil Nadu	SKU 28992	EU267905	EU267101	EU267091
5	*B. procumbens* (Gravely et Mayuranathan) Plowes	Maruthuvamalai hills, Kanyakumari district, Tamil Nadu	SKU 28638	-	HM366932	HM366938
6	*B. truncato-coronata* Sedgewick	Tumkur hills near Pemphanahalli village, Karnataka	SKU 28645	HM366935	HM366930	HM366936
7	*B. umbellata* (Roxb.) Haworth	Palni hills, Dindigul district, Tamil Nadu	SKU 27964	EU267901	EU267104	EU267092
8	*B. indica* (Wight et Arn.) Plowes	Satara district, Maharashtra	Kamble 2131	EU267903	EU267099	EU267089
9	*Caralluma adscendens* (Roxb.) R.Br. var. *adscendens*	Near Air port, Madurai, Tamil Nadu	SKU 27963	EU267898	EU267094	EU267082
10	*C. adscendens* var. *attenuata* (Wight) Grav. et Mayur.	Oddanchatram, Dindigul district, Tamil Nadu	SKU 27947	EU267897	EU267095	EU267083
11	*C. adscendens* var. *carinata* Grav. et Mayur.	Near Nagamalai hills, Madurai, Tamil Nadu, India	SKU 27939	EU267896	EU267096	EU267084
12	*C. adscendens* var. *fimbriata* (Wall.) Grav. et Mayur.	Kadiri, Anantapur district, Andhra Pradesh	SKU 27937	EU267900	EU267098	EU267086
13	*C. adscendens* var. *gracilis* Grav. et Mayur.	Palni hills, Dindigul district, Tamil Nadu	SKU 27945	EU267899	EU267097	EU267085
14	*C. bhupinderiana* Sarkaria	Vallanadu forest, Palayamkottai, Tamil Nadu	SKU 28472	HM366923	HM366928	HM366934
15	*C. sarkariae* Lavranos et Frandsen	Nagamalai hills, Madurai,Tamil Nadu	SKU 27965	EU267904	EU267102	EU267087
16	*C. stalagmifera* Fisher	Near Nagamalai hills, Madurai, Tamil Nadu	SKU 27968	EU267894	EU267103	EU267088
17	*Caudanthera edulis* (Edgew.) Meve et Leide	Kuyyala surroundings, Jaisalmer district, Rajasthan	SKU 31764	HM366924	HM366929	HM366935

and 0.1 per cent ß-mercaptoethanol) and incubated at 65°C for 30 mins. The solution was mixed vigourously with 500 µl of chloroform : isoamyl alcohol (24:1) and the supernatant was extracted after centrifugation at 13000 rpm. The chloroform extraction was repeated twice. The supernatent (~400 µl) was mixed with 0.6 volumes of ice-cold isopropyl alcohol and incubated in ice for 10 mins. The precipitate was collected by centrifugation at maximum speed. The pellet was washed with 70 per cent ice-cold ethanol and air dried. The DNA pellet was finally suspended in 100 µl TE buffer (10 mM Tris-HCl, 1mM EDTA, pH 8.0) and stored at -20°C. For some samples DNA was extracted using DNeasy plant mini kit (Qiagen) according to the manufacturer's instructions.

Table 3.2: *Caralluma* Species Used from Genbank, Accession Numbers of ITS, *trnL* and *trnLF* Regions

Name	*ITS*	trnL	trnLLF
Ceropegia dichotoma	EU267906	EU120019	EU127989
Caralluma arachnoidea	AJ310785	AJ410038	AJ410039
Desmidorchis flava	AJ488789	AJ488358	AJ488359
Desmidorchis lavranii	AJ488790	AJ488362	AJ488361
Apteranthes munbyana	AJ488774	AJ488316	AJ488317
Desmidorchis acutangula	AJ488786	AJ488349	AJ488350
Australluma peschii	AJ488776	AJ488322	AJ488323
Apteranthes europaea	AJ488314	AJ488313	AJ488314
Apteranthes tuberculata	AJ488775	AJ488319	AJ488320
Apteranthes burchardii	EU267907	EU120018	EU127988
Caudanthera edulis	AJ402162	AJ402139	AJ402140
Caudanthera sinaica	AJ488782	AJ488340	AJ488341
Desmidorchis arabica	AJ488788	AJ488355	AJ488356
Rhytidocaulon macrolobum	AJ488824	AJ488463	AJ488464
Monolluma socotrana	AJ488806	AJ488409	AJ488410
Monolluma quadrangula	AJ488805	AJ488406	AJ488407
Monolluma hexagona	AJ488804	AJ488403	AJ488404
Echidnopsis squamulata	AJ488798	AJ488385	AJ488386
Echidnopsis angustiloba	AJ488796	AJ488379	AJ488380
Echidnopsis socotrana	DQ469549	-	-

PCR amplification of ITS region was done using primers ITS4 and ITS5m. The ITS product was ~700 bp in length. Chloroplast *trnL* and *trnL-F* regions were amplified using primer pairs c/d and e/f, respectively and the lengths of the amplified products were ~500 bp and ~ 400 bp respectively. PCR amplications were performed in a 25 µl volume containing 10 ng genomic DNA template, 1 µl (10 pM/µl) of both 5'and 3'end-primers, 0.25 mM of each dNTP, 1U Taq polymerase, 2.5 mM $MgCl_2$, 10× PCR buffer containing 50 mM of KCl, 10 mM of HCl. PCR was performed on a Peltier

Thermal Cycler (PTC 200, MJ Research) with an initial 1 min at 95°C followed by 35 cycles of 95 °C for 30 sec, 57°C for 45 s, 72°C for 1min, and nally 72°C for 5mins. The reaction products were electrophoresed on 1 per cent agarose gels using 0.5× Tris-Acetic acid ETDA (TAE) buffer, stained with 0.5 µg/ml ethidium bromide and visualized under UV light to ensure specic amplications before purication. Specic PCR product were excised from the gel and puried with PCR purication kit (Roche) gel puried DNA samples were directly sequenced using the same primers as above with the Big Dye Terminator kit v. 3.1 (Applied Biosystems) on Applied Biosystems 3100 Genetic Analyser.

Table 3.3: Taxa, Total Number of Characters, Parsimonious Information Sites and Models of Evolution

Item	*Number of Taxa*	*Total Characters*	*Parsimony Informative Characters*	*Model*
ITS	39	639	91	SYM+G
TrnL-trnLF	39	825	11	F81+I
trnL-trnLF (gaps coded)	39	845	20	F81+I
Combined	40	1484	111	GTR+I+G

Phylogenetic Analysis

Sequences were aligned using Kalign (Lassmann and Sonnhammer, 2005) and manually edited in BioEdit (Hall, 1999). Phylogenetic analyses was performed using PAUP v. 4.0 beta10 (Swofford, 2002), MrBayes v. 3.1.2 (Ronquist and Huelsenbeck, 2003) and Garli v. 0.951 (Zwickl, 2006). Gaps were coded by simple coding method (Simmons and Ochoterena, 2000) using FastGap v1.1 (Borchsenius, 2009). Maximum likelihood (ML) analysis was performed using Garli. ML bootstrap was performed using 100 repetitive tree searches in Garli. The resulting 100 trees were input into PAUP and the boostrap (BS) values were calculated from the 50 per cent majority-rule consensus tree. The best-fit nucleotide substitution model was selected using jModeltest v. 0.1.1 (Posada, 2008). For Bayesian analysis, two simultaneous independent runs with four Markov chains in 5 million repetitions were performed and trees were sampled every 100th generation. 20 per cent of the resulting 50000 trees were considered as burn-in and the remaining 40000 trees were summarized. Trees were visualized in Figtree v. 1.2.3 (Rambaut, 2007).

Results

Phylogeny Based on ITS Dataset

The total number of taxa and characters for different datasets are given in Table 3.2. The ITS dataset comprised of 39 taxa with 639 nucleotides of which 9 characters were parsimony informative characters. A heuristic search with 100 repetitions, random addition of sequences and TBR swapping resulted in 150 equally parsimonious trees (TL=147, CI=0.904, RI=0.948, RC=0.857, HI=0.096). A strict consensus tree of the 150 most parsimonious trees (data not shown) were basically similar in topology to the ML tree obtained in Garli. The best model selected by the

Akaike information criterion (AIC) was SYM+G. The maximum-likelihood tree with SYM+G model is shown in Figure 3.1. Bayesian posterior support (BPP) and ML bootstrap support (BS) are shown on the branches.

The taxa from India were placed in four separate clades in forming 4 genera, *Apteranthes, Boucerosia, Caralluma* and *Caudanthera* (Figure 3.1). The core *Caralluma sensu sricto (s.s.)* group related to *C. adscendens* formed a well supported clade (BPP=1; BS=100). The African *Caralluma* species *C. arachnoidea* and *C. priogonium* formed well supported sister clade to the Indian *Caralluma s.s.* clade. Another major Indian *Caralluma s.l.* clade well supported (BPP=1; BS=89) of *Boucerosia umbellata, B. lasiantha, B. crenulata, B. pauciflora* and *B. bhupinderiana* (*Boucerosia* clade in Figures 3.1–3.3). *Frerea indica* was found related to this clade but not with significant statistical support. *Apteranthes tuberosa* (syn. *Caralluma tuberosa*) and *Caudanthera edulis* (syn. *Caralluma edulis*) grouped with their respective clades with significant BPP and BS support (Figure 3.1)

Phylogeny Based on cpDNA Dataset

C. bhupinderiana and *Echidnopsis socotrana* used in the ITS analysis were not used in the cpDNA analysis. *C. bhupinderiana* could not be used because its *trnL* sequence could not be obtained in full length. The cpDNA region was quite homogeneous, but had several conserved gaps which might be useful for phylogenetic reconstruction and hence the gaps were coded by the simple coding method (Simmons and Ochterena, 2000). The cpDNA dataset had 39 taxa with 845 characters of which 20 were parsimoniously informative. A heuristic search with 100 repetitions, random addition of sequences and TBR swapping resulted in 1698 equally parsimonious trees (TL=50, CI=0.959, RI=0.972, RC=0.857, HI=0.041). The best model as selected by AIC was F81+I. Bayesian phylogeny tree is shown in Figure 3.2. *Caralluma (s.s.)* and *Boucerosia* were shown in two separate clades but the BPP and BS support were very low. In the cpDNA analysis, similar to ITS, the 4 genera, *Apteranthes, Boucerosia, Caralluma* and *Caudanthera* were resolved but without any BPP/BS (values not shown) support.

Phylogeny Based on Combined ITS and cpDNA Dataset

The combined ITS and cpDNA(coded) dataset had 40 taxa with 1484 characters of which 111 were parsimoniously informative. A heuristic search with 100 repetitions, random addition of sequences and TBR swapping resulted in 2073 equally parsimonious trees (TL=189, CI=0.909, RI=0.943, RC=0.858, HI=0.091) (data not shown). Bayesian analysis of the combined dataset was performed by partitioning and applying the two different models SYM+G and F81+I for ITS and cpDNA datasets respectively. The ML tree (Figure 3.3) was similar in topology to the Bayesian tree and the strict consensus tree from the parsimony analysis. The combined dataset was resolved similar to ITS phylogenetic tree (Figure 3.1). The Indian taxa were resolved in to the clades of *Apteranthes, Boucerosia, Caralluma* and *Caudanthera* with significant statistical support.

Discussion

The choice of taxa for this study was based on the earlier work by Meve and Liede (2002). In their work, they found a well supported clade "southern" clade which comprised of genera from Southern Africa including Madagascar. The samples in the southern clade were excluded in this analysis because they formed a separate clade apart from the core *Caralluma* which are "northern" sensu Meve and Liede (2004).

From the present study it is observed that there are two separate genetic lineages of *Caralluma s.l.* within India based on ITS sequences, "*Caralluma*" clade and *Boucerosia* clade (Figures 3.1–3.3). Plowes (1995) based his classification of Carallumas on two groups, Group A - stems slender, tapering apically, inflorescences racemose, leaves usually lanceolate. Group B - stems robust, not tapering, inflorescence terminally umbellate or laterally displaced by further stem-growth, leaves broad, ovate-acute. The "*Caralluma*" clade falls in Group A and "*Boucerosia*" clade falls in Group B according to Plowes' revision.

The "*Caralluma*" clade consists of the type specimen *Caralluma adscendens*. This group has the following features (Gilbert, 1990): Stems non-rhizomatous, usually erect, pale in colour and usually 4 angled, sometimes terete, tapering at the apex. Leaves lanceolate, leaf rudiments conspicuous. The apical part of the stem bears flowers and is usually long, slender, mostly terete, whip-like often withers after flowering. Inflorescence, few-flowers (2 or more flowers), opening in succession. Flowers usually pendent. They have tufted stipular hairs, corolla usually small, campanulate, brownish-purple with vibratile fusiform cilia. Corona mostly cup-like, biseriate, often stipitate. Corpuscula flange-winged (corpusculum with a triangular wing of thin transparent tissue starting at or slightly beyond the open end of the clasping slit and terminating at the centre of the corspuculum), therefore resembling like the body of a squid, ellipsoidal, follicle pairs erect, V-shaped. This group is distributed in peninsular India and Sri Lanka. *C. subulata* Forsskål ex. Decne. an Arabian species distributed in Yemen, Saudi Arabia, Sudan etc. is closely related to the Indian *C. adscendens* (Plowes, 1995) and is also shown Figures 3.1 and 3.2. *C. sarkariae* and *C. stalagmifera* are also closely related this group by morphology group and nested within the *Caralluma* clade (Figures 3.1–3.3).

C. stalagmifera shows close affinity to *C. adscendens* var. *fimbriata* based on ITS data with good support (Figure 3.1). The morphological similarity between the two are also high. The difference between the two species are corolla characters which are darkish purple throughout with hairs on the margin in *C. stalagmifera* and corolla with transverse yellow striations and also with hairs on the margin in *C. adscendens* var. *fimbriata*. Similarly the distinguishing characters between *C. sarkariae* and other *C. adscendens* varieities is only non-pendulous flowers.

C. priogonium K. Schumann and *C. arachnoidea* (P.R.O.Bally) M.G. Gilbert which are from East Africa (Ethiopia, Kenya, Somalia and Tanzania) were found closely related to the "*Caralluma*" clade with good support in both ITS and CP datasets. *Australluma peschii* (Nel) Plowes (syn. *C. peschii* Nel) a monotypic Namibian endemic genus (Bruyns, 2002) with hairy corolla lobes groups with the core *Caralluma* clade without bootstrap and Bayesian support. In Meve and Liede's (2002) analysis it was clustered with the "southern" clade also without support. According to Plowes (1995) *A. peschii* with slender stems is related to *Caralluma* whereas Meve and Liede (2002)

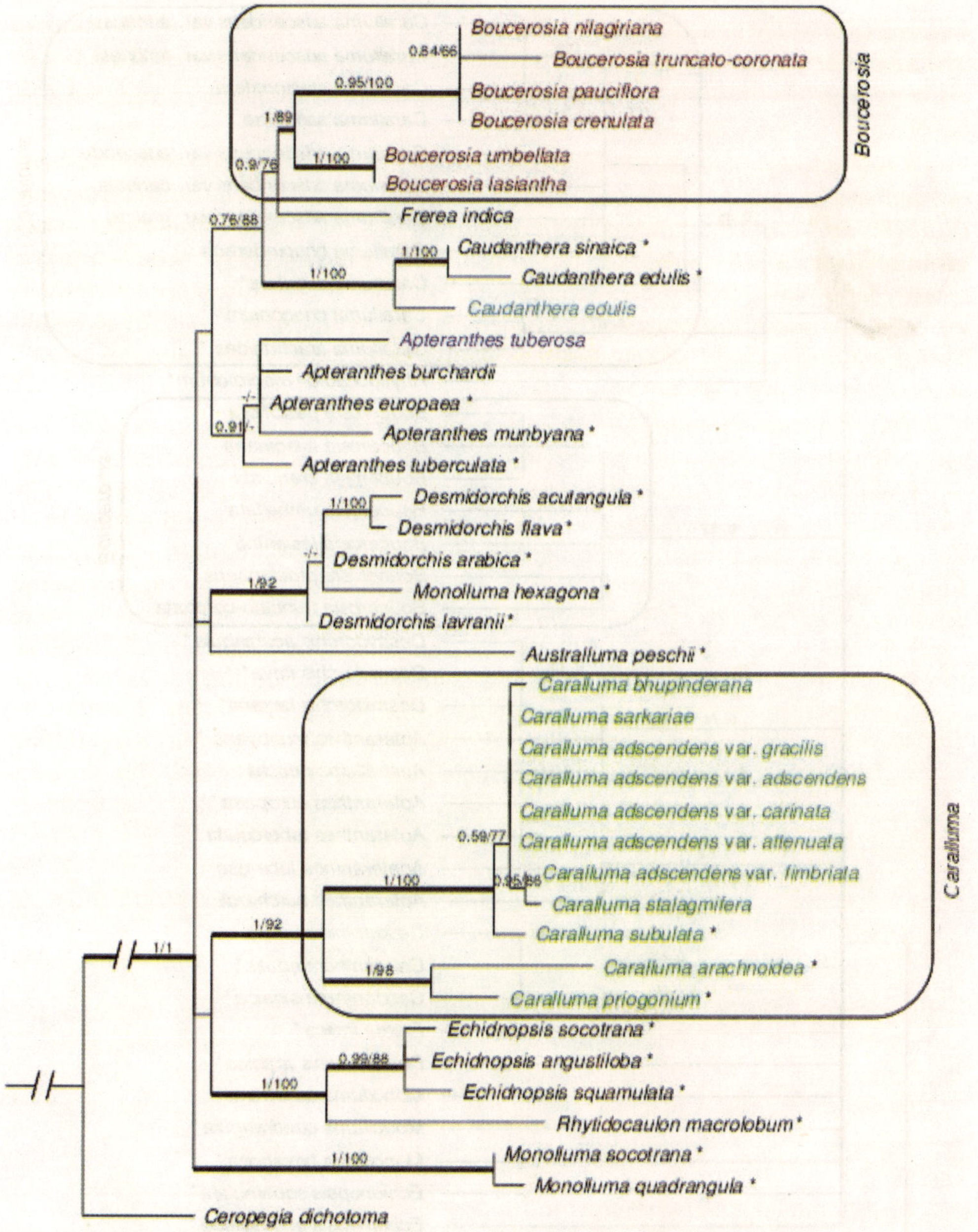

Figure 3.1: Maximum Likelihood Tree Based on ITS Sequences

Numbers beside branches indicate Bayesian posterior probabilities and ML bootstrap values (>50 per cent), in that order. Thick lines indicate branches with significant (≥0.95) posterior probability support. Sequences generated in this study are indicated with asterisk.

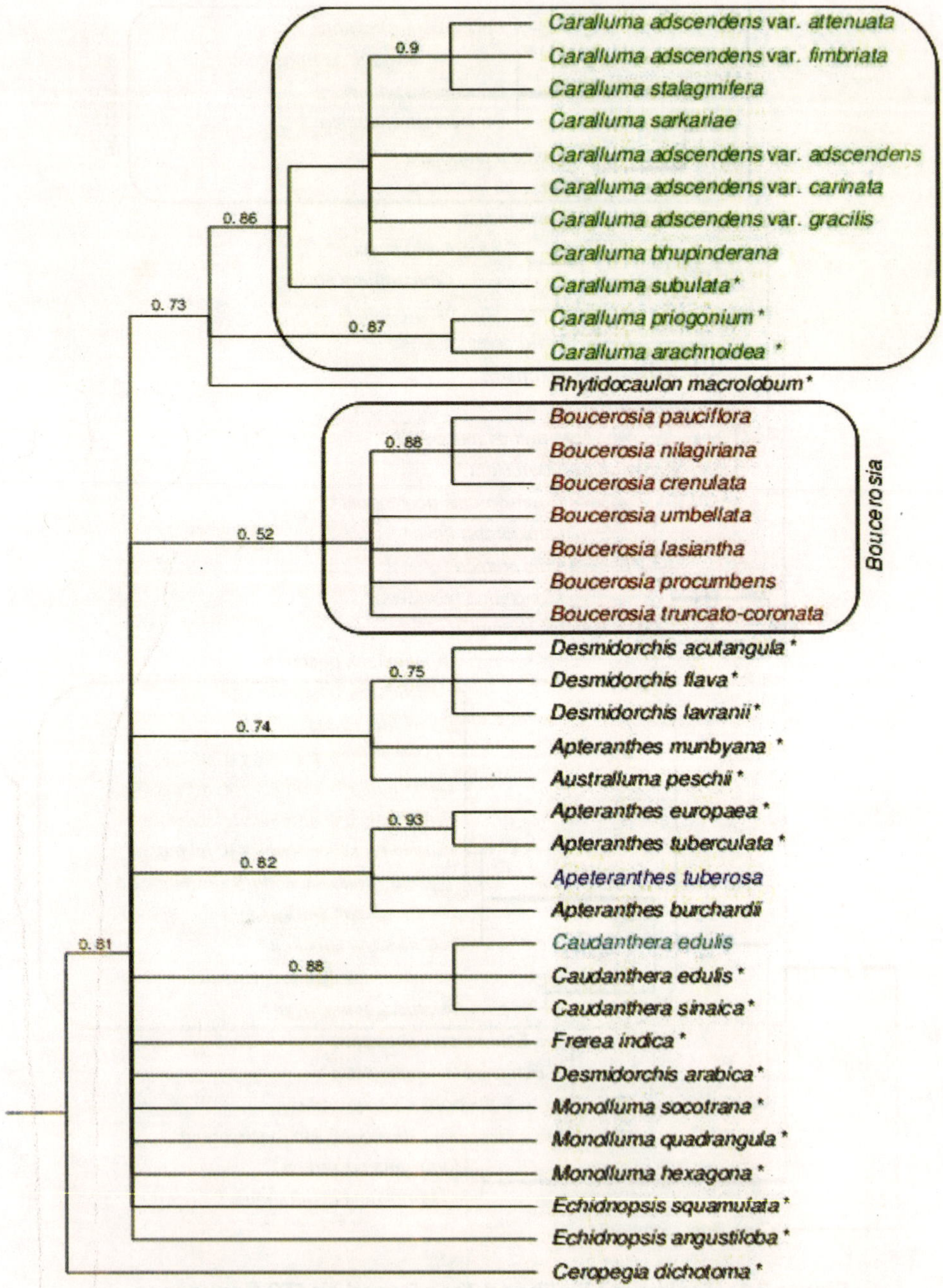

Figure 3.2: Bayesian Tree Based on cpDNA Regions

Numbers beside branches indicate Bayesian posterior probabilities. Sequences generated in this study are indicated with asterisk.

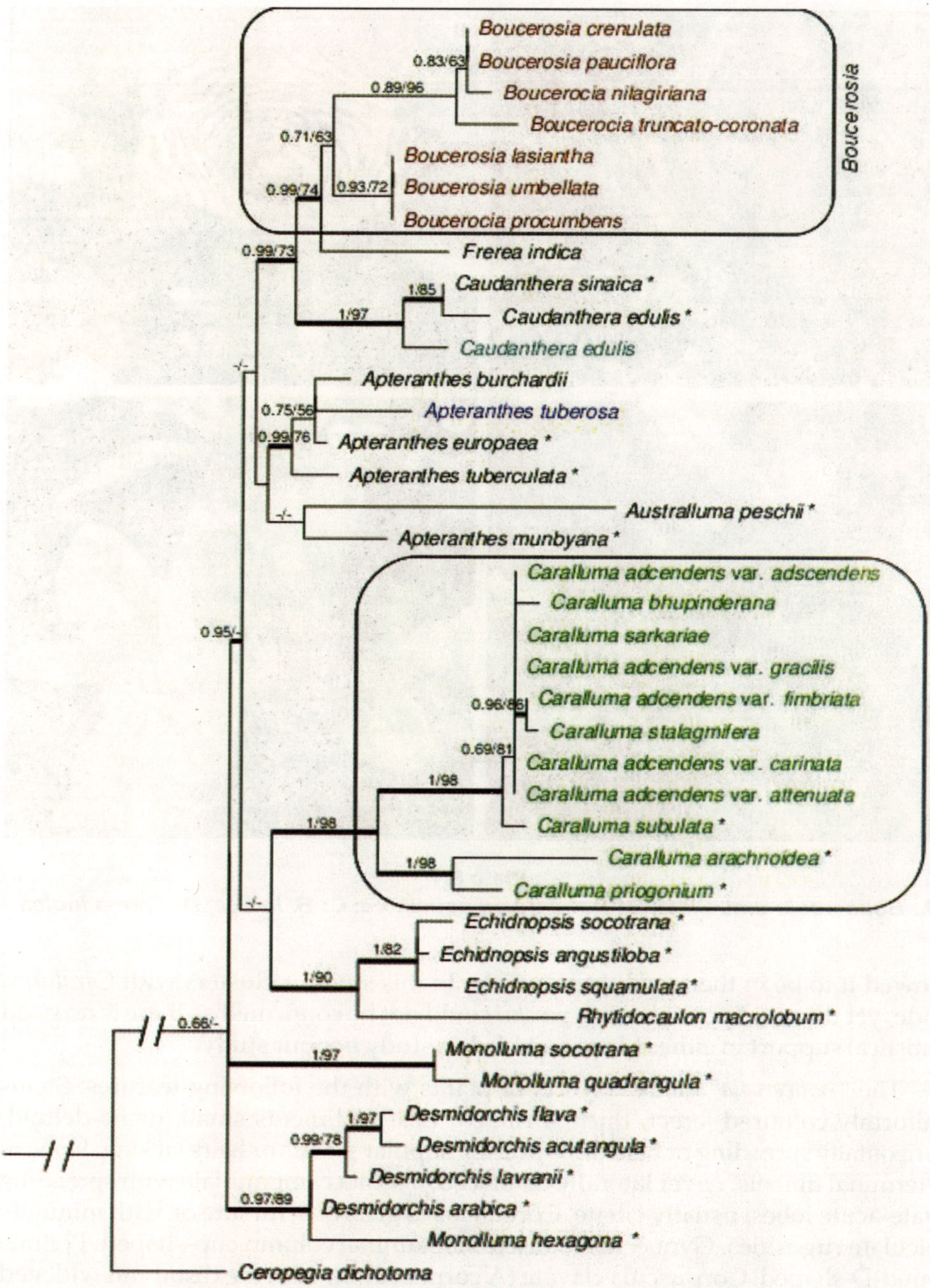

Figure 3.3: Maximum Likelihood Tree Based on ITS and cpDNA Regions

Numbers beside branches indicate Bayesian posterior probabilities and ML bootstrap values (>50 per cent), in that order. Thick lines indicate branches with significant (≥0.95) posterior probability support. Sequences generated in this study are indicated with asterisk.

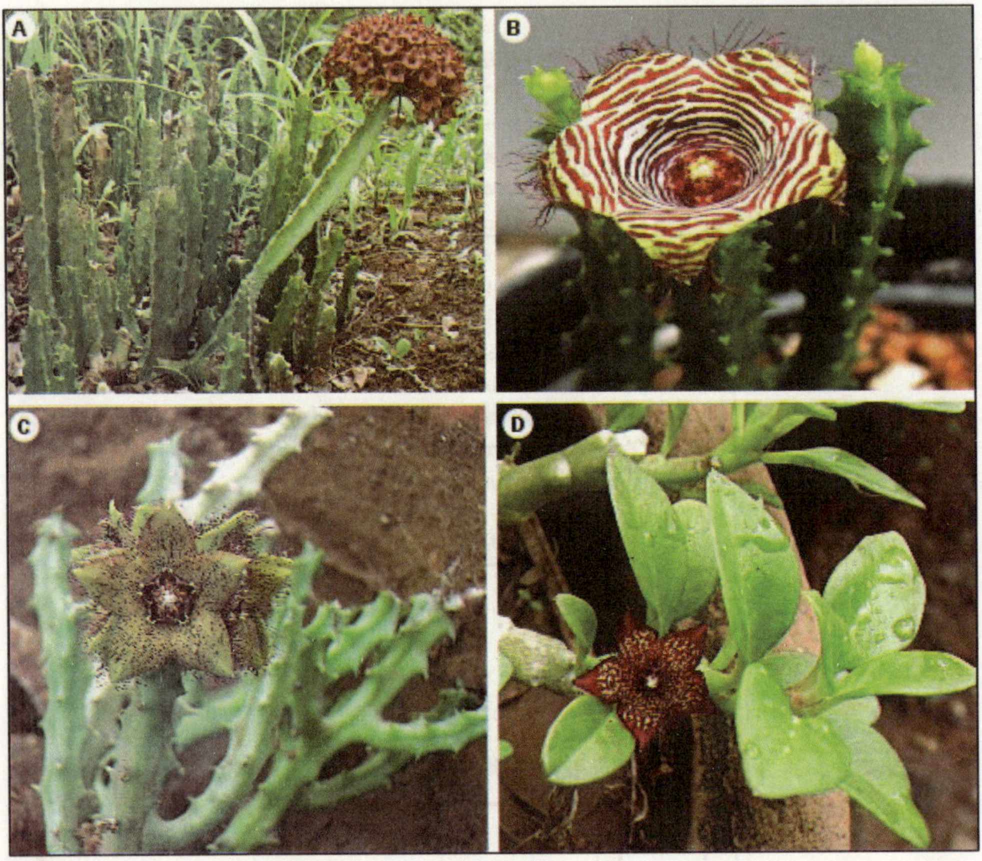

Plate 3.1
A: *Boucerosia umbellata;* B: *Boucerosia pauciflora*; C: *B. indica;* D: *Frerea indica*

showed it to be in their "southern" clade. In this study it clusters with *Caralluma* clade, yet the exact position of *A. peschii* could not be confirmed as there is no good statistical support in either Meve and Liede's study nor our study.

The "*Boucerosia*" clade consists of plants with the following features: Stems uniformly coloured, erect, thick, 4-ribbed. Leaf rudiments small, ovate-deltoid, horizontally spreading or bent downwards. Stipular glands or hairs lacking. Flowers in terminal umbels, never laterally displaced. Corolla campanulate with spreading ovate-acute lobes, usually ciliate. Corolla lobes glabrous, hirsute or with minutely spiculate rugosities. Gynoecium subsessile, staminal column cup-shaped. Pollinia round-D-shaped. Corpuscula clavate (A corpusculum with the distal end widened like a shield), flange winged. Follicles slender, subulate. The members of this clade are distributed in southern India and Sri Lanka (Plowes, 1995).

Frerea indica was subsumed into *Boucerosia* as *B. frerei* based on molecular data, the same results are observed in this analysis as well (Figure 3.1). This treatment is acceptable based on the ITS based phylogeny, but on chloroplast data (Figure 3.2), *Frerea* does not fall under *Boucerosia* clade (Figure 3.2). Therefore we propose to reinstate *Frerea* as a separate monotypic genus.

Frerea indica (syn. *Boucerosia frerei*) is a peculiar species in several aspects. It possesses well-defined leaves and most importantly fusiform underground tubers which are only present in leafy genera of Ceropegiae such as *Ceropegia*. The tubers are formed only in seed grown plants and not from stem cuttings (Sarkaria, 1980). These two characters have led to the speculation that *Frerea* is a relictual genus. But the diploid chromosome number of 44 instead of 22 suggests that it is a polyploid and a derived species (Meve, 1997). Moreover a hybrid between *Frerea* and *Caralluma europaea* has been reported (Plowes, 1995). This interbreeding proves that *Frerea* is closely related to *Caralluma*. From the molecular data in this study *Frerea* is closely related to *Boucersia* clade. Yet the morphology of solitary flowers in *Frerea* is in strong contrast to terminal clustered flowers in *Boucerosia* clade. Therefore there is a possibility that *Frerea* might be derived as a hybrid between both *Caralluma* -like ancestor and a *Boucerosia*-like ancestor. The presence of primitive characters like large leaves and tubers leads to confusing conclusions on the evolution of *Frerea* (Bruyns, 2000). These characters may be synapomorphic, acquired later in evolution rather than derived from a *Ceropegia*-like ancestor. If these characters were derived from an ancient leafy ancestor, the diversity of species with these characters *viz.* presence of leaves, tuber and succulent stems is void. Based on the present molecular data, it can be hypothesized that *Frerea* is a modern genus within the stapeliads with great level of genomic plasticity. To confirm the exact position of this genus several other genes must also be sequenced. It would be fruitful to study the evolution of functional genes especially those responsible for leaf development among *Frerea* and its relatives. Biogeographically *Frerea* must be a neoendemic in its present location in Maharashtra state in India. Considering the fact that the orgin of *Caralluma s.l.* might be in Eastern Africa (Meve, 1997), the ancestor of *Frerea* might have moved eastwards via the dry regions to India, hybridizing among themselves. Its present location which is foot hills of the Western Ghats is relatively rain fed region therefore it might have reverted to a leafy form.

The genus *Caralluma* is an interesting group because of its diversity of beautiful flowers. Several workers have attempted to classify this genus but still a convincing phylogenetic classification is lacking. Meve and Liede (2002) used several taxa of southern Africa in their study, yet the inclusion of taxa is not complete. Several important genera and species used in Gilbert (1990) and Plowes (1995) were not used probably because of unavailability of samples..

Chapter 4
In vitro Propagation

Introduction

Plant tissue culture is a technique used to grow plants or plant tissues and organs starting from a single cell or a small group of cells. This method requires some laboratory knowledge and skill as well as basic laboratory equipment. Micropropagation, the clonal production of complete plants, is commonly used to grow plants on a commercial scale. Some advantages of tissue culture and micropropagation are that many plants can be started in a small space; the plants are kept in sterile condition for research or until they are ready for either hydroponic or traditional growth.

Plants have a remarkable regenerative power, as evidenced by the relative ease with which they can be rooted, transplanted and grafted. Early attempts at growing plants *in vitro* from isolated parts were unsuccessful, because knowledge of plant nutrition and physiology was inadequate. With the discovery of essential plant hormones, some progress was made starting in the 1920s and 30s. A major advancement was made by White in 1939 with his report of continuous culture of carrot and tobacco done completely *in vitro*. Further progress was made by Folke Skoog, who discovered new and important properties of the hormone auxin. Skoog, along with Toshio Murashige, went on to develop the still widely used standard plant nutrient medium *i.e.* Murashige-Skoog (MS) medium (1962). The work begun by Kenneth Vivian Thimann in the late 1950s, which demonstrated that kinetin broke the dormancy of lateral buds, allowing them to develop as if they were at the tips of plants, paved the way for rapid advancements. From then on, new and important results were announced almost every year. Today almost any plant can be grown under laboratory control from a wide range of starting tissues.

In vitro propagation is an efficient means of *ex situ* conservation of plant diversity because with this technology many endangered species can be quickly propagated and preserved from a minimum plant material and with little impact on wild population. In view of the importance of Asclepiadaceous members in medicine and their rarity author and his team have studied methods for *in vitro* propagation.

Tissue Culture Methods

Plant Materials and Surface Sterilization

Plants of *Caralluma* and its relatives can be collected from their natural habitats and grown in garden containing pots under dry conditions. The explants may be selected from well grown tender shoots of potted plants. The shoot segments with six inter nodes are seized and washed with running tap water for 15 min. The nodes are cut (1 cm) separately and they are washed with Tween 20 (Merck, India) detergent solution (5 per cent v/v) for 5 min. After thorough washing, the surface sterilization of explants is followed by rinse with sterile distilled water 3 to 4 times to remove trace of detergent, rinsing in 80 per cent ethanol for 30 s and finally, treatment with mercuric chloride (0.1 per cent w/v) ($HgCl_2$) for 3 min duration. To remove every trace of the sterilant, the shoot material is then washed with sterile distilled water at least 4 to 5 times.

Culture Media and Culture Conditions

A culture medium containing MS (Murashige and Skoog, 1962) salts supplemented with macro-elements, micro-elements, 3 per cent sucrose and gelled with 0.8 per cent (w/v) agar. The pH of media are adjusted, to 5.8 by 1 N NaOH or 1 N HCl after adding the growth regulators. The media are steam sterilized in an autoclave under 15 psi and 121°C for 20 min. All the cultures are incubated under 80 µMol M^{-2} S^{-1} light provided with cool white fluorescent lamp for a photoperiod of 16 h at 25 ± 2°C.

Shoot Initiation and Multiplication

For shoot induction, the nodal explants are cultured on MS medium supplemented with various plant growth regulators like 6-benzyladenine (BA), Kinetin (Kn), 2-Isopentenyl adenine (2iP) and Zeatin (Zn) at different concentrations (0.5, 1.0, 2.0, 3.0 and 5.0 µM) either individually or in combination with indole-3-acetic acid (IAA), indol-3-butyric acid (IBA) (or) α- naphthalene acetic acid (NAA) (0.1 and 0.5 µM). The effects of different strengths of MS media (1/4, 1/3, 1/2 and full strength), various pH levels (5.0, 5.4, 5.8 and 6.2) and different concentrations (50, 100, 200 and 500 mg/l) of ascorbic acid (AA) on morphogenesis are also assessed using optimal concentrations and combinations of BA (8.87 µM) and IAA (2.85 µM). All the cultures are subcultured on to the fresh medium after every four weeks. The frequency with which explants produced shoots, the number of shoots per explant and the shoot length are recorded after six weeks of culture. Shoots with 5 cm in height are separated and individual shoots are transferred for rooting to half-strength MS medium containing different concentrations of NAA (α-naphthalene acetic acid), IAA (indole-3-acetic acid) and IBA (Indole-3-butyric acid). The cultures are incubated under 16 h photoperiod for 30 days until the micro shoots developed the roots.

Acclimatization and Transplantation of Plantlets

The well grown rooted plantlets are removed from the culture tubes and washed with tap water to remove traces of agar. Then, the plantlets are planted onto plastic cups containing a mixture of finely chopped peat mass and sterilized garden manure in 1:1 ratio. The plastic cups are covered with transparent polythene cover to maintain humidity until the development of new rudimentary leaves for 20 days. Then, the plastic cups are transferred to green house and polythene covers are removed. Quarter strength MS major salts solution poured with 7 days intervals up to 40 days of hardening and followed by pouring of tap water. Hardened plants are transferred to pots containing mixture of garden soil and forest humus (1:1 ratio). The pots are watered two days interval under green house condition.

Results and Discussion

Succulent plants differ from their leafy relatives in that they have the ability to retain water longer. They fall into several categories that, while different, all share the same characteristic of being frugal with the moisture they absorb from the soil. When cultured *in vitro*, they must have been supplied with special nutrition because they are having specialized physiological adaptations. Even many successors already standardized the succulent plant tissue culture and multiplied the plants for mass propagation through *in vitro* techniques. *In vitro* propagation of *Caralluma edulis* was reported by Kaur *et al.* (1992). Rathore *et al.* (2008) carried out micropropagation of *Caralluma edulis*. They cultured nodal segments of *Caralluma edulis* on MS medium + 0.25 mg/l BAP + 0.25 mg/l Kn + 0.1 mg/l IAA + Additives and reported that 10-11 shoots were produced with in three to four weeks. Aruna *et al.* (2009) reported micropropagation in three different varieties of *Caralluma adscendens* – *C. adscendens* var. *adscendens*, *C. adscendens* var. *attenua*ta and *C. adscendens* var. *fimbriata*. They cultured nodal segments of three varieties and reported that MS medium + 8.87 μM BAP gave best response (Figure 4.1A, B). Rhizogenesis was reported on half strength MS medium + 0.54μM NAA (Figure 4.1B, C). Kiranmai (2008) has standardized potential multiplication protocol for *Boucerosia pauciflora* with optimum cytokinin concentration for shoot multiplication 7.2 μM BAP and for rooting 1.2 μM IAA.

An efficient protocol has been developed for *in vitro* propagation of *Caralluma sarkariae* by Sreelatha *et al.* (2009). They produced optimal callus for regeneration from mature intermodal explants on MS medium with various concentrations of auxins. They also reported that maximum number of shoots were regenerated from the callus on MS medium + 2 mg/l BAP + 0.5 Kn + 0.5 mg/l NAA.

An efficient protocol was described by Ugraiah *et al.* (2011) for the rapid *in vitro* multiplication of *Caralluma bhupenderiana*, via enhanced axillary bud proliferation from nodal explants collected from young shoots of six-months-old plant. The physiological effects of growth regulators [6-Benzyladenine (BAP), kinetin (Kn), 2-Isopentyl adenine (2iP), zeatin (Zn), indole-3-acetic acid (IAA), indole-3-butyric acid (IBA)], different strengths of Murashige and Skoog (MS) medium and various pH levels on *in vitro* morphogenesis were investigated. The highest number (8.40 + 0.50) of shoots and the maximum average shoot length (3.2 ± 0.31 cm) were recorded on MS medium supplemented with BAP (8.87 μM) at pH 5.8. Rooting was best achieved on

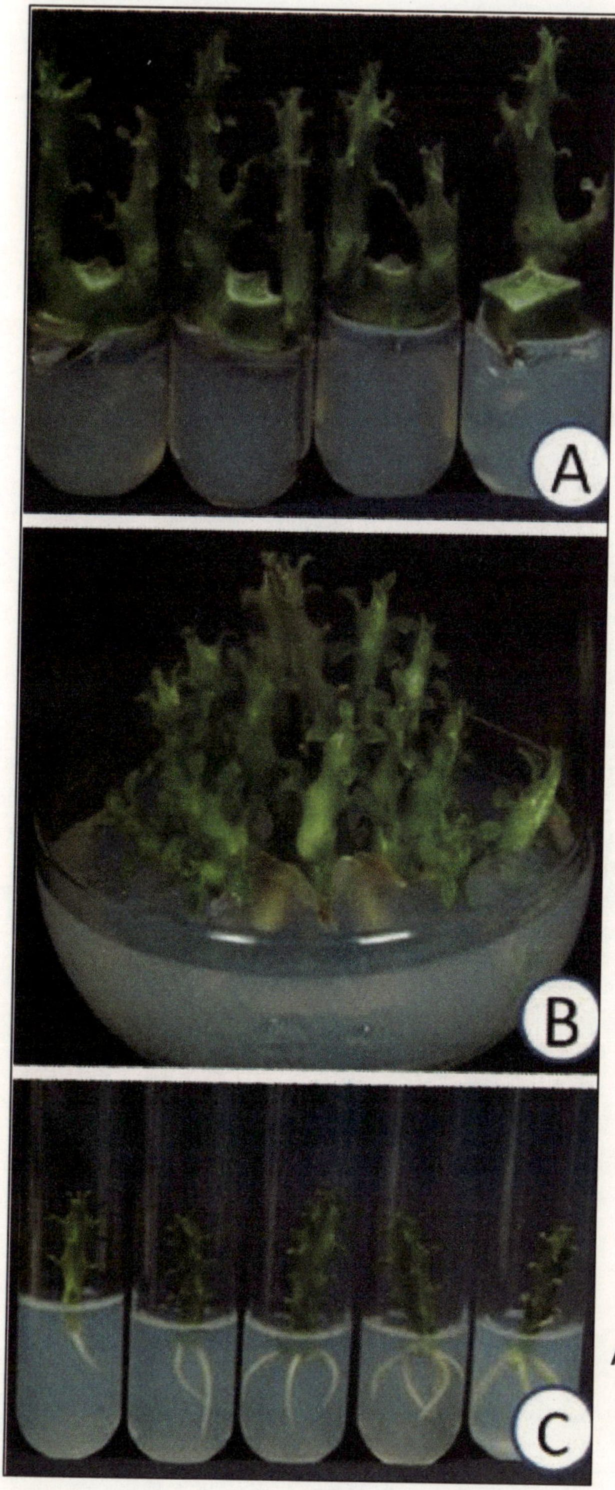

Figure 4.1
A: Sprounting of nodal explants *in vitro Boucerosia lasiantha*;
B: Multiple shoot initiation of *Boucerosia lasiantha;*
C: Root induction

half-strength MS medium augmented with NAA (2.69μM). The plantlets regenerated *in vitro* with well-developed shoot and roots were successfully established in pots containing peat mass and garden manure in 1:1 ratio and grown in a greenhouse with 80 per cent survival rate. The regenerated plants did not show any immediate detectable phenotypic variation.

Nodal explants of mature plants responded on MS medium supplemented with BAP 3 mg/l in *Boucerosia truncato-coronata* respectively. For *Boucerosia indica* MS medium fortified with BAP (2 mg/l) + NAA (0.5 mg/l) was found best for regeneration. In majority of the members half strength MS medium fortified with IBA 1 mg/l or NAA 1 mg/l was effective for better rooting.

Conclusions

We have established a direct *in vitro* culture system for many *Caralluma* species including *Caralluma adscendens* and its varieties, *Caralluma bhupinderiana*, *Caralluma sarkariae*, *Caralluma stalagmifera*, *Boucerosia indica*, *Boucerosia lasiantha*, *Boucerosia pauciflora*, *Boucerosia truncato-coronata*, and *Boucerosia umbellata*, which should enable the large-scale nursery production of these valuable medicinal plants for the conservation and mass multiplication. The outline of protocol offers a potential system for improvement, conservation and micropropagation of all these Indian stapeliadas from nodal explant. MS medium containing BA (2.20 - 8.87 μM) is the best for shoot proliferation. The use of axillary nodes for micropropagation is beneficial than other explant types for these succulents. Half strength MS basal medium supplemented with NAA (1.50 - 2.69 μM) is the best for root induction. There are many modern applications of plant tissue culture techniques. An important application is micro propagation. This is a technique of saving endangered species of plants. It is immensely popular for mass multiplication in a shorter span of time. Thus, this technique has become popular for commercial use too. Hybrid types of explants and clones are produced for further scientific research. Plant tissue culture techniques will be very beneficial in the future for protecting endangered plant species in general.

Chapter 5
Past and Present Work

Past Work

The genus *Caralluma* was first described in 1810 by Robert Brown to include an Indian species with very characteristic elongated flowering stems. A number of other related genera were described subsequently: *Tridentea* (Haworth, 1812), *Pectinaria* (Haworth, 1812), *Desmidorchis* (Ehrenberg, 1829), *Boucerosia* and *Hutchinia* (Wight and Arnott, 1834), *Apteranthes* (Mikan, 1835), *Quaqua* (N.E. Brown, 1879), *Orbeobsis* and *Pachycymbium* (Leach, 1978), *Urmalcala* and *Rhytidocaulon* (Munster, 1990), *Australluma, Borealluma, Caudanthera, Crenulluma, Cryptolluma, Cylindrilluma, Monolluma, Sanguilluma, Saurolluma, Somalluma, Spiralluma* and *Sulcolluma* (Plowes, 1995). Indian *Caralluma* (*sensu lato*), with over 16 species and perhaps 4 genera, have been much less studied and are more diverse than is generally realized. Many new taxa have been described since Gravely and Mayuranathan (1931): These include Kumari and Subba Rao (1976), Lavranos and Frandsen (1978), Sarkaria (1980), Karuppusamy and Pullaiah (2007), Ramachandran *et al.* (2011) and Soumen Aditya (2011a,b). However, only very tentative primitive steps have been taken towards untangling the problems of overall species relationships and generic delimitation. After getting revision of the genus *Caralluma* by Gilbert (1990) and Plowes (1995), the genus is attracting the botanists in many countries. But still vast lacuna in the taxonomy of Indian *Caralluma* exist.

Caralluma adscendens (Roxb.) R.Br. (Syn. *Stapelia adscendens* Roxb.) was originally described from Coromandal coast of Peninsular India without indicating precise locality by Roxburgh. Gravely and Mayuranathan (1931) recognized a total of five varieties within this species. Mainly these varieties can be divided into 2 major groups based on whether the stems have rounded or acute angles. But Bruyns (1984) has drawn attention to the very great similarity between one of these variety *fimbriata*, and *Caralluma subulata* from Arabia and *Caralluma dalzielii* from West Africa. This could be taken to indicate that the two groups such as round and acute angles varieties merit formal recognition at least as subspecies. The status of the varieties within *C. adscendens* seems more questionable as Gravely and Mayuranathan indicated that intermediates are apparently common (Gilbert, 1990).

Following Brown, other taxonomists have also been greatly acknowledged the genus *Caralluma* for different other succulents like *Frerea*, *Stapelia* etc. (White and Sloane, 1937; Rowley 1980). *Boucerosia* was first described by Wight and Arnott to include Indian species with flowers in terminal umbels. It was used quite widely for Indian, Arabian and Mediterranean species. Brown did not attempt to recognize infrageneric grouping of the genus. Schumann (1895) has recognized three sections, *Eucaralluma* (=*Caralluma*), *Lalacruma* (=*C. gracilis*) and *Boucerosia*, but completely ignored all Southern African species and restricted the genus to East Africa northwads. White and Sloane (1937) have accounted all the species under a single genus with an uncritical compilation aimed for horticulturists but with a remarkable number of critical illustrations and listing of taxa known at the time. They described *Caralluma* as that group of species left when all the other Stapeliad genera have been delimited. Such a definition is an immediate indication that *Caralluma* sensu N. E. Brown is likely to be a heterogeneous assemblage of taxa only dubiously related to each other.

Leach and Plowes (1966) divided the genus into a series of a informal groups. These can now be seen to be of limited value, they include some glaring anomalies. They recognized many of the names conspecifics to each other and also many species did not have collections and preserved specimens. The main practical strength of these groupings is that they are largely geographically based and thus they have picked out, partly, some major groupings, at least some of which deserve generic status.

As long as all the present species of *Caralluma* remain in that genus, the name *Caralluma* has no relevance as a guide either to their phylogenetic relationships or to their overall appearance. Gilbert (1990) reviewed the genus *Caralluma* and the species it still included; this was a notable contribution to the overall understanding of this genus and its various species complexes, but he restricted the *Caralluma* for long stemmed racemose flowering species together with those that had compact umbellate cluster of flowers, either as subgenera or as other infra-generic aggregations. This treatment, however, does not appear to be based on any strong unifying factors that justify keeping all these disparate taxa grouped in one or two genera only (Plowes, 1995).

Plowes in 1995 strongly proposed 17 genera. Indian species of *Caralluma* were placed in 4 different genera including a *Caralluma* and *Boucerosia*, the additionally added the new generic names for Indian *Caralluma* such as *Cryptolluma* (=*Caralluma edulis*) and *Borealluma* (=*Boucerosia tuberculata*). He has erected many genera that are based on monotypic. But recent taxonomists (Meve and Liede, 2002) greatly opposed the Plowes view on the delimitation of names for genus *Caralluma*.

The history of Indian *Caralluma* started in 1795 by Roxburgh, who described the first species as *Stapelia adscendens*, currently recognized as *Caralluma adscendens*. Then, Haworth (1812) has described *Boucerosia umbellata*. The chronological order of Indian *Caralluma* descriptions are given in Table 5.1. At present about 16 accepted taxa with eleven varieties (infraspecific) taxa were identified so far. Many of the previously described genera and species were recognized as synonyms for existing taxa.

Table 5.1: Chronological Order of Descriptions of Indian *Caralluma*

Sl.No.	Caralluma Species	Year	Author	Place of Collection
1.	*Stapelia adscendens*	1795	Roxburgh	Coromandel India
2.	*Caralluma umbellata*	1812	Haworth	South India
3.	*Caralluma crenulata*	1830	Wallich	Segain on the Irrawady, Myanmar
4.	*Boucerosia pauciflora*	1834	Wight	Palayamkottai, Tamil Nadu
5.	*Hutchinia indica* (*Boucerosia indica*)	1834	Wight and Arnott	Indian peninsula
6.	*Boucerosia campanulata*	1850	Wight	Unknown locality, India
7.	*Boucerosia diffusa*	1850	Wight	Coimbatore
8.	*Boucerosia lasiantha*	1850	Wight	Nuggur hills, Madras
9.	*Boucerosia edulis*	1862	Edgeworth	Multan and Sindh
10.	*Caralluma tuberculata*	1892	N.E. Brown	Punjab and Baluchistan
11.	*Boucerosia truncato-coronata*	1921	Sedgewick	Hubli, Dharwar
12.	*Caralluma stalagmifera*	1925	Fischer	Vandalur near Madras
13.	*Caralluma adscendens* var. *fimbriata*, var. *attenuata*, var. *carinata*, var. *geniculata*, var.*gracilis*	1931	Gravely and Mayuranathan	Tamil Nadu
14.	*Boucerosia procumbens*	1931	Gravely and Mayuranathan	Aramboli hills, Kanyakumari dt.
15.	*Caralluma nilagiriana*	1976	Kumari and Subba Rao	Nilagiri hills, Tamil Nadu
16.	*Caralluma sarkariae*	1976	Lavranos and Frandsen	Madurai, Tamil Nadu
17.	*Caralluma bhupenderiana*	1980	Sarkaria	Palayamkottai, Tamil Nadu
18.	*Caralluma stalagmifera* var. *longipetala*, var. *intermedia*	2007	Karuppusamy and Pullaiah	Madurai, Tamil Nadu. Gooty, Anantapur
19.	*Caralluma moorei*	2011	Aditya	East coast of Southern India
20.	*Caralluma sarkariae* var. *longipedicellata*	2011	Aditya	Madurai, Tamil Nadu
21.	*Caralluma adscendens var. bicolor (=Caralluma bicolor)*	2011	Ramachandran	Coimbatore, Tamil Nadu

List of Genera Related to Indian *Caralluma*

1. **Apteranthes J.C. Mikan (= *Borealluma* Plowes)**
   a) *Apteranthes tuberculata* (Plowes ex N.E. Brown) Meve et Liede = *Caralluma tuberculata* N.E. Brown

2. **Boucerosia Wight et Arnott**
   a) *B. crenulata* (Wall.) Wight et Arnott = *Caralluma crenulata* Wall.
   b) *B. diffusa* Wight = *Caralluma diffusa* (Wight) N.E.Brown
   c) *B. indica* (Wight et Arnott) Plows = *Hutchinia indica* Wight et Arnott = *C. indica* (Wight et Arnott) N.E.Brown
   d) *B. lasiantha* Wight = *Caralluma lasiantha* (Wight) N. E. Brown
   d) *B. pauciflora* Wight = *Caralluma pauciflora* (Wight) N.E.Brown
   e) *B. procumbens* (Gravely et Mayuranathan) Plowes = *C. procumbens* Gravely et Mayuranathan
   f) *B. truncato-coronata* Sedgewick = *Caralluma truncato-coronata* Gravely et Mayuranathan= *Caralluma nilagiriana* Kumari et Subba Rao
   g) *B. umbellata* (Haworth) Wight et Arnott = *Caralluma umbellata* Haworth (*B. frerei* (Rowley) Meve et Leide = *Frerea indica* Dalz. – we excluded from the current enumeration because of the leafy tuberous succulent, not forming umbellate flowers on stem tip)

3. ***Caralluma* R. Brown**
   a) *Caralluma adscendens* (Roxb.) N.E. Browm = *Stapelia adscendens* Roxb.
   b) *C. adscendens* var. *attenuata* (Wight) Gravely et Mayuranathan = *Caralluma attenuata* Wight
   c) *C. adscendens* var. *carinata* Gravely et Mayuranathan
   d) *C. adscendens* var. *bicolor* (Ramachandran *et al.*) Karup., Ugraiah et Pullaiah = *C. bicolor* Ramachandran *et al.*
   e) *C. adscendens* var. *fimbiata* (Wallich) Gravely et Mayuranathan = *Caralluma fimbriata* Wallich
   f) *C. adscendens* var. *gracilis* Gravely et Mayuranathan
   g) *C. bhupinderiana* Sarkaria
   h) *C. geniculata* (Gravely et Mayuranathan) Meve et Liede = *C. adscendens* var. *geniculata*
   i) *C. moorei* Aditya
   j) *C. sarkariae* Lavarnos et Frandsen
   k) *C. sarkariae* var. *longipedicellata* Aditya
   l) *C. stalagmifera* C.E.C. Fischer

m) *C. stalagmifera* var. *intermedia* Karup. et Pullaiah

n) *C. stalagmifera* var. *longipetala* Karup. et Pullaiah

4. Caudanthera Plowes
(= Cryptolluma Plowes)

a) *Caudanthera edulis* (Plowes ex Edgew.) Meve et Liede = *Boucerosia edulis* Edgew.

Vernacular Names

It is postulated that the word *Caralluma* originates from the Telugu vernacular 'kar' or 'karu'- 'allam'. 'Kar' or 'karu' means forest or wild and 'allam' means ginger. But this name could not be found among the Telugu people today.

The local names of *Carallumas* are based either on their habitat, shape, association or some such characteristics. The follicles of some of the plants are likened to the hare ('Kundelu') ears ('Chevulu or Chevi') or horns ('Kommulu' or 'Kommu'). Thus, *C. stalagmifera* and members with a similar appearance, like *C. adscendens* var. *fimbriata*, are commonly called as "Kundeti Kommulu" in Telugu. Even the Tamil name "Muyal Kombu Chedi" gives the same meaning. *C. adscendens* var. *fimbriata* is called as "Makad Sing" in Marathi, meaning "monkey's horn". The leaves of the smaller members of the 'indica' group are likened to the ears of smaller animals like mouse and are called "Eluka Chevulu" (Henry *et al.*, 1987; Gravely and Mayuranathan, 1931; Ram Gandhi, 1999). In the Anantapur district the name 'kalabanda'(Hooker, 1885) is the name most commonly used, though elsewhere it seems to be confined to aloes and agaves. It means literally "a dweller among rocks". *Boucerosia tuberculata* is called "Churungli" or "Panchungli" in the Sunderbani area, Jammu, literally meaning "four-fingers" or "five-fingers". This name aptly describes the way these finger-like projections poke out of the grass in habitat (Kirtikar and Basu, 1935; Ram Gandhi, 1999).

The most widespread name for some of the *Boucerosia* in Tamil Nadu is "Kallimuliyan". This is perhaps because of their association with *Euphorbias*, which are referred to as "Kalli" (succulents) in Tamil. In some areas, the above-mentioned words are corrupted to "Kallivan" and "Iluvan". Since *Boucerosia umbellata* is eaten by only the Oddan caste in Salem district of Tamil Nadu, it is called "Oddan Kallivan" (Gravely and Mayuranathan, 1931; Henry *et al.*, 1987; Ram Gandhi, 1999)

Other associations give rise to other names. In Tirupattur region of Tamil Nadu, *Carallumas* are likened to *Cissus quadrangularis* because of the squarish nature of stem, which is called as "Pirandai" in Tamil. So they are called "Puliyam pirandai or Pulicham pirandai" which literally means "Sour *C. quadrangularis*". The sour taste of some of these plants also gets them the name of "Pulicha thanda" (sour stick) in Palghat area and "Pulichan" (sour thing) in Pollachi area. Stronger attributes given to some of them are "Kallukudainchan" and "Kallumudayan" (that which pierces the rock) in Tirunelveli area (Gravely and Mayuranathan, 1931; Henry *et al.*, 1987). Some part of Dindigul district in Tamil Nadu local tapoos named the Carallumas as "Iluvaan, Elumaan, pulichaan and uppampulichaan". At Hospet in the Bellary district the Kanarese were found to combine the Kanarese word 'huli' with the Telugu word "chinta", both meaning tamarind, and to use the resulting 'hulichinta' (Brown,1892) for *Caralluma*. In Jaisalmer area, Rajasthan *Caudanthera edulis* is called as 'Pimpa'. Small stemmed *Boucerosias* like *B. indica* and *B. pauciflora* are called as "Sirupirandai" in Madurai district of Tamil Nadu.

Uses of Carallumas

In literature, we come across only two uses for the *Caralluma*. While some of these are reported to be edible, few of them are accredited with medicinal properties. The following is an account of the uses of Carallumas.

Edible Uses

Caralluma edulis, as the name suggests, is edible. It is reported that the young shoots of this plant are sold in the market at Jaisalmer. They are described as acidic in taste (Bhandari, 1978).

Some of the *Carallumas* like *C. adscendens, C. attenuata, C. fimbriata, C. edulis, C. indica* are reported to be useful as vegetable (Cook, 1905; The Wealth of India, 1950).

Caralluma tuberculata occurs wild and is also reported to be cultivated throughout Pakistan. This plant is claimed to be eaten raw or cooked as a vegetable (Ahmad, 1988, 1993). This plant is reported to be eaten by people in Punjab as a vegetable (Chunga), either cooked or pickled. It is also supposed to be eaten by goats and other herbivores. It has a bitter sour taste.

The smaller plants of the indica group like *Boucerosia truncato-coronata, B. indica* and *B. pauciflora* are often eaten raw by the locals, especially the shepherds and goatherds as well as their goats. They are not so bitter; rather, they have a sourish taste. The larger forms of *Boucerosia* do not seem to be eaten at all except by the Oddans of Coimbatore and Salem districts, who first cook them.

Historical Uses

Caralluma use is well recorded in Ayurveda and Unani records dating back to centuries ago. Many references to *Caralluma* as food are found throughout a vast historical search of archived literature. Thus toxicity is a taboo. Some species however have toxic compounds and for any one interested in buying *Caralluma* they need to be very sure of their source. Interestingly enough we find numerous cures for ailments ascribed to *Caralluma*, *e.g.*, Diabetes mellitus, Rheumatoid arthritis, Leprosy, Ascariasis, used for Blood purification.

Indian Contribution

Mayuranathan was the first Indian to conduct a survey of *Carallumas* in India along with Gravely. They described 12 species and 5 varieties of *Carallumas*. (Gravely and Mayuranathan, 1931).

Jagadish S. Sarkaria, in the past three decades, has traveled extensively in the field and studied the Indian *Carallumas* in detail. He is credited with the discovery of two new species – *C. bhupinderiana* and *C. sarkariae*. He feels that there are still at least two more plants that need to be described. He is the founder of the "Indian Society of

Cactii and Succulents". He was responsible for the development of "National Cactus and Succulent Botanical Garden and Research Centre" at Chandigarh.

Dr. Ram Gandhi of New Delhi, a doctor by profession and a hobbyist, is the first Indian to write the book entitled "*Carallumas* of the Indian Subcontinent" (Ram Gandhi, 1999). This book is with colour photographs of different *Carallumas* but line diagrams are not informative.

Present Work

The Present investigation involved detailed survey of the dry areas of eight Indian states namely Tamil Nadu, Andhra Pradesh, Karnataka, Orissa, Jammu and Kashmir, Rajasthan, Maharashtra and Gujarat. Frequent field visits were carried out in all the study areas in various seasons to record flowering and fruiting nature of genus *Caralluma*.

Field Study

During the course of present study (2007-2011), intensive field visits were carried out in different seasons covering almost all the important dry areas in different regions of India for collection of species belonging to the genus *Caralluma* of sub-family Asclepiadoidae of Apocynaceae. Field trips include pre-monsoon, monsoon and post-monsoon periods to procure different developmental stages of plants, *i.e.*, vegetative, flowering and fruiting. Collections were made from a wide range of habitats, *i.e.*, foot of the hills, open scrub areas, road side etc. The specimens were collected in quadruplicate. Relevant field data such as habit, habitat, flower colour and aroma, associated plants, abundance, general distribution, local names and economic importance of the individual species were collected. Information on medicinal uses of some plants was collected from local inhabitants. Field numbers were given for every specimen collected and all the above information was recorded carefully in the field itself. Photographs of all plants and general vegetation types were also taken during field work. Many of our photographs have been sent to Stapeliad database maintained by Cactus and Succulent Society of America (CASSA) (http://www.stapeliads.info/serv/core.s3) and can be viewed by taxonomists and stapeliad lovers.

Preparation of Herbarium

Standard universally accepted methods prescribed by Santapau (1955) and Jain and Rao (1977) in herbarium preparation have been followed. The specimens were collected in well-tied thick polythene bags to avoid desiccation and to protect from withering. Preparation of herbarium of the *Caralluma* is very difficult because of its succulent nature. The quadrangular succulent stems were cut vertically length wise, processed in alcohol with a pinch of Mercuric chloride ($HgCl_2$) for a few minutes to prevent the fungal infection. Dipping the plant in mercuric chloride is called dry method. Immediately they were placed in between the blotting papers with the help of forceps. These were tied properly with the help of iron plant pressers. Next day, the blotting papers were changed and the specimens were spread properly in such a way that their physical appearance is not changed. The spread specimens were once again placed in iron pressers and this process is continued till the specimens were completely dried.

The poisoned, well pressed and dried specimens were pasted with fevicol on standard herbarium sheets measuring 42 X 28 cm. The specimens were stitched wherever necessary. Labels with all relevant information such as botanical name, family, locality, altitude, date of collection, collector's name etc. were affixed on the right hand bottom corner of herbarium sheets.

Modern identification methods were followed for the identification of collections, consulting in the initial stages various floras of Hooker (1885), Gamble (1915-35), Matthew (1983), Henry *et al.* (1987), Jagtap and Singh (1999), State floras like Flora of Andhra Pradesh (Pullaiah and Moulali, 1997), Flora of Karnataka (Sharma *et al.*, 1984), Flora of Orissa (Saxena and Brahmam, 1995), Flora of Maharashtra (Almeida, 2001), Flora of Bihar Analysis (Singh *et al.*, 2001), Flora of Rajasthan (Shetty and Singh, 1991) etc., district Floras like Flora of Anantapur (Pullaiah and Yesoda, 1989), Flora of Kurnool (Venkata Raju and Pullaiah, 1995), Flora of Krishna (Lakshminarayana *et al.*, 1997), Flora of Medak (Pullaiah *et al.*, 1997), Flora of Visakhapatnam (Venkateswarlu *et al.*, 1972, Subba Rao and Kumari, 2002), Flora of Adilabad (Pullaiah *et al.*, 1992), Flora of Guntur (Pullaiah *et al.*, 2000), Flora of Nizamabad (Pullaiah and Ravi Prasad rao, 1995), Flora of Ranga Reddi (Pullaiah and Mohammed, 2000), Flora of Nellore (Suryanarayana and Sreenivasa Rao, 2001), Flowering plants of Chittoor (Madava Chetty *et al.*, 2008), A contribution to the flora of Prakasam (Bhairavamurthy and Mohan, 1991), Flora of Kolhapur (Yadav and Sardesai, 2002), Flora of Palghat (Vajravelu, 1990), Flora of Nasik (Lakshminarasimhan and Sharma, 1991) etc. and also other relevant research papers.

Preliminary identification was verified with the authenticated specimens at Madras herbarium, Coimbatore (MH), Central National Herbarium, Howrah (CAL) and Herbarium of Botanical survey of India, Pune (BSI).

Final identifications were made after carefully dissecting the floral parts of the specimens under Olympus binocular microscope. Various dissected floral parts were affixed on a small adhesive paper board and placed it in a small pocket and it turn it is affixed on the left hand bottom side of the concerned herbarium sheet. Illustrations were drawn after critical study. After identification, the mounted herbarium sheets were kept in the Herbarium of Department of Botany, Sri Krishnadevaraya University, Anantapur (SKU) for future use and reference. A second set has been deposited in Madras Herbarium (MH), Botanical survey of India, Coimbatore and third set has been deposited in Central National Herbarium (CAL), Botanical survey of India, Howrah. Fourth set has been kept as stock.

Ethnobotanical study of genus *Caralluma* was also carried out during the field visits by enquiring the local inhabitants on the uses of *Caralluma* species.

During the field visit, observations were made for the *Caralluma* species such as habit, habitat, habit association, flowering and fruiting phenology, population variation and frequency, population overlapping with other species of *Caralluma*, reproductive capacity of population and threatening factor for *Caralluma* diversity.

Table 5.2: Periodical Field Trips Conducted for *Caralluma* Collection all Over India during the Years 2007–11

Sl.No.	*Place Visited*	*State*	*Date*	*Species Collected*	*Total Voucher Numbers*
1.	Bhupoor, Pavagada	Karnataka	24-02-08	*Caralluma adscendens* var. *attenuata, C. adscendens* var. *fimbriata, Boucerosia umbellata*	3
2.	Soudatti, Dhawar	Karnataka	26-03-08	*Caralluma adscendens* var. *fimbriata*	2
3.	Gooty	Andhra Pradesh	23-04-08	*Boucerosia lasiantha, Caralluma adscendens* var. *fimbriata, C. stalagmifera* var. *intermedia*	5
4.	Madurai	Tamil Nadu	04-05-08	*Caralluma adscendens* var. *attenuata, C. stalagmifera* var. *stalagmifera, C. sarkariae, C. stalagmifera* var. *longipetala, C. adscendens* var. *carinata*	8
5.	Vallanadu, Tirunelveli	Tamil Nadu	05-05-08	*Boucerosia pauciflora, Caralluma bhupinderiana*	3
6.	Kottaram hills, Kanyakumari	Tamil Nadu	07-05-08	*Caralluma geniculata, Boucerosia procumbens*	2
7.	Sirumalai, Palani hills, Varathamanthi dam, Dindigal	Tamil Nadu	08-05-08	*Caralluma stalagmifera* var. *stalagmifera, C. adscendens* var. *adscendens, C. adscendens* var. *carinata, C. sarkariae, C. adscendens* var. *gracilis, Boucerosia umbellata*	7
8.	Kurdimalai, Madukarai, Coimbatore	Tamil Nadu	10-05-08	*C. adscendens* var. *attenuata, Boucerosia nilagiriana*	3
9.	Halumalleswar, Lokadal, Chitradurg	Karnataka	14-06-08	*Caralluma adscendens* var. *attenuata, C. adscendens* var. *adscendens, C. adscendens.* var. *fimbriata, Boucerosia lasiantha*	12
10.	Pavagada hills	Karnataka	18-06-08	*Boucerosia lasiantha, Caralluma stalagmifera* var. *stalagmifera, C. adscendens* var. *fimbriata*	4
11.	Penchalakona,Nellore dt.	Andhra Pradesh	12-07-08	*Boucerosia indica*	1
12.	Kalasamudram	Andhra Pradesh	19-07-08	*C. adscendens* var. *attenuata, Boucerosia lasiantha, Caralluma adscendens* var. *fimbriata*	3
13.	Vellore	Tamil Nadu	02-08-08	*C. stalagmifera* var. *stalagmifera*	1
14.	Thiruvannamalai	Tamil Nadu	04-08-08	*Boucerosia diffusa*	2
15.	Sukunda, Mohrikaluva, Ganjam	Orissa	29-08-08	*Caralluma adscendens* var. *adscendens*	2

Contd...

Table 5.2–*Contd...*

Sl.No.	*Place Visited*	*State*	*Date*	*Species Collected*	*Total Voucher Numbers*
16.	Muchukotakanam,Tadipatri, Bugga, Srisailam, Mallelathertham	Andhra Pradesh	08-09-08	*C. adscendens* var. *attenuata, C. adscendens* var. *fimbriata, C. stalagmifera* var. *stalagmifera*	7
17.	Sunderbahni	J&K	08-11-08	*Apteranthus tuberculata*	1
18.	Kuyyala, Jaisalmer	Rajasthan	14-11-08	*Caudanthera edulis*	1
19.	Pemmanalli,Tumkur hills	Karnataka	29-11-08	*Caralluma stalagmifera* var. *stalagmifera, Boucerosia umbellata, Boucerosia truncato-coronata*	6
20.	Thuthukudi	Tamil Nadu	17-01-09	*Caralluma bhupinderiana*	2
21.	Mavatur, Penukonda, Madakasira	Andhra Pradesh	28-01-09	*C. stalagmifera* var. *stalagmifera, C. adscendens* var. *attenuata, Boucerosia umbellata, Boucerosia lasiantha*	4
22.	Diveghat, Pune	Maharashtra	23-07-09	*Caralluma adscendens* var. *fimbriata*	1
23	Yellapur, Patchapur	Karnataka	26-07-09	*C. adscendens* var. *fimbriata*	1
24.	Shahupuri,Gurhathwadi, Sangli dt.	Maharashtra	27-07-09	*C. adscendens* var. *fimbriata*	4
25.	Rani bavi, Nagasane, Gundlakona water falls, Kadapa dt.	Andhra Pradesh	24-10-09	*Caralluma adscendens* var. *attenuata, C. stalagmifera* var. *stalagmifera, Boucerosia umbellata*	4
26.	Rayapur, Kullur forest, Nelapattu bird sanctuary, near Tada, Nellore dt.	Andhra Pradesh	25-10-09	*Boucerosia indica, Caralluma adscendens* var. *attenuata, Caralluma stalagmifera* var. *intermedia*	7
27.	Chandragiri forest hills, Bakarapeta, Udayapalyam, Pileru, Chandragiri, Chittoor dt.	Andhra Pradesh	27-10-09	*Boucerosia umbellata, B. indica, Caralluma adscendens* var. *attenuata, C.adscendens* var. *attenuata, C. adscendens* var. *fimbriata*	7
28.	Kuyyala, Jaisalmer (dt), Bilad, Jodhpur, (dt.)	Rajasthan	10-11-09	*Caudanthera edulis*	2

Contd...

Table 5.2–*Contd...*

Sl.No.	*Place Visited*	*State*	*Date*	*Species Collected*	*Total Voucher Numbers*
29.	Penukonda	Andhra Pradesh	20-05-10	*Boucerosia umbellata*	3
30.	Punganoor, Tiruvannamalai	Andhra Pradesh, Tamil Nadu	13-06-10	*Boucerosia indica, Caralluma stalagmifera, Boucerosia diffusa*	3
31.	Coimbatore, Madhukkarai hills and Maruthamalai hills	Tamil Nadu	19-7-10	*C. adscendens* var. *attenuata, C. adscendens* var. *bicolor, Boucersia umbellata, B. truncato-coronata*	8
32.	Sirumalai hills, Dindigul dt.	Tamil Nadu	23-9-10	*C. adscendens* var. *adscendens, C. stalagmifera, C. sarkariae, Boucrosia pauciflora, Boucerosia umbellata*	10
33.	Megamalai hills, Theni dt.	Tamil Nadu	24-5-11	*C. adscendens* var. *carinata, C. sarkariae, C. sarkariae* var. *longipedicellata, Boucerosia pauciflora, Boucerosia umbellata*	13
34.	Maruthuvamala hill, Aramboli hills Kanyakumar dt.	Tamil Nadu	10-8-11	*C. geniculata, C. adscendens* var. *gracilis, Boucerosia procumbens*	6
35.	Yercaud, Pakkoda point, Salem dt.	Tamil Nadu	12-9-11	*Boucerosia umbellata*	2

The representative specimens were collected from all the fields and preserved in the form of herbarium. Table 5.2 gives a list of *Carallumas* recorded in India and their places of availability.

Visit to other Indian Herbaria

Authors visited the following herbaria to study the specimens of *Caralluma* species

1. Central National Herbarium, BSI, Howrah – CAL
2. Madras Herbarium, BSI, Coimbatore – MH
3. Herbarium, BSI, Pune – BSI
4. Herbarium, BSI, Dehra Dun – BSD
5. Herbarium, Forest Research Institute, Dehra Dun - DD
6. Herbarium, Industrial Section, Indian Museum – Kolkata - BSIS
7. Herbarium, National Botanical Research Institute (NBRI) – Lucknow – NBG
8. Blatter Herbarium, St. Xavier College, Mumbai - BLAT

Visit to Botanical Gardens

Authors visited Botanical Gardens at the following places.

1. Indian Botanic Garden, Howrah. To our surprise we found that not even a single *Caralluma* plant is available at Indian Botanic Garden.
2. National Botanical Research Institute – Lucknow
3. National Cactus and Succulent Botanical Garden and Research Centre – Chandigarh. After the demise of Dr. J.S. Sarkaria this garden is not maintained well. Most of the plants are on the verge of extinction.

Authors have donated live specimens of all the species to several Botanic gardens including the above.

Distribution

Carallumas are distributed from the Mediterranean to East Indies. *Carallumas* are found in Southern Europe, Iran, Iraq, African countries like Kenya, Somalia, Sudan and Ethiopia, Arabian countries like Oman, UAE and Yemen and Asian countries like Afghanistan, Pakistan, India, Nepal, Burma and Sri Lanka (Meve and Liede, 2002).

Carallumas are distributed throughout India and its neighbouring countries. In the North, *C. staintonii* is seen in Nepal whereas *Apteranthus tuberculata* is seen in Jammu (Figure 5.1) extending into Pakistan. In the East, *Boucerosia crenulata* has been reported from Guwahati, Assam, though, originally described from Myanmar. In West, *Caudanthera edulis* is seen in Jaisalmer, Rajasthan (Figure 5.8) extending into Pakistan. *Caralluma aucheriana* was given misleadingly by Jagtap and Singh (1999) for *Caralluma tuberculata*. Many following investigators also mentioned this species in Indian distribution, but it is originally Arabian species wrongly quoted in many works as Indian species. In the present study also this species is not found in India.

C. adscendens var. *fimbriata* has been reported from Maharashtra, Western Madhya Pradesh into adjacent Rajasthan. The southern peninsula has majority of the species, Tamil Nadu, possessing maximum number of species of *Boucerosia* and *Caralluma* (Figures 5.2–5.7).

Taxonomy

The earlier accounts indicate that *Caralluma adscendens* is variable and widely distributed species; at least six distinct morphoforms have been recognized. In the three varieties, *viz.* var. *adscendens, attenuata* and *fimbriata*, that have long been known and have hitherto been regarded as distinct species (Gamble, 1919), the stem is squarish in section with the sides usually slightly hollowed and the angles always rounded. Another three varieties have acute angles *i.e.* var. *carinata, gracilis* and *geniculata*. Bruyns (1987) suggested that variable forms of African *Caralluma* complex taxonomically still needs to be answered because of this complex has never been revised as a whole. Egyptian *Caralluma europaea* complex have been revised based on the morphology and karyology studies by Meve and Heneidak (2005). Meve and Liede (2002) attempted molecular taxonomy of this group, they stated that *C. adscendens* var. *geniculata*, could be raised to species level (*Caralluma geniculata*) based on their molecular data.

Genus *Boucerosia* was first discovered in 1834 by Wight and Arnott with flowers in terminal umbels. It was used quite widely for Indian, Arabian and Mediterranian Stapeliad species until N.E. Brown (1892), who included *Boucerosia* under the genus *Caralluma*, perhaps overwhelmed by the variety of species being discovered latter in Southern India combined with coronal variations, stem characters, striations and hairiness patterns on flowers. Brown made no attempt to recognize infrageneric groupings of the taxa. Schumann (1895) recognized three sections under *Boucerosia* which are *Eucaralluma* (=*Caralluma*), *Lalacruma* (=*Caralluma gracilis*) and *Boucerosia*, but completely ignored that subgenus *Boucerosia* is restricted only to Southern India, Sri Lanka and Myanmar.

Boucerosia truncato-coronata was described by Sedgewick in 1921 near Hubli in Dharwar district of Karnataka. The type specimen was not preserved in any herbaria and also protologue has not mentioned any types. Based on Sedgwick, Gravely and Mayuranathan (1931) have included the taxon in their monograph of Indian *Caralluma*. Later, Kumari and Subba Rao (1976) have described a new species of South India *Caralluma* (*Boucerosia*) *nilagiriana* from Nilgiri hills, which is closely related to *B. tuncato-coronata*. They have given obvious differences between these two allied species and also they have provided the line drawings for their new species. After Brown (1810), the genus has not got any attention of taxonomists, but the first review on *Caralluma* and its segregates came in 1990 by Gilbert, he has segregated the succulent

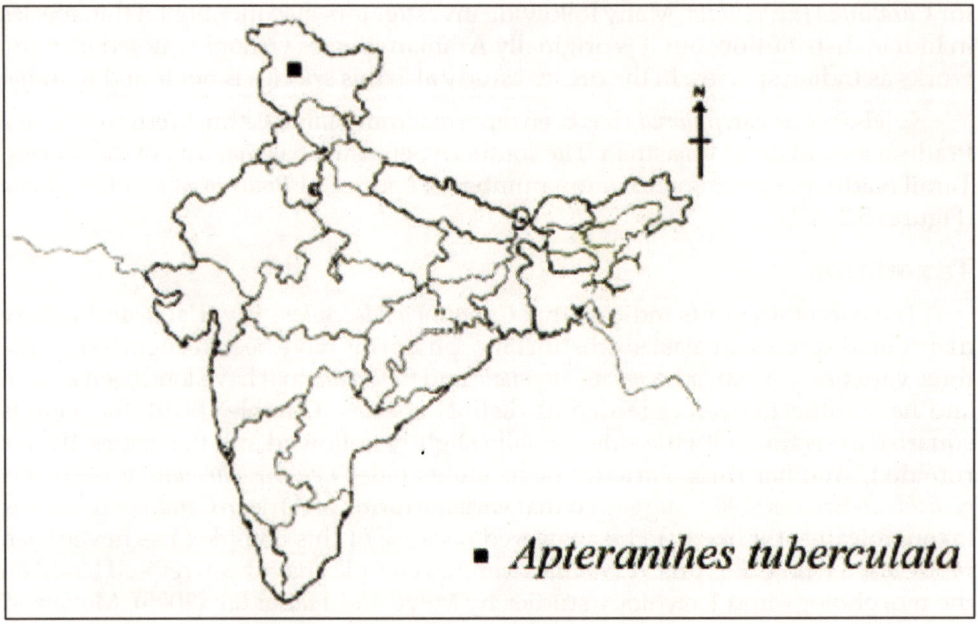

Figure 5.1: Map Showing Distribution of the Genus *Apteranthes* in India

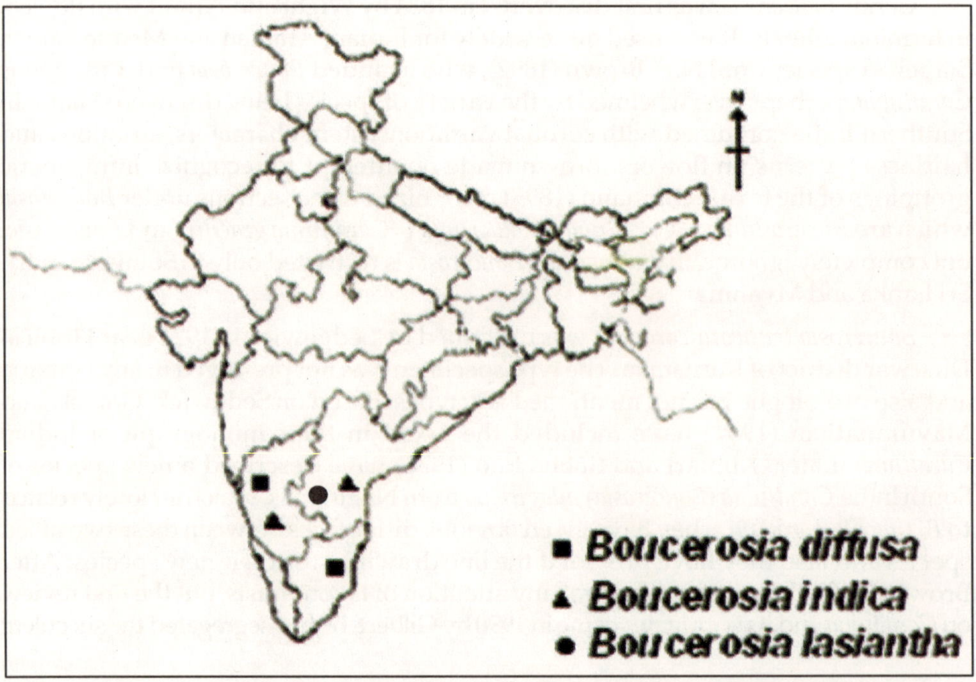

Figure 5.2: Map Showing Distribution of the Genus *Boucerosia* in India

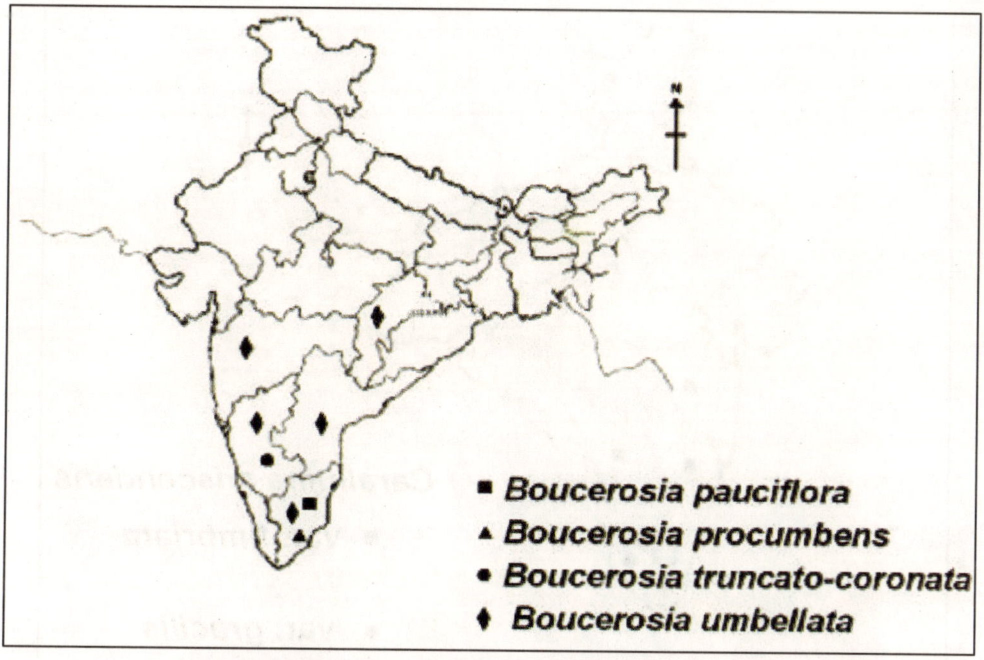

Figure 5.3: Map Showing Distribution of the Genus *Boucerosia* in India

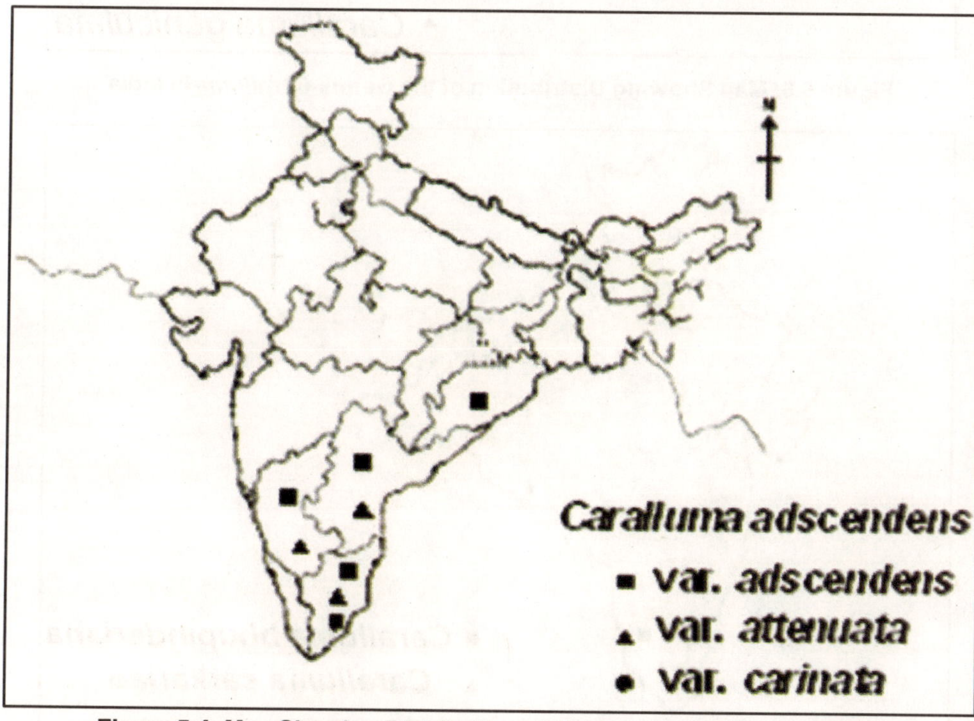

Figure 5.4: Map Showing Distribution of the Genus *Caralluma* in India

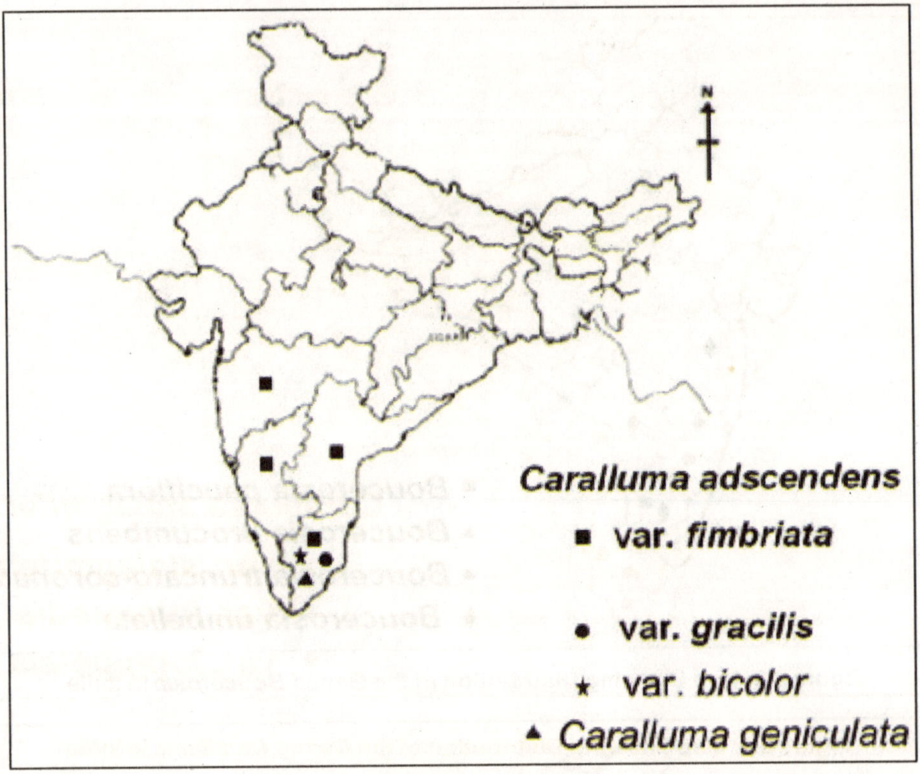

Figure 5.5: Map Showing Distribution of the Genus *Caralluma* in India

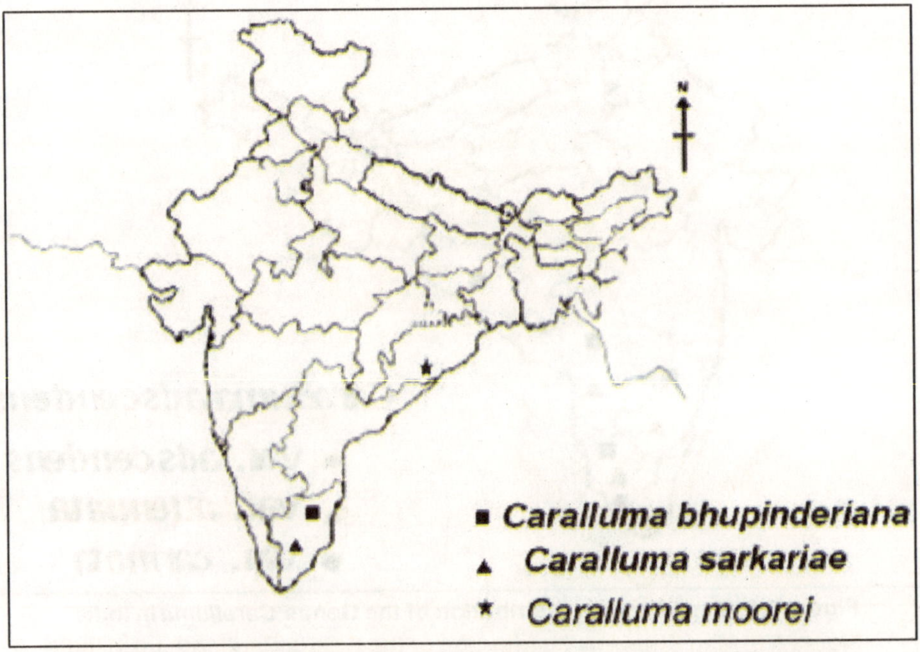

Figure 5.6: Map Showing Distribution of the Genus *Caralluma* in India

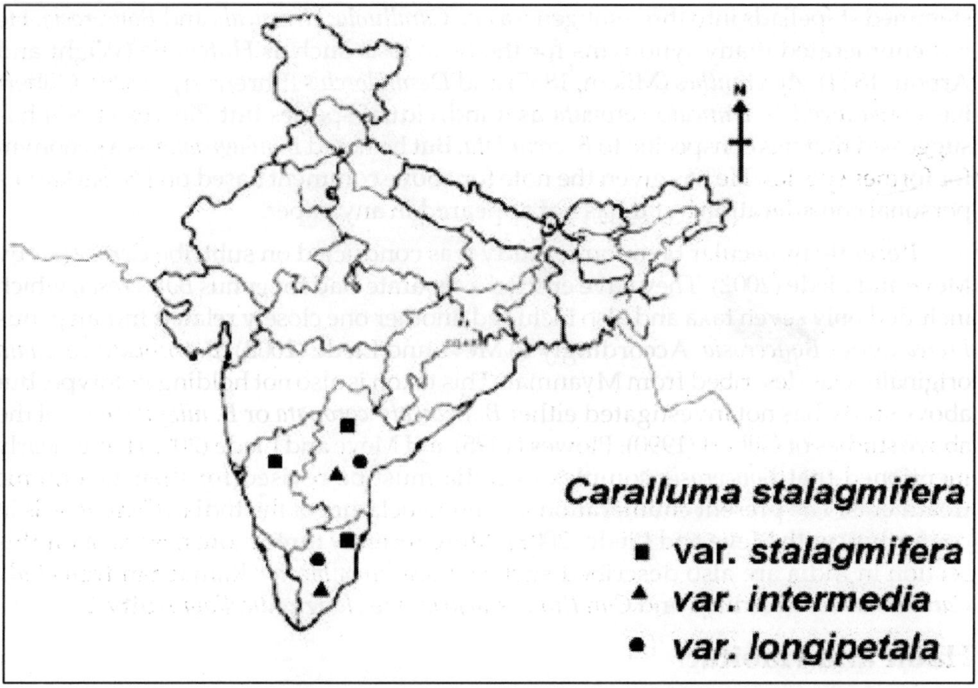

Figure 5.7: Map Showing Distribution of the Genus *Caralluma* in India

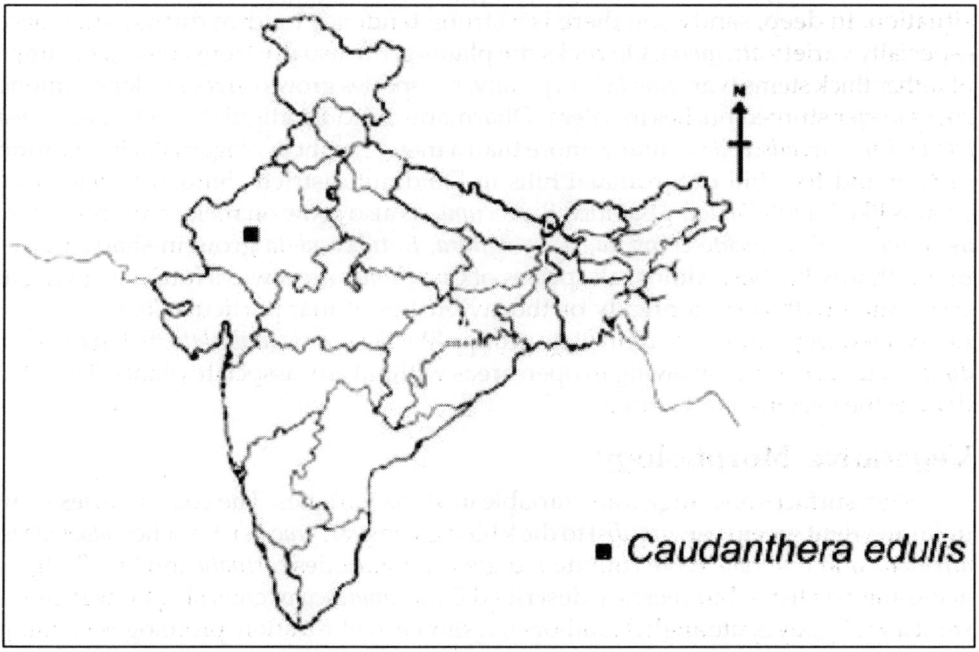

Figure 5.8: Map Showing Distribution of the Genus *Caudanthera* in India

stemmed stapeliads into three subgenera *viz. Caralluma, Urmalcala* and *Boucerosia*. He has enumerated many synonyms for the *Boucerosia* such as *Hutchinia* (Wight and Arnott, 1834), *Apteranthes* (Mikan, 1835) and *Desmidorchis* (Ehrenberg, 1829). Gilbert has considered *B. truncato-coronata* as a individual species but Plowes (1995) has suggested that it is conspecific to *B. crenulata*. But he noted *B. nilagiriana* as a synonym for former species. He has given the note for above comment based on J.S. Sarkaria's personal consideration but it has not appeared in any paper.

Recently molecular taxonomic study was conducted on subtribe *Ceropegiae* by Meve and Liede (2002). They have erected a separate clad for genus *Boucerosia*, which included only seven taxa and also included another one closely related Indian genus *Frerea* under *Boucerosia*. Accordingly to Meve and Liede (2002), *B. truncato-coronata* originally was described from Myanmar. This taxon is also not holding holotype. But above study has not investigated either *B. truncato-coronata* or *B. nilagiriana*. All the above studies of Gilbert (1990), Plowes (1995) and Meve and Liede (2002) have clearly mentioned that *Boucerosia* complex of India must be revised for their taxonomic treatments. The present enumeration and nomenclature of the Indian *Caralluma* is in conformity with Meve and Liede (2002). More recently three more new taxa for this section in India are also described such as *Caralluma bicolor* Ramachandran *et al., Caralluma moorei* Aditya and *Caralluma srakariae* var. *longipedicellata* Aditya.

Habit and Habitat

As is typical for most *Carallumas, Caralluma adscendens* prefers shaded stands such as the base of thorny bushes (Jonkers and Walker, 1993). The individuals nevertheless vary considerably in their general habit depending on the edaphic situation. In deep, sandy soil there is a strong tendency to form diffuse stem base especially variety *attenuata*. On rocks the plants grow usually from compact clumps of rather thick stems (var. *gracilis*). Typically, the species grows on rocky slopes among rocks under stunted bushes in Salem, Dharmapuri and Dindigul districts. *Caralluma adscendens* var. *adscendens* attains more than a meter height in Nagamalai in Madurai district and foot hill of Sirumalai hills in Dindigul districts. Similarly *Boucerosia* groups like *B.umbellata, B. lasiantha, B. procumbens* also grow on rocky crevices where as *B. indica, B. truncato-coronata, B. pauciflora, B. tuberculata* grow in shady places under thorny bushes. Almost all species of *Carallumas* are always found growing in association with certain prickly or thorny bushes of that particular habitat. Very rarely a few populations of umbellate groups like *Boucerosia umbellata, B. lasiantha, B. diffusa*, etc., are found growing in open areas without any associate plants. Table 5.3 depicts the various associations.

Vegetative Morphology

Stem surfaces and angles are variable in all six varieties. The colour varies from uniform bright green (var. *gracilis*) to dark blue green (var. *gracilis*). Varieties *adscendens, attenuata* and *fimbriata* have rounded angles and varieties *carinata* and *gracilis* have acute angled stems. But recently described *Caralluma bicolor* consists of lower stems stout and slightly acute angled (authors not shown in illustration, protologue contains

Table 5.3: Habitat Association

Plants Name	*Associated Plants*	*Soil Type*
C. adscendens var. *adscendens*	*Prosopis chilensis* *Commiphora berryi* *Canthium parviflorum* *Carissa spinaram* *Catunaregum spinosa* *Dyschoriste madurensis* *Barleria noctiflora*	Sandy loam, Red soil
C. adscendens var. *attenuata*	*Prosopis chilensis* *Balanites aegyptiaca* *Acacia leucophloea* *Barleria buxifolia*	Sandy loam, Clay soil, Black soil
C. adscendens var. *bicolor*	*Acacia planifrons* *Heteropogon contortus* *Euphorbia antiquorum* *Leucas tenuiflorum* *Tephrosia purpurea*	Red sandy soil on Rocky boulders
C. adscendens var. *carinata*	*Carissa spinaram* *Commiphora berryi* *Tephrosia purpurea* *Barleria buxifolia* *Barleria cristata* *Euphorbia antiquorum*	Red sandy soil
C. adscendens var. *fimbriata*	*Canthium parvifloram* *Prosopis chilensis* *Euphorbia caducifolia* *Catunaregum spinosa* *Phoenix loureirii*	Red sandy soil
C. adscendens var. *gracilis*	*Prosopis chilensis* *Euphorbia antiquorum* *Didymocarpus tomentosus* *Catunaregum spinosa* *Sansevieria roxburghiana*	Red sandy soil with rocky substratum
C. bhupinderiana	*Commiphora berryi* *Barleria cristata* *Barleria noctiflora* *Securinega leucopyrus* *Gmelina asiatica* *Allmania nodiflora*	Red soil
C. geniculata	*Endostemon viscosus* *Euphorbia antiquorum* *Cissus quadrangularis*	Red sandy soil on Rocky boulders
C. stalagmifera var. *stalagmifera*	*Prosopis chilensis* *Opuntia dillenii* *Barleria buxifolia* *Justicia tranquebariensis* *Dyschoriste madurensis* *Pentantropis capensis*	Red sandy soil
C. stalagmifera var. *longipetala*	*Barleria buxifolia* *Kalanchoe pinnata* *Blepharis maderaspatana*	Red sandy soil

Contd...

Table 5.3–*Contd...*

Plants Name	*Associated Plants*	*Soil Type*
C. stalagmifera var. *intermedia*	*Prosopis chilensis* *Acanthospermum hispidum* *Ziziphus oenoplia*	Red sandy soil
C. sarkariae	*Barleria cristata* *Barleria noctiflora* *Dyschoriste madurensis* *Prosopis chilensis* *Cissus quadrangularis*	Clay soil
C.sarkariae var. *longipedicellata*	*Barleria cuspidata* *Commiphora berryei* *Euphorbia antiquorum* *Dichrostachys cinerea* *Carissa spinarum*	Sandy-loamy soil
Caudanthera edulis	*Ziziphus mauritiana* *Cymbopogon* sp.	Clay Sandy soil
Boucerosia diffusa	*Commiphora berryi* *Prosopis chilensis* *Carissa spinarum*	Red soil
Boucerosia indica	*Hemionitis australis* *Selaginella wightii* *Cyanotis tuberosa* *Cissus quadrangularis*	Rocky crevices
Boucerosia pauciflora	*Commiphora berryi* *Ziziphus oenoplia* *Asparagus racemosus* *Prosopis chilensis* *Barleria noctiflora*	Red sandy soil
Boucerosia procumbens	*Catunaregum spinosa* *Euphorbia antiquorum* *Fluggea leucopyros* *Phyllanthus reticulatus* *Cymbopogon martinii*	Red sandy soil
Boucerosia truncato-coronata	*Indigofera linnaei* *Sida cordata* *Euphorbia fusiformis* *Kalanchoe pinnata*	Red soil
Apteranthus tuberculata	*Dodonaea viscosa* *Cymbopogon coloratus*	Clay soil, rocky boulders
Boucerosia umbellata	*Canthium parviflorum* *Euphorbia antiquorum* *Euphorbia caducifolia* *Catunaregum spinosa* *Gmelina asiatica* *Barleria buxifolia* *Tephrosia purpurea* *Barleria cristata* *Kalanchoe pinnata* *Cissus quadrangularis* *Prosopis chilensis* *Hyptis suaveolens* *Cymbopogon martinii* *Heteropogon contortus*	Red soil on rocky substratum

only floral axis, but it is clearly cylindrical). In *Caralluma edulis* stem is rounded with minutely grooved. In *Boucerosia* group, the size of stem varies *i.e.,* except *Boucerosia pauciflora, B. indica* and *B. truncato-coronata,* in all other species of this group having equal size of stem and toothed angled stem. A few populations of *B. umbellata* stems obviously are winged at all four corners as seen in Wight's illustration.

Floral Morphology

Variability in flower morphology of *C. adsendens* is higher than typically found in widespread *stapeliads,* and has therefore hampered a sound taxonomic treatment. The increasing availability of plant material has demonstrated infraspecific variability, where almost every population shows its own features (the many illustration published by Gravely and Mayuranathan, 1931). Especially with regard to frequently occurring differences in corolla structure, size and ciliation, a wealth of information has been given (see floral key). However, several distinct tendencies that support infraspecific differentiation have to be considered. Inner coloration of the corolla surface is predominantly purple, but creamy yellow coloration is found in var. *gracilis.* Dense purple-red transverse stripes or streaks are found in all the six varieties of *C. adscendens* but each variety has different patterns and amount of striation (Plate 5.1). Flower size is small in var. *gracilis* but rather larger in var. *carinata.* Amount of hairiness of the petals also varied in all six varieties (Plate 5.1).

Microscopic studies of the corolla epidermis of samples were conducted that revealed a characteristic separation between the varieties and its populations. Varieties *attenuata, fimbriata, adscendens* showed homogeneously isodiametric with slightly convex to dome-shaped papillate (bottle-neck like) cells (Plate 5.2). However in the varieties like *gracilis, bicolor* and *carinata,* heterogeneous cells mingled with papillate-apiculate cells on the corolla epidermis were found (Plate 5.2). The very smooth and tiny periclinal wall lacks a pleated cuticle but they are topped by mighty papilla-like structure showing a varicose to prickly surfaces. Corona structures and their coloration are rather similar in all the varieties. The corona is normally purplish; however in varieties *fimbriata* and *attenuata* it is occasionally yellowish-brown. Shape and size of pollinia are also greatly differing in all six varieties (Plate 5.3).

Morphologically, there are quantitative differences between all the six varieties. Typically the corolla epidermis of those samples is more strongly sculptured with markedly convex outer epidermal wall specifically in each variety. The amount of papillate sculpture serves as demarcation line between the varieties. The present study is comparable with *Caralluma europaea* complex (Meve and Heneidak, 2005).

Taxonomically significant variation in chromosome sizes in stapeliads have been reported by Albers and Meve (2001) at the tribe level, Meve and Liede (2001) at genus and species level and Meve and Heneidak (2005) at infraspecific level. Even within species, however, chromosome length varies around 0-2 per cent. The ca. 10 per cent deviation found between the two varieties *C. adscendens* is then not significant at all, and falls within the variation range which can be expected on species level.

Plowes (1995) suggested that the *C. adscendens* complex in India may segregate species level. This has not been questioned by succeeding *Caralluma* investigators. Considering the high vegetative, floral and chemical variability, the diploidy and tetraploidy, and the narrow and nearly discontinuously distribution, the treatment of the complex as variable species. The acute angled varieties (var. *carinata* and *gracilis*) is having tetraploid (autoploid) chromosomes, which is taxonomically significant but these populations are not overlapping anywhere in natural condition. Another acute angled variety *geniculata* might have originated independently with its habitats due to geographical isolation. Hence, this variety may be considered as separate species as supported by Meve and Liede (2002). All other rounded angle varieties might be considered as ecotypes which are exhibiting overlapping populations sometimes. The differences between the varieties are really pronounced between rounded angled and sharp angled. However, the fairly high number of characters concerned point to a considerable degree of separation.

Variations in Carallumas

Caralluma

This is a small group consisting of 6 species and 11 varieties, all found in Southern India. Of the southern species only *Caralluma adscendens* var. *fimbriata* distributed far wide, having been recorded from Myanmar in the East, Sri Lanka in the South and Maharashtra, in the West of India. This is the most variable group of succulents. Another variable species is *Caralluma stalagmifera* which is also distributed along the foot hills tracts of Eastern Ghats from the Visakhapatnam in the north of Andhra Pradesh to the south of Ramnathapuram district in the Tamil Nadu state. The southern members are usually found growing in open shrubby areas with other semi-xerophytic vegetation. The shrubs are catching the plumes and the seeds that drop at their bases, to allow them to germinate and grow. These shrubs give the Carallumas shade, support and some protection from grazing animals. This allows some of these Carallumas to grow up to heights of 100 cm.

Caralluma adscendens (Roxb.) R.Br. (Syn. *Stapelia adscendens* Roxb.) was originally described from Coast of Coromandal area of Peninsular India without indicating precise locality by Roxburgh. Gravely and Mayuranathan (1931) recognized a total of six varieties within this species. Mainly these varieties can be divided into 2 major groups based on whether the stems have rounded or acute angles. But Bruyns (1984) has drawn attention to the very great similarity between one of these varieties *fimbriata*, and *Caralluma subulata* from Arabia and *Caralluma dalzielii* from West Africa. This could be taken to indicate that the two groups such as round and acute angles varieties merit formal recognition at least as subspecies. The status of the varieties within *C. adscendens* seems more questionable as Gravely and Mayuranathan indicated that intermediates are apparently common (Gilbert, 1990).

The earlier accounts indicate that *Caralluma adscendens* is variable and widely distributed species at least six distinct morphoforms have recognized in the three varieties, *viz.* var. *adscendens s.str.*, *attenuata* and *fimbriata*, that have long been known and have hitherto been regarded as distinct species (Gamble, 1919). The stem is

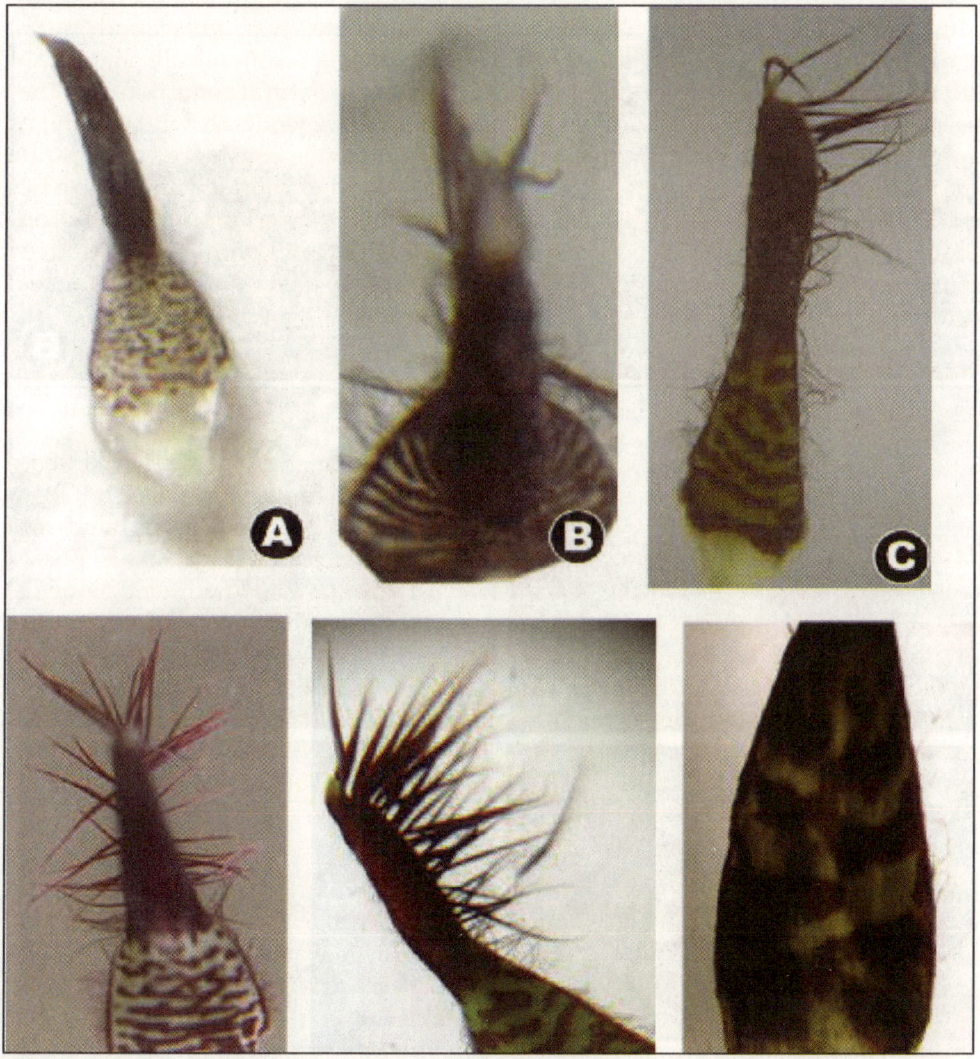

Plate 5.1: Diversity Patterns of Striations or Streaks on Petals of *Caralluma adscendens* Group

A: ***Caralluma adscendens*** var. ***adscendens***; B: ***Caralluma adscendens*** var. ***attenuata***; C: ***Caralluma adscendens*** var. ***carinata***; D: ***Caralluma adscendens*** var. ***fimbriata***; E: ***Caralluma geniculata***; F: ***Caralluma adscendens*** var. ***gracilis***.

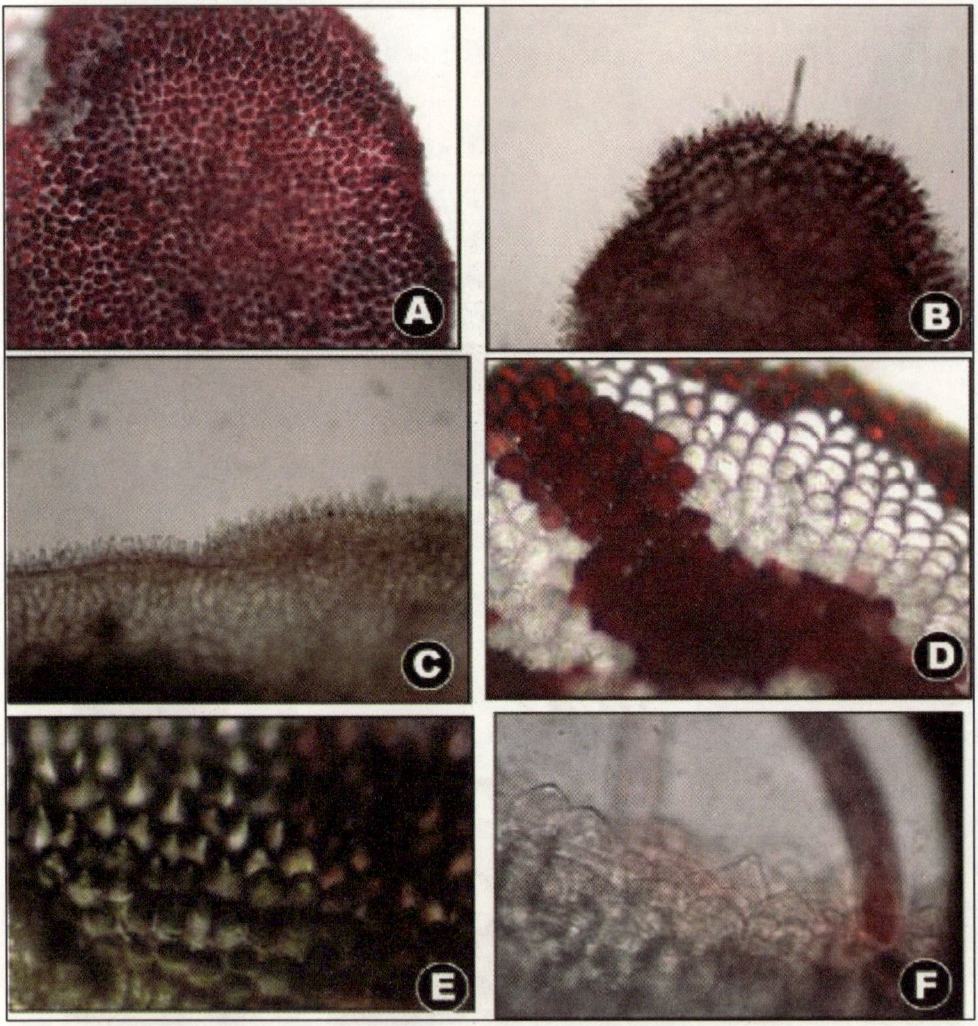

Plate 5.2: Microscopic Studies of the Corolla Epidermis of *Caralluma adscendens* Group

A: ***Caralluma adscendens*** var. ***adscendens***; B: ***Caralluma adscendens*** var. ***attenuata***' C: ***Caralluma adscendens*** var. ***carinata***; D: ***Caralluma adscendens*** var. ***fimbriata***; E: ***Caralluma geniculata***; F: ***Caralluma adscendens*** var. ***gracilis***.

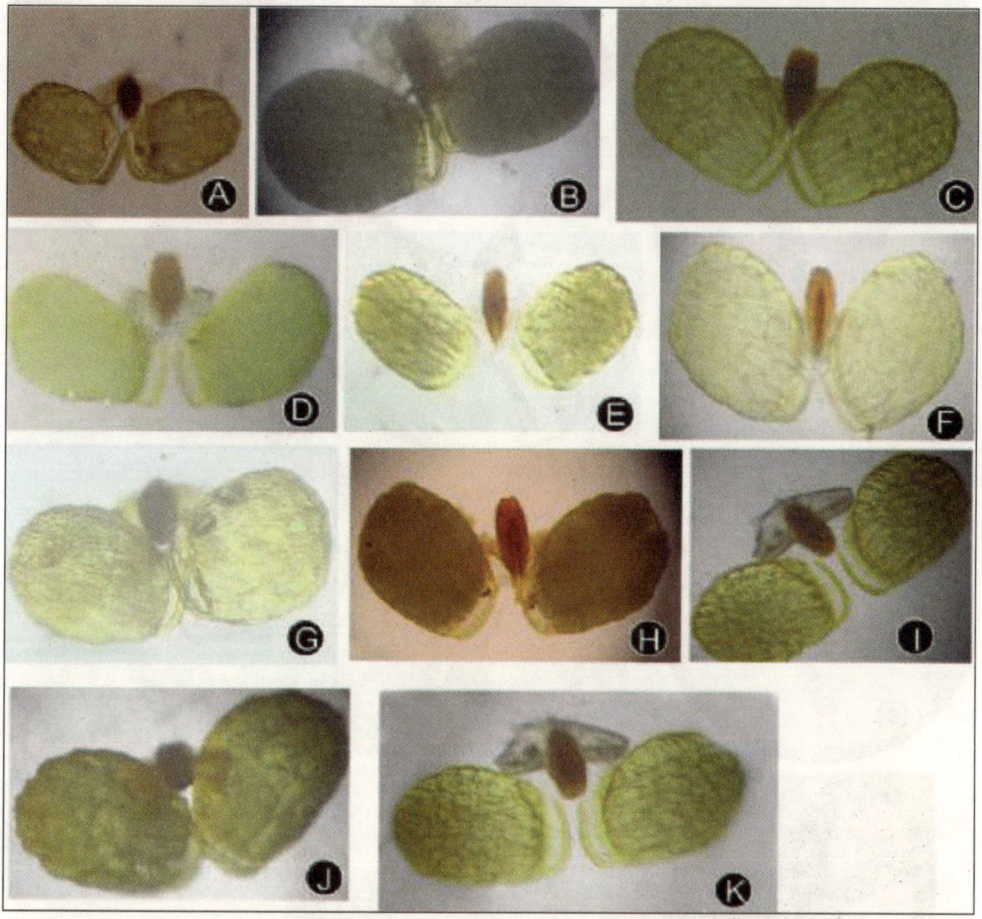

Plate 5.3: Pollinial Diversity in *Caralluma* Group

A: *Caralluma adscendens* var. *adscendens*; B: *Caralluma adscendens* var. *attenuata;* C: *Caralluma adscendens* var. *carinata*; D: *Caralluma adscendens* var. *fimbriata*; E: *Caralluma geniculata*; F: *Caralluma adscendens* var. *gracilis*; G: *Caralluma bhupinderiana*; H: *Caralluma sarkarieae;* I: *Caralluma stalagmifera* var. *stalagmifera*; J: *Caralluma stalagmifera* var. *intermedia*; K: *Caralluma stalagmifera* var. *longipetala.*

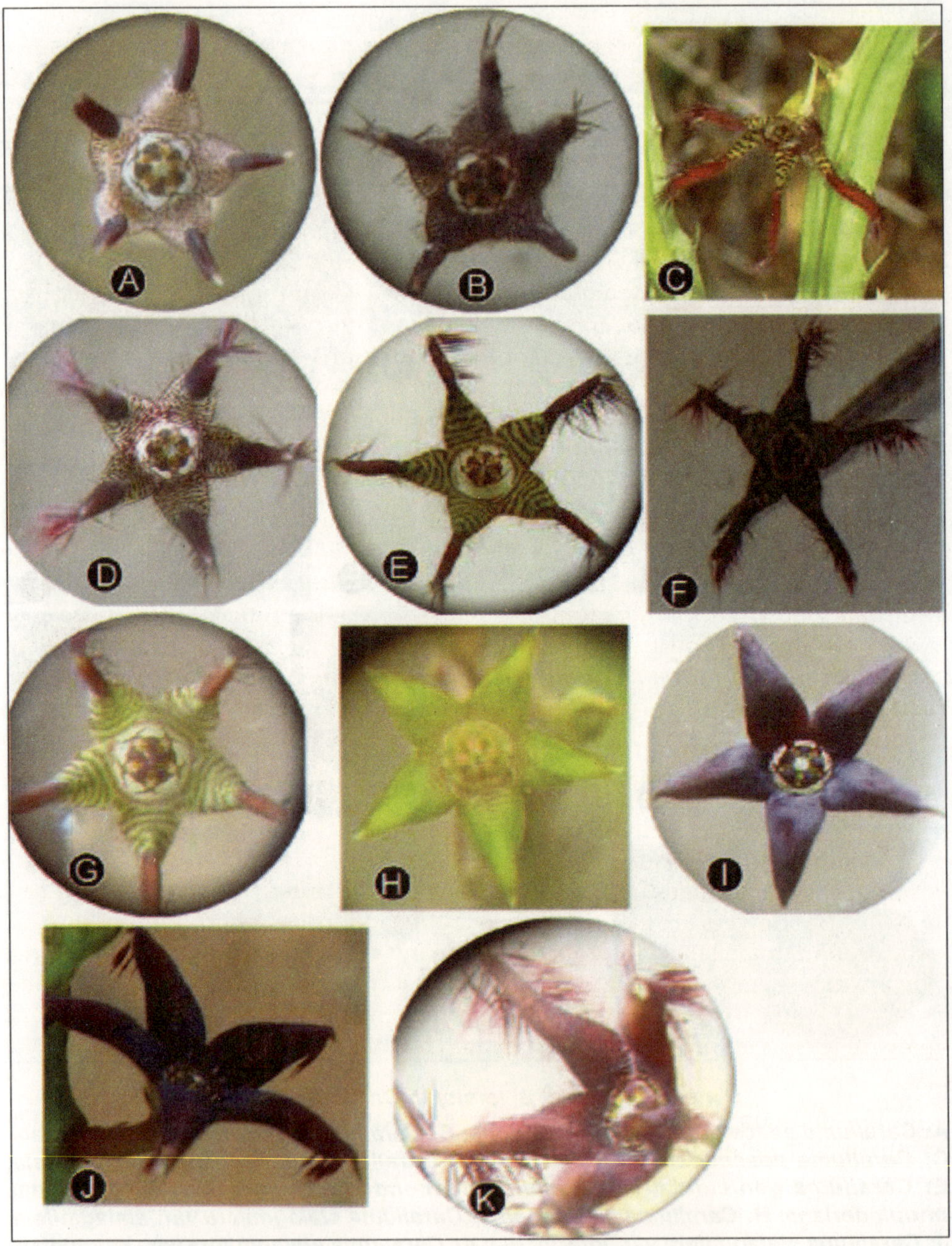

Plate 5.4: Floral Diversity in *Caralluma* Group

A: *Caralluma adscendens* var. *adscendens*; B: *Caralluma adscendens* var. *attenuata*; C: *Caralluma adscendens* var. *carinata*; D: *Caralluma adscendens* var. *fimbriata*; E: *Caralluma geniculata*; F: *Caralluma adscendens* var. *gracilis*; G: *Caralluma bhupinderiana*; H: *Caralluma sarkarieae;* I: *Caralluma stalagmifera* var. *stalagmifera*; J: *Caralluma stalagmifera* var. *intermedia*; K: *Caralluma stalagmifera* var. *longipetala*.

squarish in section with the sides usually slightly hollowed and the angles always rounded. Another three varieties have acute angles *i.e.* var. *carinata, gracilis* and *bicolor* which are distributed in narrow ranges in Tamilnadu. Gravely and Mayuranathan (1931) have suggested to use classification of three varieties partly in the flower morphology and partly in the stem morphology. But these characters unable to hold in herbarium specimens of these groups, because of these are succulent genera. There is considerable floral (but also vegetative) variability in *C. adscendens* (Plate 5.4), quite often even between plants of single populations, but almost always between different populations. These circumstances have stimulated many taxonomists and regional florists to describe morphotypes, ecotypes or varieties or forms. The diversity of *C. adscendens* in Tamil Nadu is indeed higher than other states of Peninsular India. Even though in many places, overlapping populations are exhibiting among these varieties. Bruyns (1987) suggested that variable forms of African *Caralluma* complex taxonomically still needs to be answered because of this complex has never been revised as a whole. In this circumstance only now a few new species were described by taxonomists such as *Caralluma moorei* and *Caralluma bicolor*.

Caralluma stalagmifera also shows considerable variations in its morphological and floral characters (Plate 5.4). Recently Karuppusamy and Pullaiah (2007) have segregated two distinct varieties in this species. Natural hybrids also have already been reported from many places (Gravely and Mayuranathan, 1931). *Caralluma sarkariae* is reported only from the type locality of Madurai district in Tamil Nadu so far. In that species, range of variations from its floral features such as hairiness and striation patterns were reported (Adithya, 2009). This could be the result of hybridization between the related taxa in natural habitats where mixed populations of *C. stalagmifera* and *C. adscendens* var. *adscendens* occur.

Boucerosia

Members of the genus *Boucerosia* are succulent plants with stems which are leafless or with ephemeral vestigial leaves. The stems are erect, trailing or decumbent in habit. The flowers are campanulate or rotate, odorous or non-odorous and are produced in umbellate cymes of a few to many at the tip of the stems. The genus *Boucerosia* is separated from the genus *Caralluma* mainly by the umbellate terminal cymes. This genus is very popular with succulent plant growers and enthusiasts and many of its species are edible and are eaten by the indigenous people of Southern India.

The common species *Boucerosia umbellata* Haw. is the best-known of the genus, occurring in habitats in the semi-arid, dry rocky regions of Peninsular India. Many natural variants of *B. umbellata* occur in the three states of Andhra Pradesh, Karnataka and Tamil Nadu.

Previous publications have described *B. umbellata* as having glabrous petals, but none of the specimens collected from Andhra Pradesh and Karnataka have glabrous petals. All flowering specimens examined had varying degrees of variation in their flowers, particularly in the hairiness of the petals (Plate 5.5) and coronal characters.

In the Palni hills of Tamil Nadu an interesting population of *B. umbellata* was discovered with glabrous petals (Plate 5.5a). The flowers were entirely different from those collected at other localities. Flowers were unpleasantly scented and large number of pollinators, like domestic flies are seen visiting the flowers. This population was associated with some tall grasses like *Cymbopogon martinii* and *Heteropogon contortus* (Table 5.3). The stapeliads grew exposed on the rocky surface between large boulders.

In Andhra Pradesh a much-branched *Boucerosia* sp. with flowers having hairy petals was collected, which was later identified as *Boucerosia lasiantha*. Wight (1850) has described this species and presented a clear illustration of its very clear differences with *B. umbellata*. Gravely and Mayuranathan subsequently transferred it into synonymy with *B. umbellata*. Gamble however retained the taxon as originally described based on specimen collected from the Gooty hills of Anantapur district in Andhra Pradesh. Later Indian Floras and revisionary works on the genus also treated this species as synonymous with *B. umbellata*. Examination of the preserved specimens of the two taxa revealed that one cannot be distinguished from the other. However living specimens examined exhibit marked variations of flower colour, number of flowers in the umbels, branching pattern of the peduncle, the hairiness of the petals, the stem length, the leaf scars and protuberances. It is therefore evident that *B. lasiantha* is clearly a good species in its own right as it was originally described.

B. lasiantha is usually associated with the leafless succulent shrub *Euphorbia caducifolia*. The populations inhabit rocky crevices among large boulders. *Ziziphus oenoplia* was the other thorny shrubs which appeared to be associated with this species. In other parts of Andhra Pradesh many variants of *B. umbellata* and *B. lasiantha* were found.

On the road sides of Penukonda in Andhra Pradesh, large-flowered specimens intermediate between *B. lasiantha* and the original *B. umbellata* were collected. Petals do not have strong hairiness similar to *B. lasiantha*, but short hairs along the lobe margins and the inner half face of the petals, with attractive reddish purple striations on the inner side of the campanulate corolla. The plant association of the population is entirely different from *B. lasiantha*, as there were large numbers of thorny bushes growing together with the species.

At regular intervals we examined the flowering and fruiting behaviour of the above-mentioned three populations from the Palni hills of Tamil Nadu, West North West (W.N.W.) of Madurai; and in Andhra Pradesh: the Gooty hills, north of Anantapur and Penukonda, south of Anantapur. Every five week we visited the area and noted the fruit developmental changes. We observed with interest the development of the fruit.

We observed that *B. lasiantha* from the Gooty hills develops follicles immediately after blooming in the months of June to September. Fertilisation and ovary development was studied and the maturation of the fruits was found after 60 days, when the follicles grow to about 7 cm in length. Flowers are densely hairy on the inner face of the petals and are non-odorous. The yellow striations or bands are not prominent, Pollinating *Drosophila*-like small dark flies and large *Diptera* flies were frequently observed around the open flowers. In the Penukonda and Palni hills populations antheses was noted only during the dry summer months from May to July, after which the unfertilized ovary stalks dry up, with only the fertilized ovary stalks

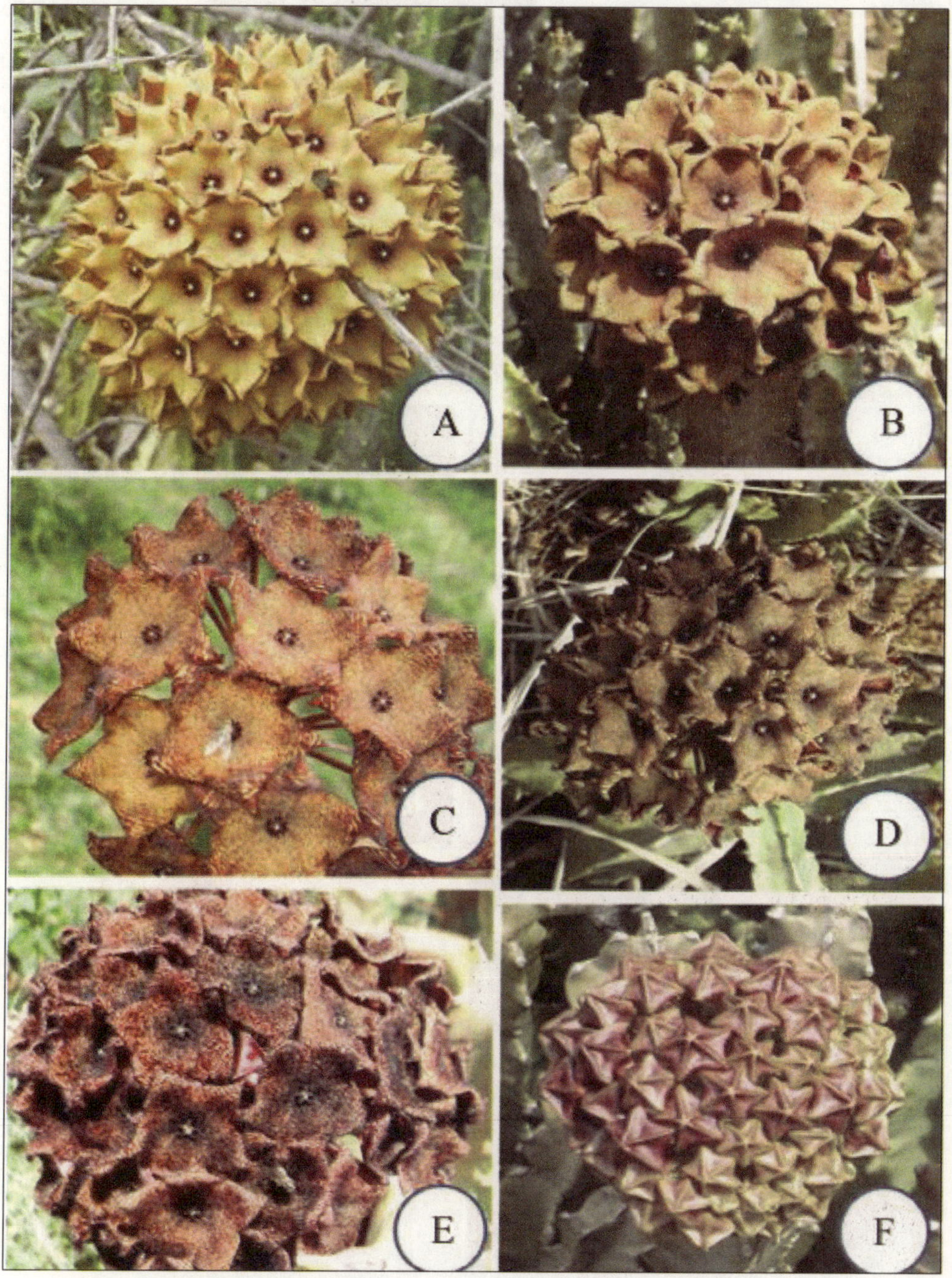

Plate 5.5: Floral Diversity in *Boucerosia umbellata*
A–E: Different types of floral color and striations; F: Flower buds.
(Karuppusamy *et al.*, 2012)

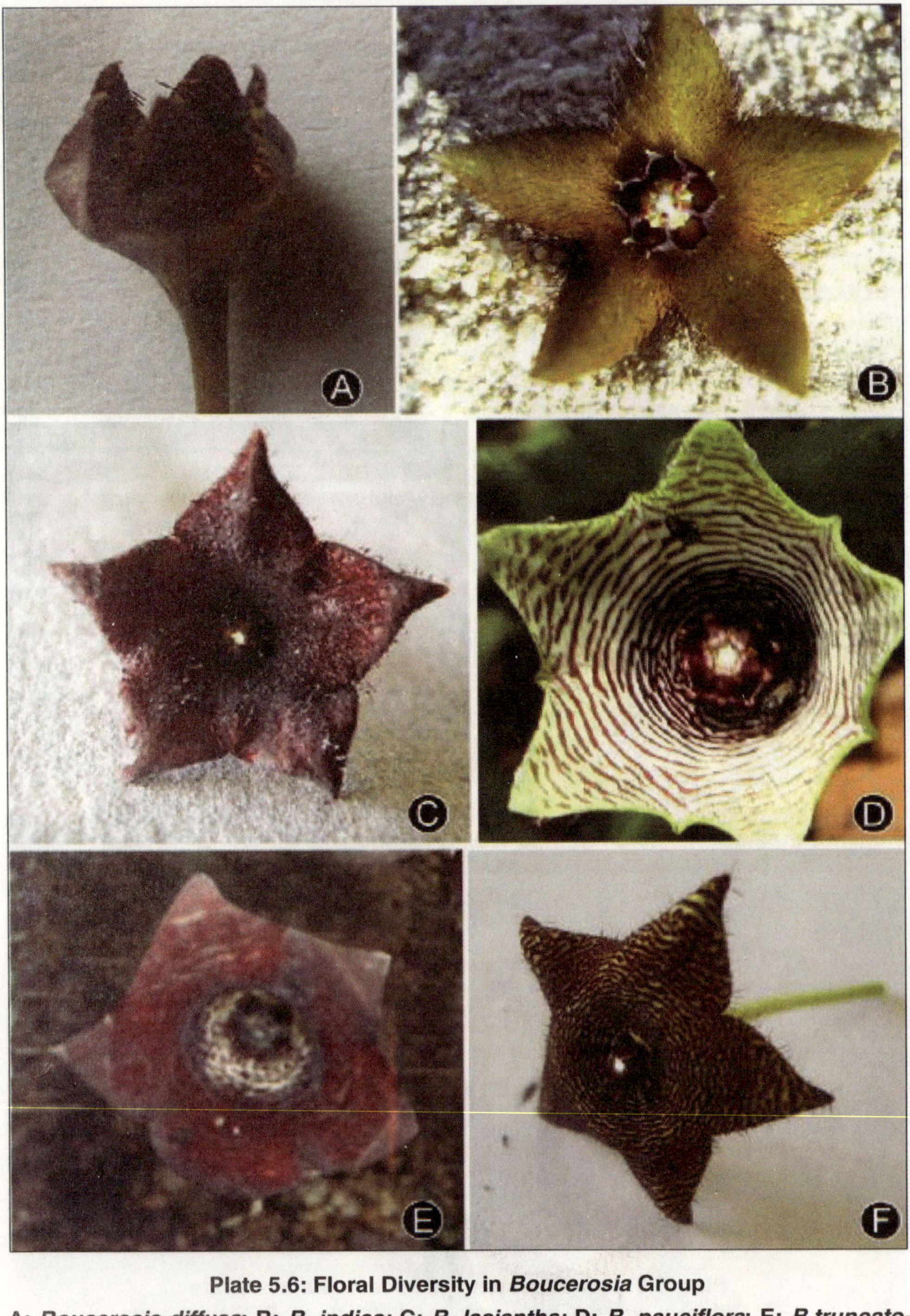

Plate 5.6: Floral Diversity in *Boucerosia* Group

A: *Boucerosia diffusa*; B: *B. indica;* C: *B. lasiantha;* D: *B. pauciflora*; E: *B.truncato-coronata;* F: *B. umbellata.*

remaining dormant for about three months. The monsoon season commences in July-August and after the initial rain shower the ovary stalk become rigid and the young, greenish ovary begins to protrude from out of the calyx lobes. In the middle of October, at the height of the rains, all of the ovary stalks grow rapidly and the follicles grow to about 5 cm long. All populations observed revealed that only two or three follicles developed from each inflorescence. All the follicles matured and ready to dehisce by the end of rainy season in January.

Boucerosia umbellata was described from the Coromandal coast of India by Adrian Haworth. But no type specimen was designated for the species. Many workers believed the original description of *B. umbellata* might have been made from a Sri Lankan specimen. It was observed that the flowers from the southernmost population from the Palni hills have glabrous petals as described by Haworth but northern plant variants from Karnataka and Andhra Pradesh have hairs on the inner faces of the flowers. Both these varieties are highly attractive when flowering, but have a foul odour when in full bloom, a lot of natural pollinator housefly-like *Diptera* are attracted by the flowers. *B. lasiantha* also has a very attractive inflorescence and is suitable as an ornamental. It does not have any perceptive smell.

Hairy flowered specimens of *Boucerosia* were collected from rocky areas of Karnataka and identified as *B. diffusa*. All local Floras have recorded only a few populations of this species in Southern India, but it is frequently found all over the Karnataka and Tamil Nadu states. Vegetative morphology of the species is very similar to *B. umbellata* but the growth form is distinct in the occurrence of underground suckers and a much-diffuse stem growth. Leaf scars are very protruberent and produce a spine-like rank along the four rows of the rims of the stems. Flowers are large, sweet scented, dark reddish purple coloured, without striations on the inner face of the corolla, hairs are present only on the margins of corolla lobes.

While searching for *Boucerosias* in Karnataka, another species was encountered which was identified as *B. truncato-coronata*. This species was described as early as 1908 by Sedgewick. After its original description, it appears that no other literature is available on the species. Indian Red Data Book recorded this species to be possibly extinct from its habitat. Originally the species was collected from Bombay Presidency, near Dharwar now in Karnataka. No specimen was preserved in any of the Indian Herbaria. The population located comprised of weak stemmed plants among the rocky crevices at Pemmonahalli village near Tumkur. The plant was small with large umbels of 6–10 flowers in cymes on tips of the stems. On enquiry with the local people, they informed that the plant is edible, particularly in the month of August. Cultivation in our collection has ensured this rare plant's future survival.

More recently Ram Gandhi brought out a book on *Carallumas* of the Indian subcontinent. In this book, he recorded that *Boucerosia truncato-coronata* was collected near Bangalore but its identity was not confirmed because he did not see the plant's flowers. We could locate plants of this species in flowering. *B. truncato-coronata* is ornamentally an important and sought-after species due to its attractive flowers and miniature succulent habit.

Boucerosia nilagiriana is a similar species and was described from Nilgiri hills of Tamil Nadu by Kumari and Subba Rao. After the original type collections, until the present, no more collection has been made of this species. Later botanists like Meve and Liede (2002) have treated the species as being conspecific with *B. truncato-coronata*. Ram Gandhi has treated both the species separately in his book.

The state of Tamil Nadu has three other endemic species of *Boucerosia*, these are *B. indica*, *B. pauciflora* and *B. procumbens*. All the three species were collected from various localities during different field visits including type localities. *B. pauciflora* is a common but tiny species and occurs in all of the southern districts of Tamil Nadu. During the months of October–December plants in flower can be seen in many thorny bushes along the road sides of the Tirunelveli, Dindigul, Madurai, Pudukottai, Sivagangai and Ramanathapuram districts of Tamil Nadu. *B. indica* is rare in the dry localities of the foothills of the Eastern and Western Ghats and it was difficult to collect flowering specimens in natural habitat. Garden specimens bloom with beautiful flowers at regular intervals of August–October and February–April every year. In the present study, this species was collected with flowers in the month of November from Nellore and Chittoor districts of Andhra Pradesh.

The rarest of the *Boucerosia* species is *B. procumbens*. Its ecology and growth habit are entirely different from other Boucerosias. We located this species at Maruthuvamalai hills of Kanyakumari distict in Tamil Nadu. It has long trailing stems, sometimes exceeding up to 3 meters. The morphology of the species varies completely from other Boucerosias: they have no prominent leaf scars on the stem and the edges of the stems are sharp with square angles. This species grows mainly near seasonal streamlets in rocky crevices on the dry hills. The variations in Indian Boucerosias were elaborately reported recently by Karuppusamy (2011).

Propagation

Propagation of Boucerosias may be achieved from cuttings or from seed. Seed is generally difficult to obtain but, if available, they are easy to grow. It should be borne in mind that in the wild the germination of Boucerosias seed takes place in the small agglomerations of leaf litter that collect under perennial thorny bushes or in rocky crevices. As with all stapeliad seed germination is rapid between 1 and 7 days after planting and those that have not germinated within 15 days may be assumed infertile. The seedlings initially grow slowly and develop a well established rootstock later. It is advisable to plant the seedlings out into large containers as soon as they are firm enough to handle comfortably.

Many of the Indian Boucerosias may be propagated by stem cuttings. Those which produce adventitious roots will nearly always root since the succulent plant body remains alive until the roots develop and are well established. In the case of the small Boucerosias *viz. B. pauciflora, B. indica* and *B. trucato-coronata* plants, the underground branched stem sucker profusely. They may be cut into pieces, which should readily root and develop. They will extend the new green stems after a few days.

Early workers on the genus in India advised that their own contributions were only initial steps towards understanding the genus and that further advances would not be possible without a far-reaching study of living material. The more recent literature by Meve and Leide is indeed based to some extent on studies of living material but their extremely scanty distribution maps and the sparse ecological information, led those authors to conclude that the relationships between the various species were 'beyond comprehension'. The consequent lack of any attempt at assessing how the genus 'fits together' in the region makes it clear that Gravely and Mayuranathan should have been more forthright. For, with very good reason, they should have stressed that detailed field studies are the only way in which the genus will be properly understood and that the study of herbarium material and cultivated specimens alone cannot add substantially to our knowledge of this complex and yet fascinating group within the giant stapeliad family.

Chapter 6
Systematic Enumeration

Key to the Genera of Indian *Caralluma* (*Sensu lato*)

1. Flowers single or paired; arising in axils of leaves 2
1. Flowers in umbel; arising terminal apex of stem 3
2. Flowers hairy .... **Caralluma** (*sensu stricto*)
2. Flowers glabrous .... **Caudanthera**
3. Flowers in umbel; arising at apical portion of stem .... **Boucerosia**
3. Flowers in umbel; arising at sub-apical portion of stem .... **Apteranthes**

Apteranthes J.C. Mikan in Nov. Act. Nat. Cur. 17: 594. 1835.

= *Borealluma* Plowes, Haseltonia 3: 63. 1995.

Type: *Borealluma munbyana* (Decaisne) Plowes

Erect succulent plants with flowers in successive sub-apical portion on opposite sides of the stem, leaving two sets of pedicel scars; stem uniformly green, 4-angled; angles toothed.

Apteranthes tuberculata (N.E. Br.) Meve et Liede in Plant Syst. Evol. 34: 199. 2002. *Caralluma tuberculata* N.E.Br. in Gard. Chron. Ser.3. 12: 370, 1892; Type: Pakisthan (Baluchistan), Nullee Salt range, *Stocks* 596 (K, holo.); Gravely and Mayuranathan in Bull. Madr. Govt. Mus. n.s. N.H. 4(1): 20. 1931; Bruyns in Bradleya 4: 33-37. 1986; Gilbert, in Bradleya 8: 15. 1990. *Caralluma plicatiloba* Lavranos in J. South Afr. Bot. 28: 211. 1962. *Caralluma aucheriana* (Decne.) Gilbert in Bradleya 8: 18.1990; Jagtap and Singh, Fasc. Fl. India 24: 208. 1999. *Boucerosia aucheriana* Decne in

DC. Prodr. viii. 649. 1844; Hooker f. Fl. Brit. India 4: 78. 1883. *Borealluma tuberculata* (N.E. Br.) Plowes in Haseltonia 3: 63. 1995.

Pant wholly glabrous, 7-15 cm high; stem 8-12 mm thick, 4-angled; angles toothed. Flowers crowded into small umbels at the sub-apical portion of the stems, dark purple-brown or blackish-purple; pedicel ca 2.5 mm long; calyx ca 4 mm long, ovate-lanceolate, acute; corolla ca 1 cm in diameter, rotate with a very short campanulate tube; lobes 0.5-1 cm long, ca 0.5 cm broad, oblong-lanceolate, subobtuse with inflexed apiculus margins reflexed, covered with small tubercles, the back glabrous and smooth; outer corona of 10 erect subulate teeth, about 0.5 cm long, formed by each of the 5 lobes being divided almost to the base into 2 slender teeth; inner corona of 5 linear lobes incumbent on the backs of the anthers and not produced beyond them (Plate 6.1, Figures 6.1, 6.2).

Distribution: INDIA (Jammu and Kashmir and Punjab).

Abundance: A very few populations on top of Laleda plateau, near Sunderbani.

Flowering and fruiting: January-June.

Chromosome number: 2n = 22 ((Khatoon and Ali, 1993; Albers, 1981).

Etymology: From the Latin word 'tuberculatum' means a small bump or swelling. This species is bearing swelled projection on the leaf scar (tubercle).

Specimens Examined

Jammu: Jammu dt., Laleda plateau, Sunderbani, 8.11.2008, A.Ugraiah 31763 (SKU).

Panjab: Camp Kathawai, salt range, 21-5-1928, Bis Ram 835 (DD).

World: Pakistan.

Uses: Fresh stems of this species are edible and are sold as a vegetable in local vegetable shops at Sunderbani in India.

Nomenclatural Notes: Bruyns, in Bradleya 4/1986, subsumed *Caralluma plicatiloba* as a synonym under *Caralluma tuberculata* based on Ali's figure in Flora of Pakistan (1983). He omitted to mention that Ali gives the flower colour as being dark purple (Arabian *B. plicatiloba* has yellow flowers with scattered purple-brown rugosities). Because of the differences in stem type and flower colour between the Indian and Arabian plants, and also because a remarkably variable population recently discovered in Dhofar, Oman, by Dr. Ian McLeish, judgement on the validity of sinking *B. plicatiloba* is reserved until more material is available for study; it is consequently transferred here at the specific level. In view of the great geographic discontinuity between these two taxa it seems reasonable to expect that they are likely to have evolved to a point where some level of taxonomic recognition is warranted for each of the two populations. If the comparatively small gap between the population of *B. tuberculata* on the Pakistan/North India border, and that of *B. staintonii* in nearby Nepal, was capable of permitting the evolution of two distinct species, than the greater disjunction between the Asian and Arabian populations reinforces the likelihood that each of these now differs in some significant respect; they have

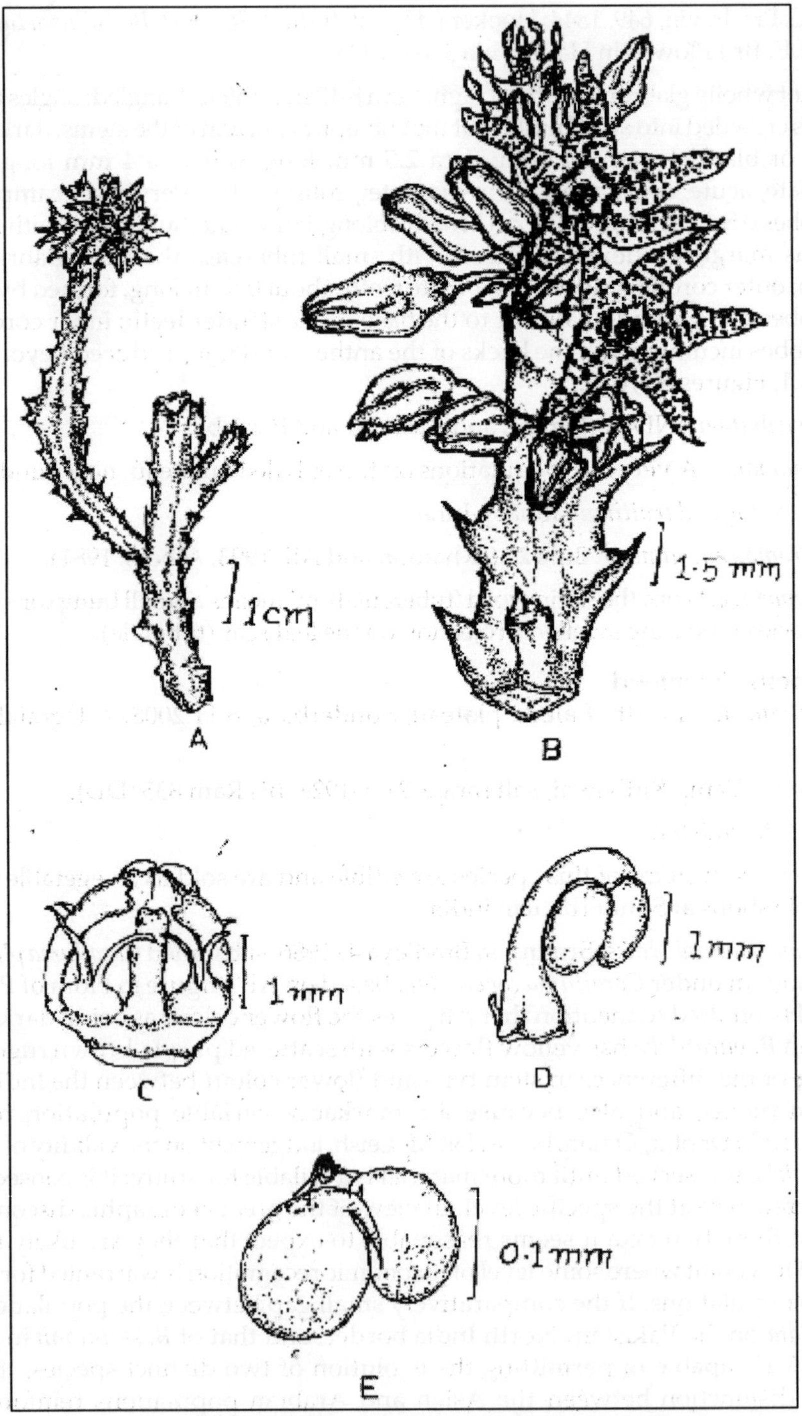

Figure 6.1: ***Apteranthes tuberculata*** **(N.E.Br.) Meve et Liede**
A: Habit; B: Inflorescence; C: Corona; D: Inner coronary lobe with anther; E: Pollinia

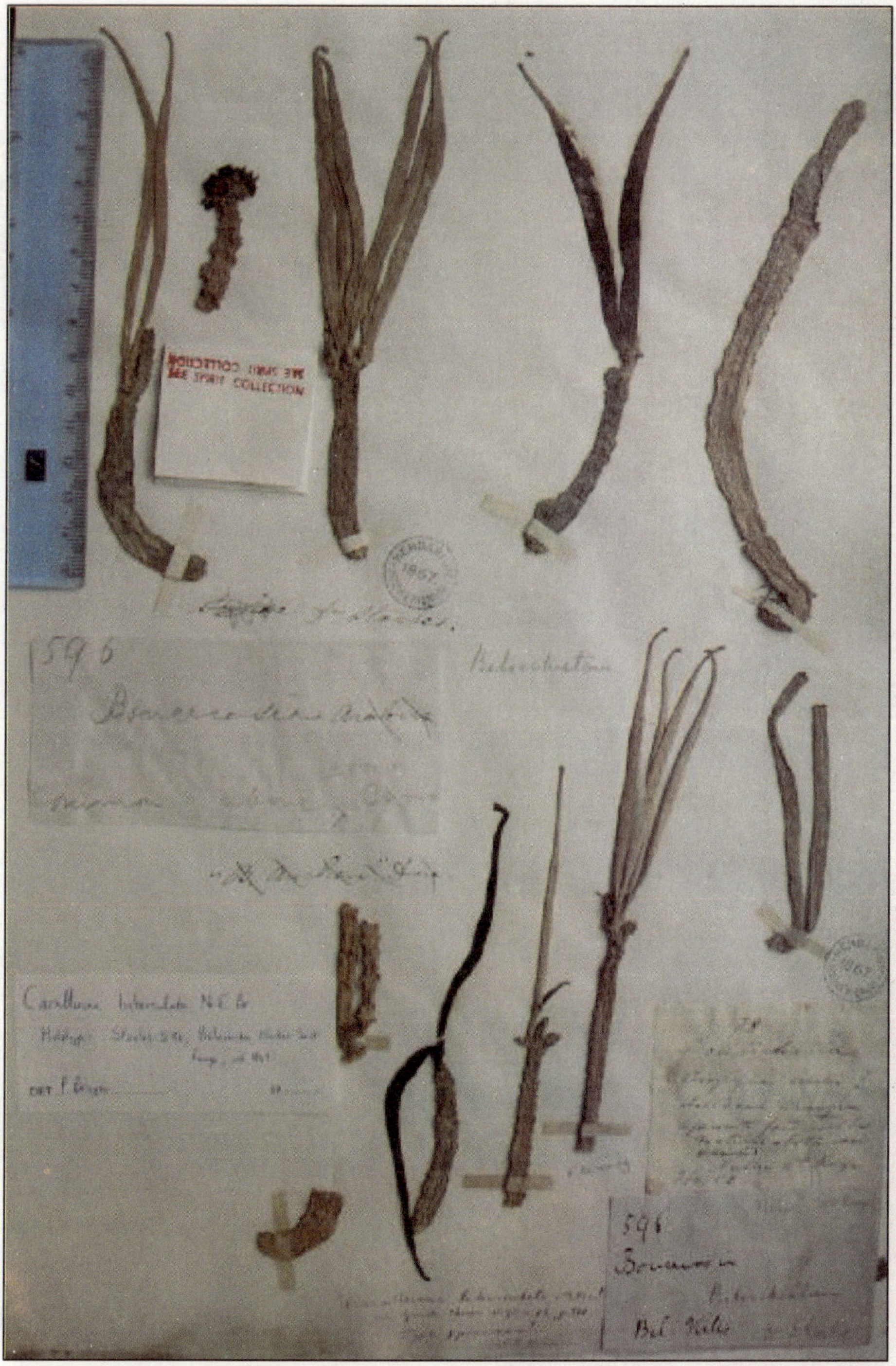

Figure 6.2: Type Specimen of *Apteranthus tuberculata* (N.E.Br.) Meve et Liede (=*Caralluma tuberculata* N.E.Br. in Gard. Chron. Ser. 3.12: 370.1892; Type: Pakistan (Baluchistan), Nullee salt range, Stocks 596 (K, Holo))

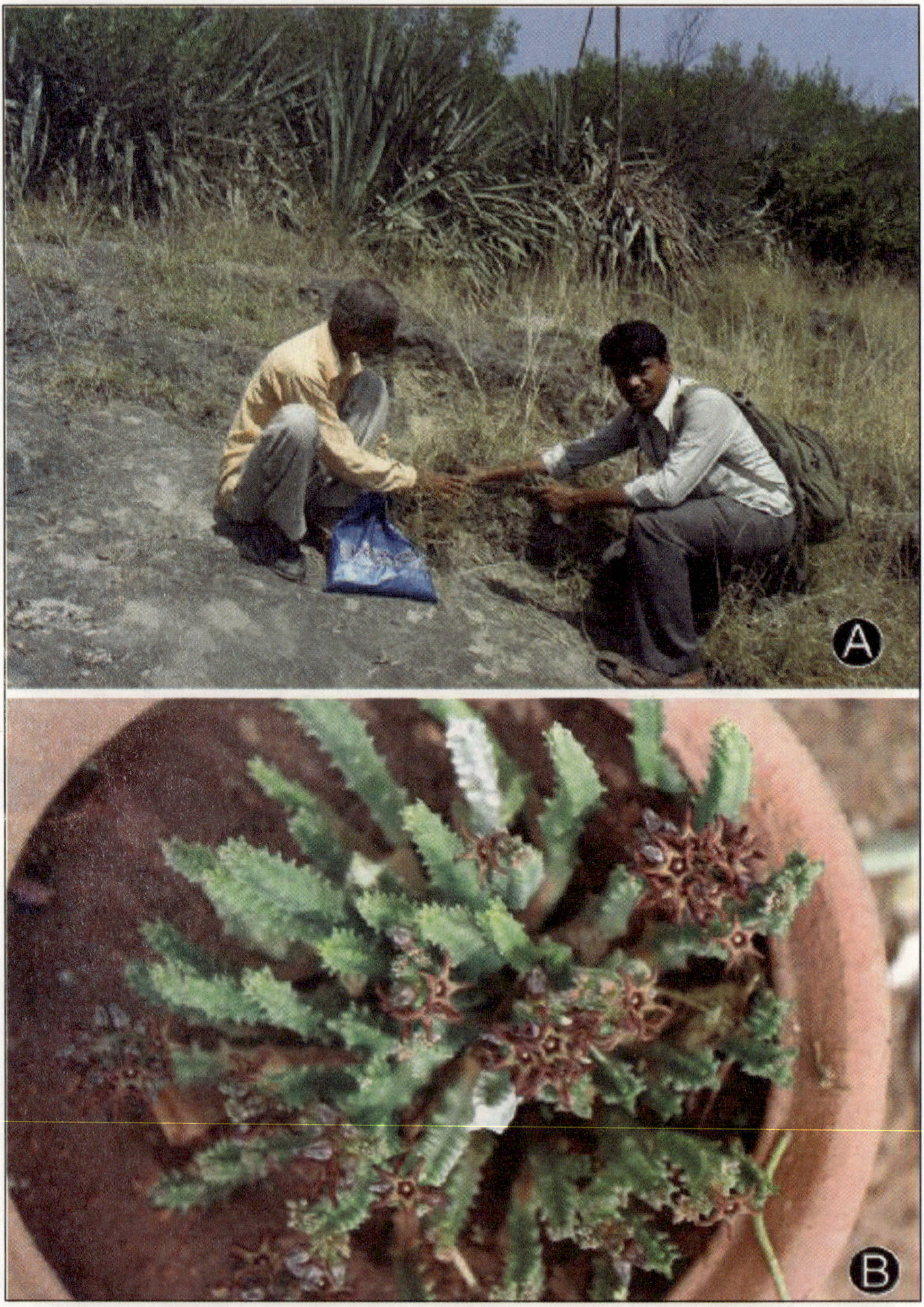

Plate 6.1: *Apteranthus tuberculata* (N.E.Br.) Meve et Liede
A: Natural habitat; B: Plant grown in garden in flowering stage

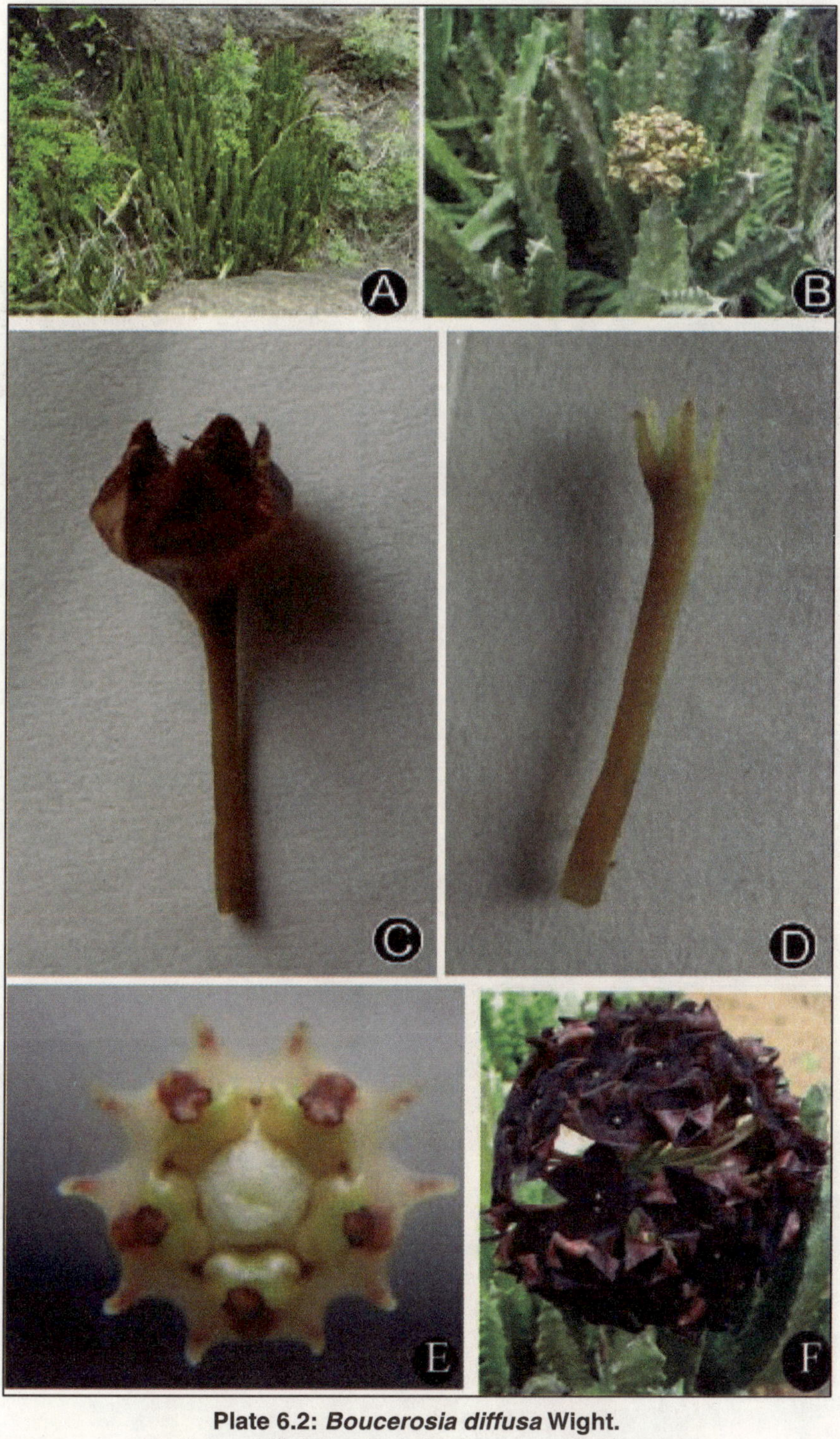

Plate 6.2: ***Boucerosia diffusa*** **Wight.**
A: Natural Habitat; B: Inflorescence; C: Flower;
D: Pedicel with sepals; E: Corona; F: Inflorescence

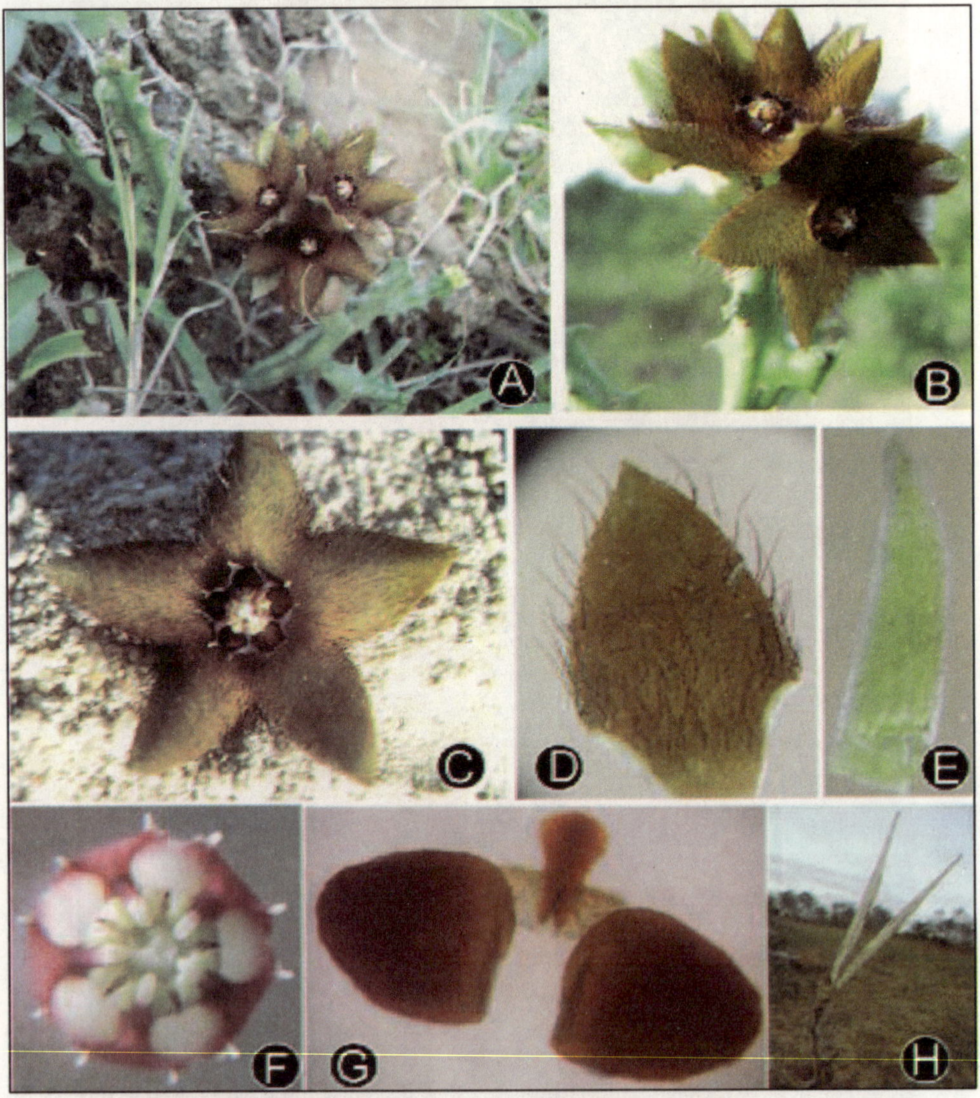

Plate 6.3: ***Boucerosia indica*** **(Wight et Arn.) Plowes**
A: Natural habitat; B: Inflorescence; C: Flower; D: Petal; E: Sepal; F: Corona; G: Pollinia; H: Fruit

presumably had a longer period of separation during which evolutionary forces could operate. Such isolation normally results in visible morphological divergence in members of the Stapelieae.

The spatial differences between the three taxa from Nepal, India, and Arabia on the one hand, and *B. munbyana* on the other, suggest that their long separation in time and space caused by this very large geographical gaps should have enabled evolutionary divergence to continue to a point where they are now possibly not compatible in the same genus: their phylogenetic relationship consequently requires more intensive study. Gilbert (1990) placed these three species together in his subgenus *Urmalcala*, with the type species given as *Caralluma tuberculata* N. E. Brown, because he found that their combination of characters "seemed to exclude them from each of the other subgenera". For this present study, it was felt better to utilize a different generic name and a different type speices in case more detailed studies later revealed a necessity to separate *B. munabyana* from the eastern taxa, in which case *Urmalcala* would be available for those.

Molecular studies by Meve and Liede (2002, 2004) have demonstrated the convenience of accepting many of Plowes segregates including *Apternathes*. The arrangement of subtribe Stapeliinae with 36 genera (Meve and Liede, 2004), 8 of which are segregates of the *Caralluma* complex: *Caralluma* R.Br. (c. 27 taxa; Africa, Arabia, India); *Apteranthes* Mikan (c. 8 taxa; South and Southeastern, Mediterranean, Canary Islands, Northwestern Africa, Arabia, Western and Central Asia); *Boucerosia* Wight and Arn. (c.7 taxa; Southern Asia); *Caudanthera* Plowes (c. 3 taxa; Africa, Arabia, Southeastern Asia). *Apteranthes* Mikan is currently accepted to include about seven African taxa and one Northwestern Indian taxa (Villalba, 2006)

Boucerosia **Wight et Arnott**
Contr. Bot, Ind.:34. 1834.

Type: *Caralluma umbellata* Haworth

Plants small to medium-sized, stems erect, sprawling or pendent, with epicutaneous branching. Latex watery. Leaves semi-persistent, ovate to lanceolate, with short scattered 1-celled crystalline marginal cilia; stipular glands or hairs lacking. Flowers in terminal umbels, never laterally displaced. Corolla campanulate with spreading ovate-acute lobes, usually ciliate; lobes surfaces glabrous, hirsute, or with minutely spiculate rugosities; gynostegium subsessile, staminal column cup-shaped; pollinia round-D-shaped; corpuscle clavate, flange-winged. Follicles slender, subulate.

World Distribution: Confined to southern India and Sri Lanka.

Key to Species

1. Stems extensively branched; corolla campanulate 2
1. Stems loosely branched; corolla rotate or campanulate 5
2. Flowers glabrous 3
2. Flowers hairy 4

3. Plants procumbent; stem growth continued from immediately below the base of umbel .... *B. procumbens*
3. Plants erect; stem growth normal, peduncle branched .... *B. umbellata*
4. Corolla campanulate, hairy; outer corona lobed .... *B. lasiantha*
4. Corolla campanulate, hairs along the margin only; outer corona annular .... *B. diffusa*
5. Corolla with clubbed hairs, confined to margin between tips of lobes 6
5. Corolla with simple hairs on the surface 7
6. Outer corona 5-lobed; top truncate with minute horns or teeth at each end .... *B. truncato-coronata*
6. Outer corona 10-lobed; horn–like appendages widely spreading .... *B. crenulata*
7. Umbels reduced to 1–3 flowered .... *B. pauciflora*
7. Umbels clustered 6–15 flowered .... *B. indica*

Boucerosia crenulata (Wall.) Wight et Arn. Contrib. Ind. Bot. 34. 1834; Hooker f. Fl. Brit. India 4: 78. 1883; Plowes in Haseltonia 3: 59. 1995; Meve and Liede in Plant Syst. Evol. 234: 200. 2002. *Caralluma crenulata* Wall. Pl. As. Rar. 1: 6. 1830. Type: tab. 7 of protologue based on plant collected by Wallich, Burma, Segain on right bank of Irrawady, opposite Ava, cult. in Calcutta; Gravely and Mayuranathan in Bull. Madr. Govt. Mus. n.s. N.H. 4(1): 21-22. 1931; Gilbert in Bradleya 8: 16. 1990; Jagtap and Singh in Fasc. Fl. India 24: 199-200. 1999. *Desmidorchis crenulata* (Wall.) Decne in Ann. Sc. Nat. 9: 266. 1838.

Stems fleshy, branched, erect, quadrangular, ca. 40 cm tall, equal thickness through out. Flowers in branched umbellate cymes, densely flowered; peduncles terete, ca 2 cm long, ca 2.5 mm in diam., glabrous; bracts thin, 3-4 x 0.5 mm, linear, apex acute, glabrous; pedicels terete, 1-3 cm long, ca 1mm in diam., glabrous. Calyx five lobed, divided up to base, lobes ca 3.5 x 1.5 mm, oblong-elliptic, apex acuminate, glandular within, glabrous. Corolla rotate, ca 1.5 cm across; corolla tube ca 1.5 mm long; lobes 5, ca 5 x 4.5 mm, ovate, apex acute, with long scattered hairs all over the inner surface, glabrous without. Corona staminal, biseriate; outer five lobed, ca 1.5 x 1 mm, with two horn like appendages widely separated from each other, appendages ca 0.5 mm long, attached on the back of anther arising from its base; inner five-lobed, very small, usually pointed and often more or less trifid, incumbent on the anthers. Stamens five, ca 1.5 mm long; pollinia five, pollen masses solitary in each anther cell, yellow, waxy, ca 360 x 331.2 μm with pellucid layer attached by light-brown caudicles 28.8-43.2 μm long, ca 57.2 μm wide, to a dark-brown corpuscle ca 216 μm long and ca 115.2 μm wide. Gynostegium ca 2.5 mm long. Follicles single, ca 7 x 0.6-0.7 cm, cylindric, apex acute, glabrous; seeds many, ca 9.5 x 4.5 mm, ovate-oblong, base rounded, brown with light-brown margin, 1-1.5 mm wide; coma silky-white, 2-3 cm long.

Jagtap and Singh (1999) reported this species from Andhra Pradesh, Maharashtra and Tamil Nadu. However during our survey we could not locate this species in these states. There is only one herbarium specimen in MH while there are no herbarium specimens in any of the other Indian Herbaria. All those specimens which were earlier referred to *Boucerosia crenulata* (=*Caralluma crenulata*) have been identified and confirmed as *Boucerosia umbellata* (=*Caralluma umbellata*).

Specimens Examined

Tamil Nadu: Adakkam, Gamble 32876 (MH).

World: Myanmar.

Etymology: From the Greek 'crenulate', meaning with small, rounded teeth. The corolla of the flower of this species have crenulate margin.

Boucerosia diffusa Wight, Icon. Pl. Ind. Orient. 4(4): 14, t. 1599. 1850; Type: Tab. 1599 of protologue based on material from India, Coimbatore; Hooker f. Fl. Brit. India 4: 78. 1883; Plowes in Haseltonia 3: 59. 1995; Meve and Liede in Plant Syst. Evol. 234: 200. 2002. *Caralluma diffusa* (Wight) N. E. Br. in Gard. Chron.12: 369. 1892; Gamble, Fl. Pres. Madras. 2: 862. 1923; Gravely and Mayuranathan in Bull. Madr. Govt. Mus. n.s. N.H. 4(1): 25-26. 1931; S.R. Srinivasan in Henry *et al.*, Fl. Tamil Nadu Analy. 2: 81. 1987; Gilbert in Bradleya 8: 16. 1990; Jagtap and Singh in Fasc. Fl. India 24: 200. 1999; Ramachandran *et al.*, in J. Threatened Taxa 3(3): 1622. 2011.

Stems fleshy, branched; branches erect, stout, 75 cm tall, four-angled, nearly equal thickness throughout; internodes 6–12 mm long and 5–15 mm in thickness, glabrous. Leaves absent, leaf scars present, appendage like growth at nodes on angle portions. Flowers many, terminal, in umbellate cymes, usually 30-35-flowered; bracts ca 1.5 mm long and 1.0–1.5 mm in diam., glabrous. Calyx 5-lobed, divided up to base, surface of the lobes hairless, but the dark streaks are minutely papillose, lobes ca 3 × 1 mm, lanceolate, apex acute, glabrous. Corolla campanulate, ca 2.5 cm dia.; corolla-tube ca 5 mm long; lobes 5, ca 3 × 2 cm, ovate, apex acute, margin ciliate, glabrous. Corona staminal, biseriate; outer annular, arising from the base of stamens, closely intact, five lobed, ca 2.5 × 1.5 mm, with two horn-like appendages widely separated from each other; inner variable, ca 1 mm long, linear, arising from the inner side of outer corona, overlapping anther-lobes. Stamens 5, ca 2.5 mm long; pollinia masses solitary in each anther cell, yellow, waxy, with pellucid layer attached by a light-brown caudicles and dark-brown corpuscle. Gynostegium ca 1.5 mm long. Follicles paired, linear-lanceolate, tapering towards apex, glabrous. Seeds glabrous, 7-10 x 3-3.5 mm, oblong, base rounded, margin dark brown, coma silky, 3-5 cm long (Plate 6.2, Figure 6.3)

Distribution: This is distributed in sacred hill in Thiruvannamalai and Coimbatore district in Tamil Nadu.

Abundance: Luxuriant population.

Flowering and fruiting: April–September.

Chromosome number: 2n = 22 (Navaneetham and Sampathkumar, 1984).

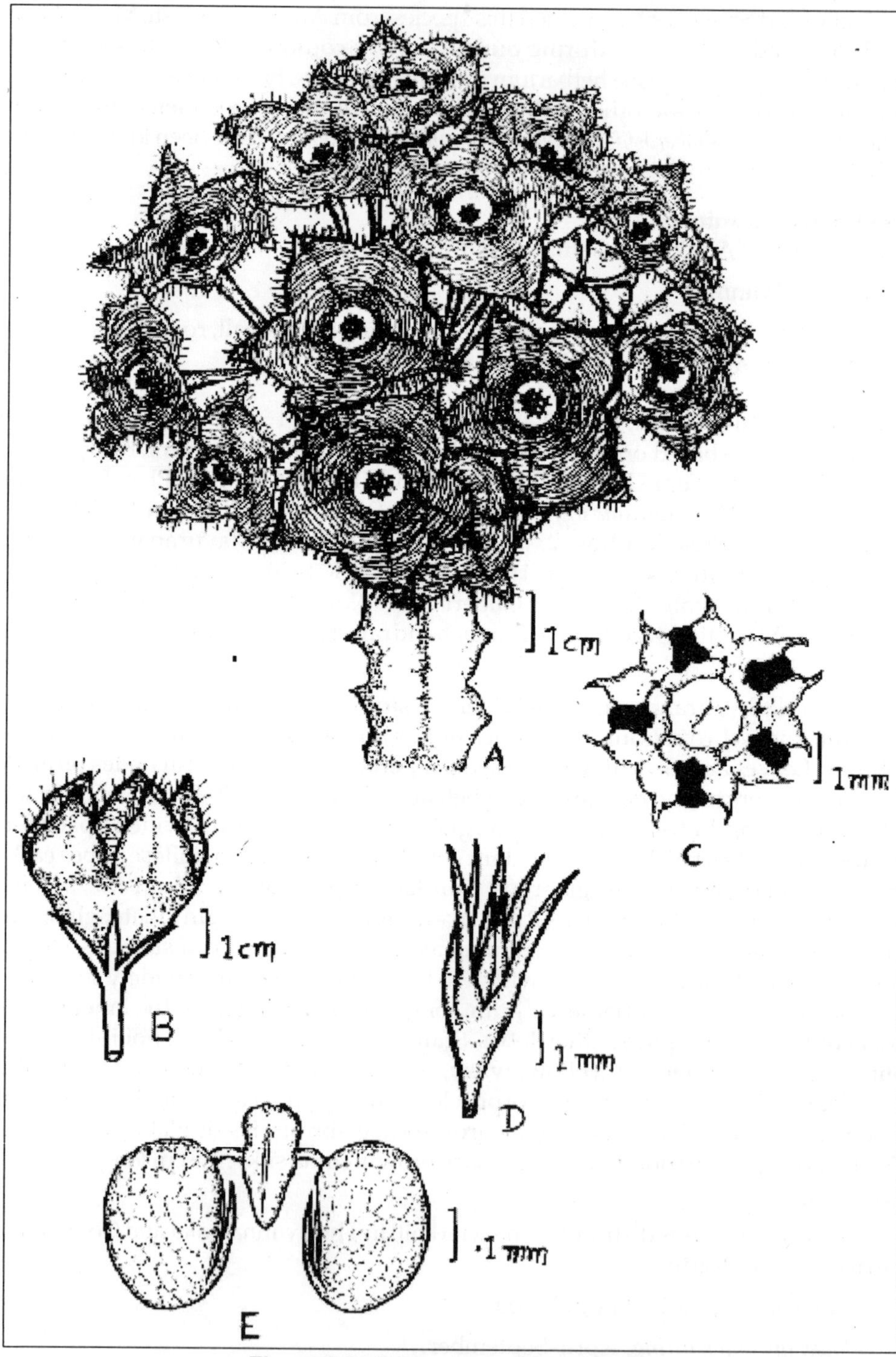

Figure 6.3: ***Boucerosia diffusa*** **Wight**
A: Habit; B: Flower; C: Corona; D: Sepals with gynoecium; E: Pollinia

Etymology: From the Greek 'diffusa' means loosely spreading; the branches of the plants are loosely spreading on the ground for specific epithet.

Specimens Examined

Tamil Nadu: Thiruvannamalai dt., Arthanaareeswarar sacred hill, 4.8.2008, A. Ugraiah 31752 (SKU); Coimbatore dt., Kalpatti, Atamalai slope, 1850 ft, 28-9-1910, C.E.C. Fischer 2258 (CAL); slope of Anamalai, 650m, 31.8.1962, C.P.Sreemadhavan 136 (MH); N. Slope of Karupparayan hills near Coimbatore, 31.10.1963, C.P. Sreemadhavan 957 (MH).

Myanmar (Burma): Pyarobeve, upper Burma, Sept 1887, H. Collett 87 (CAL).

Notes: This species was described based on collections from dry hills of Coimbatore district in Tamil Nadu. There are a few specimens collected from Coimbatore hills and deposited in MH. We surveyed all the hill ranges of Coimbatore, but we failed to locate. However we could locate luxuriant populations in Thiruvannamalai district. Ramachandran *et al.* (2011) also reported its occurrence in Madukkarai hills in Coimbatore district in Tamil Nadu.

Uses: The succulent stems are used as a vegetable by local people.

Boucerosia indica (Wight et Arn.) Plowes in Haseltonia 3: 59. 1995. *Hutchinia indica* Wight et Arn. Contrib. Bot. Ind.: 34. 1834; Type: India, Madras Presidency; near Madras. Wight, Ic. v.2, p.4, t. 355.1842. *Boucerosia hutchinia* Decne. in DC. Prodr. 8:649. 1844; Hooker f. Fl. Brit. India 4: 78. 1883; Meve et Liede in Plant Syst. Evol. 234: 200. 2002. *Caralluma indica* (Wight et Arn.) N.E.Br. in Gard. Chron. 2: 369. 1892; Gamble Fl. Pres. Madras 2: 862. 1923; Gravely and Mayuranathan in Bull. Madr. Govt. Mus. n.s. N.H. 4(1): 23. 1931; S.R. Srinivasan in A.N. Henry *et al*. Fl. Tamil Nadu Anal. 2: 81.1987; Gilbert in Bradleya 8: 16.1990; Jagtap and Singh, Fasc. Fl. India 24: 203.1999; Hanumanthappa in Pullaiah and Ali Moulali Fl. Andhra Pradesh 2: 583. 1997.

Plant herbaceous, erect, 12 cm to 18 cm tall, Stems fleshy, irregularly branched, quadrangular, tapering towards base, stout in middle; internodes small, 2–6 mm long and 2–4 mm across, glabrous. Leaves small, ca 1.5 x1 mm, triangular, acute at apex, dentate margin, glabrous. Flowers terminal in umbellate cymes, usually 5-8 flowered; pedicels terete, 7 mm long, glabrous. Calyx 5-lobed, divided up to base, lobes ovate-oblong, apex acute, glabrous. Corolla rotate, ca 8 mm long, ca 1.6 cm across; corolla-tube ca 3.5 mm long; lobes 5, ca 4.5 x 4 mm, ovate, apex acute, with slightly pointed tip, hairs present all over the corolla except tip (glabrous without), white fringed within, light brownish-yellow. Corona staminal, biseriate; outer 5-lobed, lobes erect, ca 4 mm long, light-yellow, with extreme tip purplish, with minute yellowish tooth usually present in the deep cleft between adjacent lobes; inner 5-lobed, incumbent on the anthers and not produced beyond them, 0.5–1 mm long. Stamens 5, ca 4 mm long; pollinia 5, pollen masses solitary in each anther cell, yellow, waxy, with pellucid layer attached by a light-brown caudicles and dark-brown corpuscle. Gynostegium ca 1.3 mm long. Follicles paired, 5.5-11 cm long, cylindrical, attenuate towards apex; seeds 7 x 5 mm, ovoid; coma 2-3 cm long (Plate 6.3; Figure 6.4).

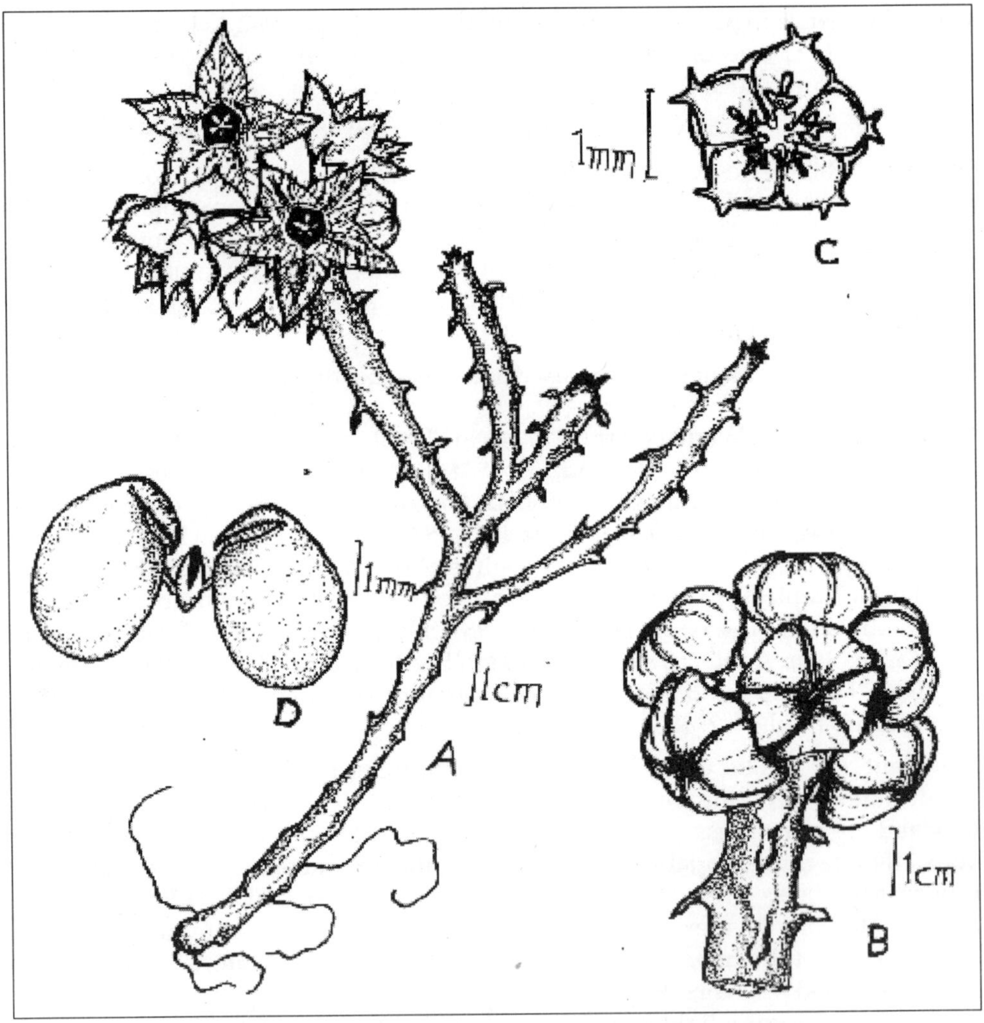

Figure 6.4: ***Boucerosia indica*** **(Wight et Arn.) Plowes**
A: Habit; B: Inflorescence; C: Corona; D: Pollinia

Distribution: Andhra Pradesh, Tamil Nadu, Karnataka.

Abundance: Discontinuous population in open scrub area of waste lands near Atapattu bird sanctuary in Nellore district and also distributed in waste lands under thorny bushes near Bakarapet in Chittoor district.

Flowering and fruiting: November–January.

Chromosome number: 2n = 22 (Ramakrishna and Afzalunnis, 1981), 2n = 44 (Navaneetham, 1980, 1981).

Etymology: For the Indian nativity.

Specimens Examined

Andhra Pradesh: Nellore dt., Penchalakona, Somasila project, 12.7.2008, A. Ugraiah 31746 (SKU); Nellore, J. S. Gamble, 32879 (MH); Chittoor dt., Bakarapet, 28.10.09, A. Ugraiah and S. Sandhya Rani 37710 (SKU); between Udayapalyam and Yerravaripalyam, 28.10.09, A. Ugraiah and S. Sandhya Rani 37711 (SKU).

Tamil Nadu: Coimbatore dt, Nellimalai R.F, 400 m, 16.10.1962, K. Ramamurthy 14787 (MH); Madras dt, J.S. Gamble, *s.n.* (MH).

Notes: This species is sparsely distributed in low lying hills and scrub forests of Eastern Ghats, particularly Nellore to south of Tirunelveli. It is poorly represented in Indian herbaria (MH Nos. 14787, 32879). Present study found this species in Nellore and Chittoor districts of Andhra Pradesh. Populations are locally vulnerable due to habitat modification and forest encroachment.

Boucerosia lasiantha Wight, Icon. Pl. Ind. Orient. 4(2): 1. t. 1286. 1848; Hooker f. Fl. Brit. India 4: 78. 1883. Type: Tab. 1286 in protologue based on plant from Nuggur Hills, Madras, India. *Caralluma lasiantha* (Wight) N. E. Br. in Gard.Chron. 12: 369.1892; Gamble Fl. Pres. Madras 2: 862. 1923; S.R. Srinivasan in A.N. Henry *et al*. Fl.Tamil Nadu Anal.2: 81.1987; Hanumanthappa in Pullaiah and Ali Moulali Fl. Andhra Pradesh 2:583.1997.

Stem fleshy, branched; branches erect, 50 cm tall, acute angled, not tapering, quadrangular. Leaves reduced, opposite decussate, sessile, deltoid, glabrous, leaf scars spine-like. Flowers terminal, in many-flowered umbellate cymes, peduncle branched; bracts ca 2–5 mm long, linear; pedicels terete, 1–2 cm long. Calyx 5-lobed, divided up to base, lobes linear, 5 mm long, apex acute, glandular within, glabrous. Corolla 5-lobed, rotate or campanulate, ca 1.5 cm long, apex acute or apiculate, dark brown colour, velvety within, long hairs on the margin and upper half. Corona staminal, biseriate; outer 5-lobed, dark-purple, truncate, ca 9 mm across; inner 5-lobed, apex acute. Stamens 5, short, ca 1.6 mm long; pollinia 5, pollen masses solitary in each anther cell, yellow, waxy. Gynostegium ca 2.6 mm long. Follicles paired, linear-lanceolate, tapering towards apex with blunt tip, glabrous. Seeds glabrous, 7-10 x 3-3.5 mm, oblong, base rounded, margin dark brown, coma silky, 3-4 cm long (Plate 6.4, Figure 6.5)

Distribution: Andhra Pradesh, Kerala.

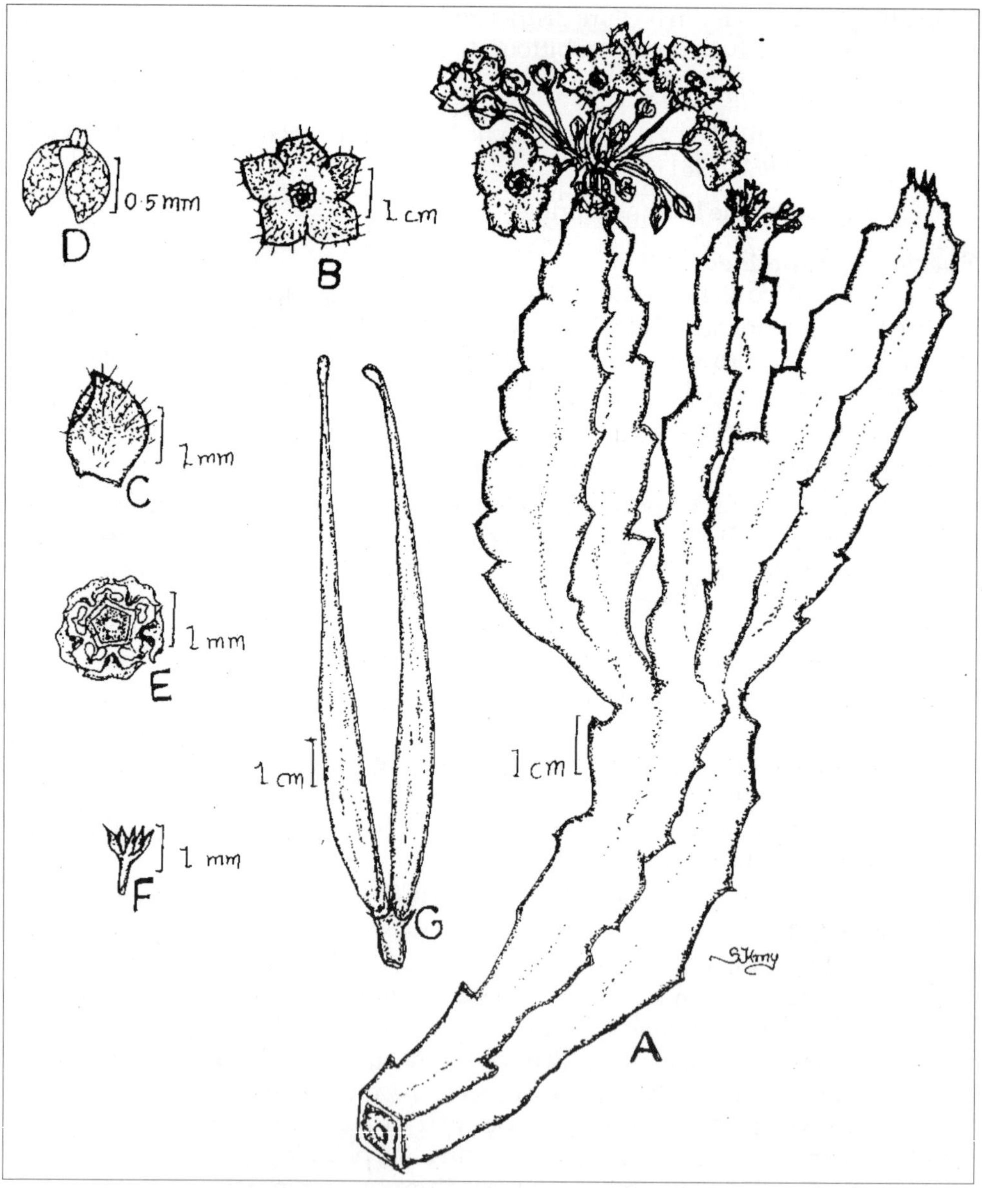

Figure 6.5: ***Boucerosia lasiantha*** **Wight**
A: Habit; B: Flower; C: Petal; D: Pollinia; E: Corona; F: Sepals; G: Fruit

Abundance: Luxuriant population in small hill area, opposite Gooty Railway station.

Flowering and fruiting: May–December.

Etymology: From the Latin 'lasiantha' means wool flower. The species is bearing wool-like velvety hairs on the inner surface of corolla lobes.

Specimens Examined

Andhra Pradesh: Anantapur dt., hills Opposite Gooty railway station, 23.4.2008, S. Karuppusamy and A. Ugraiah 31709 (SKU); Gooty foot hills, 23.4.2008, S. Karuppusamy and A. Ugraiah 31706 (SKU); Chittoor dt., Horsley hills, 24.12.2008, A. Ugraiah 31779 (SKU).

Kerala: Travencore dt., Bellyrirangan hills, E. Barner 103470 (DD)

Note: Gravely and Mayuranathan (1931) in their monograph on Indian *Caralluma* have not given occurrence of this species in India. Jagtap and Singh (1999) in their Fascicles of Flora of India and Gilbert (1990) have treated it under *Caralluma umbellata.* However Gamble (1923) has clearly mentioned the differences between these two species and its occurrence in Gooty hills in Anantapur district and hills of Chittoor district in Andhra Pradesh. We have found several populations from the same localities, *i.e.*, Gooty hills and Horsley hills. Both the populations of *C. umbellata* and *C. lasiantha* are coexisting in this area. We also found that the foul smell emanating from the flowers of *B. umbellata* is not found in *B. lasiantha.* The hairiness of the corolla lobes and much branched aerial branches in stem also vary.

Uses: The stem of this species is used as vegetable in Andhra Pradesh.

Boucerosia pauciflora Wight in Madras J. Sci. vi. t and p.473. 1837; Type: India, Madras, Palayamkottai, Wight 2429 (Kew) from South India; Hooker f. Fl. Brit. India 4: 78.1883; Plowes in Haseltonia 3: 59. 1995; Meve and Liede in Plant Syst. Evol.234: 200. 2002. *Caralluma pauciflora* (Wight) N.E.Br. in Gard. Chron. 2: 278.1892; Gamble, Fl. Pres. Madras. 2: 862. 1923; Gravely and Mayuranathan in Bull. Madr.Govt. Mus. n.s. N.H. 4(1): 22. 1931; S.R. Srinivasan in A. N. Henry *et al.* Fl.Tamil Nadu Anal. 2: 81.1987; Gilbert in Bradleya 8: 16.1990; Jagtap and Singh, Fasc. Fl. India 24:204. 1999. *Desmidorchis pauciflora* Decne. in Ann.Sci. Nat. 9: 266. 1838.

Stems fleshy, 15-20 cm high, slender, branched; branches quadrangular, internodes short, 3–12 x 2.5–6 mm, glabrous. Leaves reduced to scales, 1.2–2 x 0.5 mm, triangular, recurved, acute at apex, glabrous. Flowers terminal, umbels reduced to single flower; bracts linear, apex acute, glabrous; pedicels terete, 3–4 mm long, glabrous. Calyx 5-lobed, divided up to base, linear to linear-lanceolate, apex acute, glandular within, glabrous. Corolla rotate, ca 1 mm long, corolla–tube 5.5–6 mm long, villous within; lobes 5, triangular, apex acute, fringed or villous within, purple streaks or bands within. Corona staminal, biseriate; outer cupular, attached to staminal column, ca 2 mm long; inner 5-lobed, attached to the inner side of the outer corona, linear, triangular, elongated, inflexed over the anther, glabrous. Stamens 5, ca 4 mm long; pollinia 5, pollen masses solitary in each anther cell, yellow, waxy, with pellucid layer attached by a light-brown caudicles and dark-brown corpuscle. Gynostegium ca 3 mm long (Plate 6.5; Figures 6.6 and 6.7).

Distribution: This species is sparsely distributed in rocky crevices of foothills of Vallanadu, where it is narrowly endemic. Earlier reports noted that this species is distributed in Tirunelvely district (Wight, 1834) and Pudhukottai forests (Gravely and Mayuranathan, 1931) of Tamil Nadu.

Abundance: Very little population associated with thorny bushes.

Flowering and fruiting: September–December.

Chromosome number: 2n = 22 (Navaneetham and Sampathkumar, 1984).

Etymology: From the Greek 'pauci' means a few or small; the plant bearig a few number of flower (1-3) on the apex of the stem.

Specimens Examined

Tamil Nadu: Tirunelveli dt., 1 km from Vallanadu towards Tuticorin 5.5.2008, A. Ugraiah and S. Karuppusamy 31719 (SKU); Kalakkad-Sivanapperi forest, 27.12.1980, E. Vajravelu 76467 (MH and CAL); Sivanapperi forest, 225 m, 14.11.1962, J. Joseph 15299 (MH); Ramanathapuram dt, Ebani forest- Sivaganga, 100 m, 12.9.1965, K. Ramamurthy 24695 (MH). Sivanapperi, J. Joseph 97554 (MH).

Boucerosia procumbens (Gravely et Mayuranathan) Plowes in Haseltonia 3: 59. 1995; Meve et Liede in Plant Syst. Evol. 234: 200. 2002. *Caralluma procumbens* Gravely and Mayuranathan, in Bull. Mad. Govt. Mus. 4: 26.1931; Type: fig. 4, 13-17 in protologue based on plants from India, S. Travancore, Maruthuvamalai; S. R. Srinivasan in Henry *et al.* Fl. Tamil Nadu Anal. 2: 82. 1987; Gilbert in Bradleya 8: 16. 1990; Jagtap and Singh in Fasc. Fl. India 24: 204. 1999.

Stems fleshy branched; branches procumbent, quadrangular, creeping across the ground or on rocks, 15 mm broad, > 2 meters long and angles acute. Latex watery. Leaves small, triangular, 1.0–1.5 × 0.5–1 mm, only on young branches, leaf scars indistinctly indicated as protuberances. Flowers terminal, in umbels, but the stem commonly sends out a side shoot from the axil of a leaf immediately below and this grows so as to push the umbel to the side. Calyx 5-lobed, lobes deeply divided up to base, acute at the apex, glabrous. Corolla campanulate, lobes-5, fleshy, glabrous, lobes whitish and streaked purple; a few purple spots found on the outer sides; Corona whitish, purplish (Plate 6.6, Figure 6.8).

Distribution: Tamil Nadu (endemic)

Abundance: A very few populations occur in Maruthuvamalai and Aramboli rocky hills near Kottaram in Kanyakumari district of Tamil Nadu.

Flowering and fruiting: June–September.

Chromosome number: 2n = 22 (Ramakrishna and Afzalunnisa, 1981).

Etymology: From the Greek 'procumbens' means horizontal spreading branches with erect stem apices.

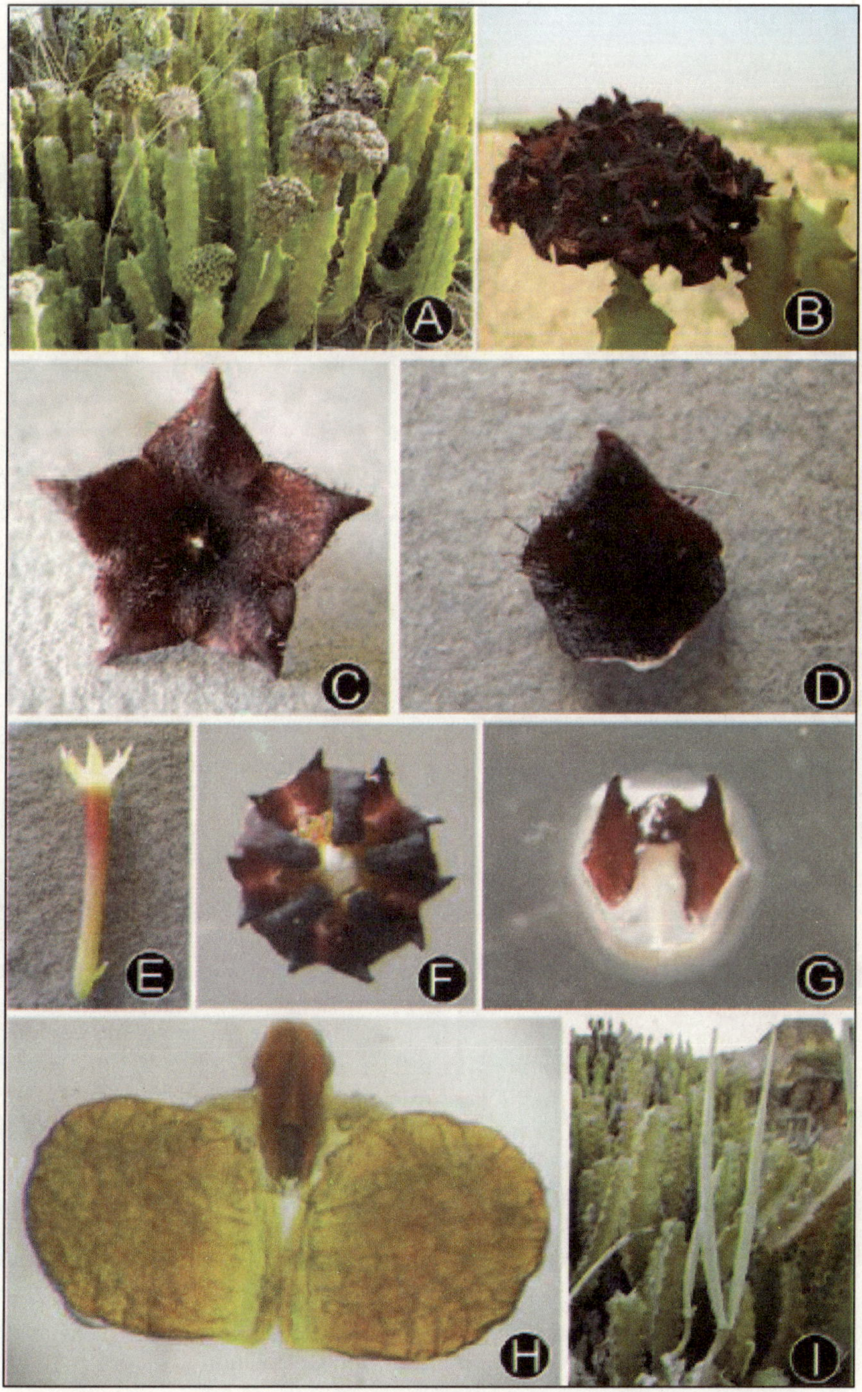

Plate: 6.4. *Boucerosia lasiantha* Wight
A: Natural habitat; B: Inflorescence; C: Flower; D: Petal; E: Pedicel; F: Corona; G: Outer corona; H: Pollinia; I: Fruit.

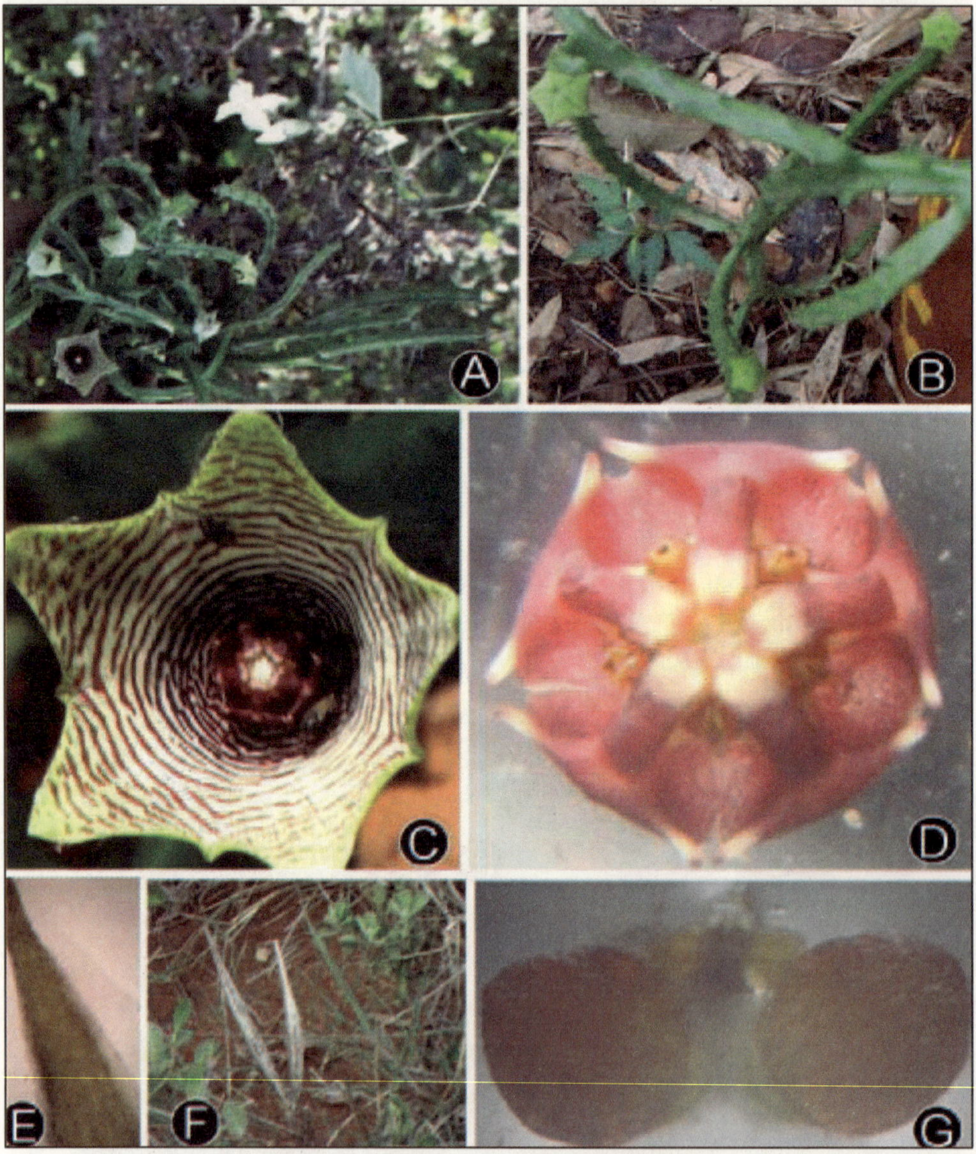

Plate 6.5. ***Boucerosia pauciflora*** **Wight**
A: Natural habitat; B: Inflorescence; C: Flower; D: Corona; E: Sepal; F: Fruit; G: Pollinia

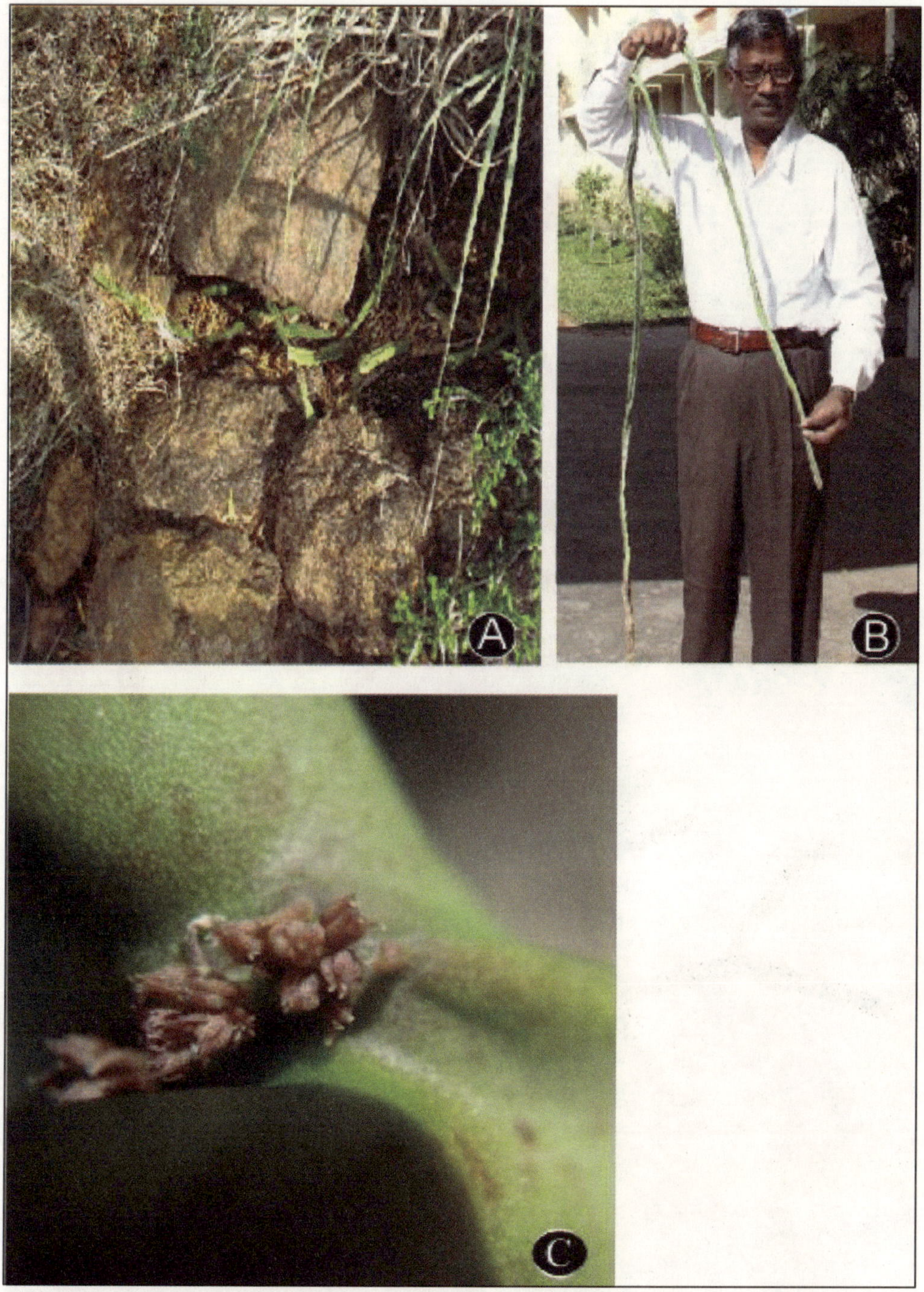

Plate 6.6. *Boucerosia procumbens* (Gravely et Mayuranathan) Plowes
A: Natural habitat; B: Author T. Pullaiah with plant; C: Habit with young buds

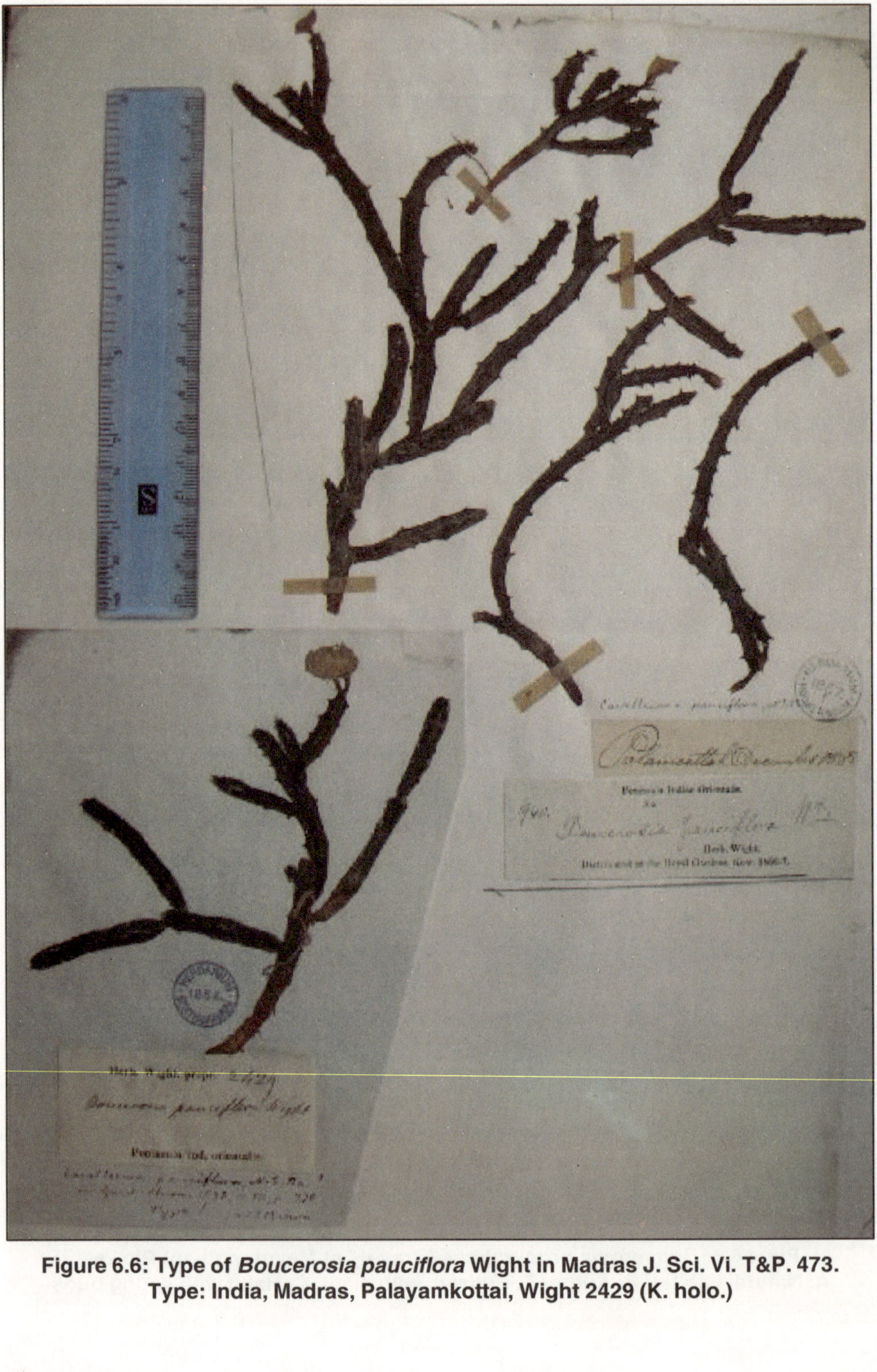

Figure 6.6: Type of *Boucerosia pauciflora* Wight in Madras J. Sci. Vi. T&P. 473. Type: India, Madras, Palayamkottai, Wight 2429 (K. holo.)

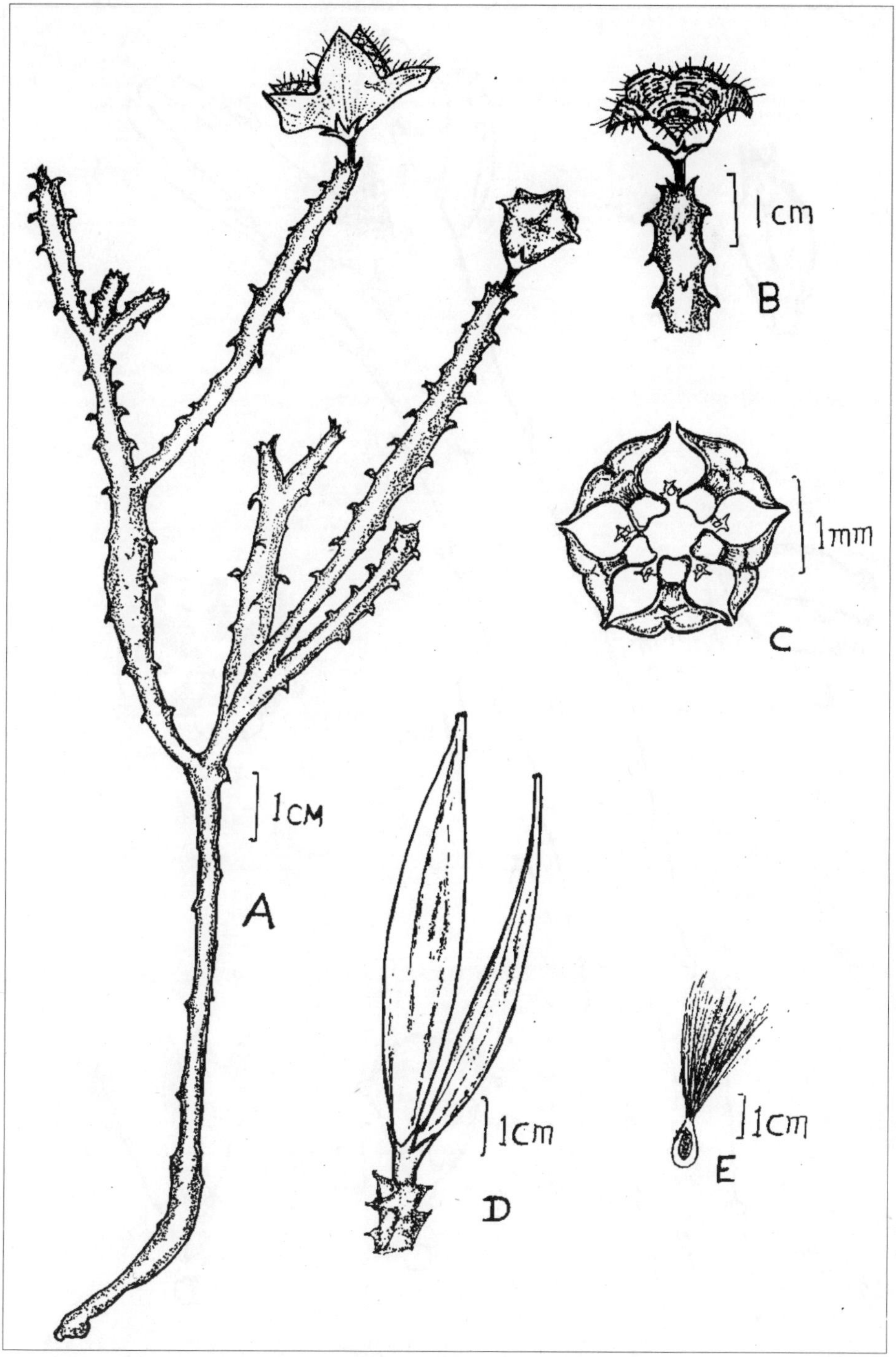

Figure 6.7: ***Boucerosia pauciflora*** **Wight**
A: Habit; B: Inflorescence; C: Corona; D: Fruit; E: Seed

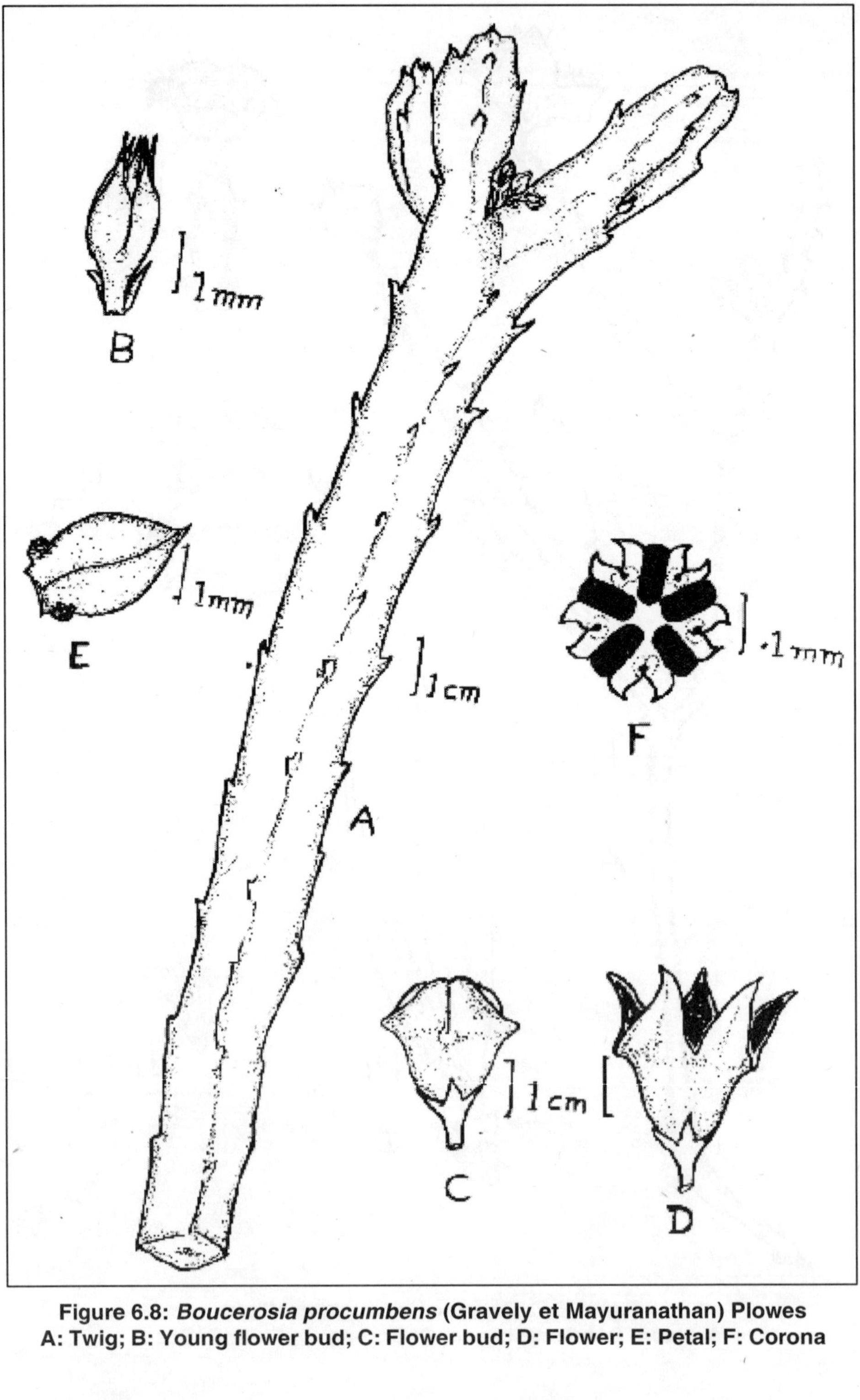

Figure 6.8: ***Boucerosia procumbens*** **(Gravely et Mayuranathan) Plowes**
A: Twig; B: Young flower bud; C: Flower bud; D: Flower; E: Petal; F: Corona

Specimens Examined

Tamil Nadu: Kanyakumari dt., Kottaram hills, Maruthuvamalai, 7.5.2008, A. Ugraiah and S. Karuppusamy 31723 (SKU).

Notes: A very few populations occur in Aramboli hills, Kalakad and Mundanthurai area of Western Ghats. This element is also endemic to Tamil Nadu. In present study we found out only from Maruthamalai hills.

Boucerosia truncato-coronata Sedgewick in J. Indian Bot. 2:125-126. 1921; Type: Hubli, Dharwar District., Carnatica region, Bombay province, India, at 2000 ft. Sept. 1919; Plowes in Haseltonia 3: 59.1995. *Caralluma truncato-coronata* (Sedgewick) Gravely et Mayuranathan in Bull. Mad. Govt. Mus. 4: 21.1931; Gilbert in Bradleya 8: 16.1990; Jagtap and Singh, Fasc. Fl. India 24: 207. 1999; Santapau and Irani, in Univ. Bomaby Bot. Mem. 4: 22. 1962; Sharma *et al*. Fl. Karnataka 165. 1984. *Caralluma nilagiriana* Kumari et Subba Rao in J. Bombay Nat. Hist. Soc. 73: 199-200. 1976; S. R. Srinivasan in Henry *et al*., Fl. Tamil Nadu Anal. 2:82. 1987. Type: India, Tamil Nadu, Nilagiri dist., between Anaikalty and Ebanad, cult. Coimbatore, Subbarao and Kumari 39262 (CAL, holo.; MH, iso.).

Plants growing in clumps, up to 15 cm high, with subterranean runners, spreading by suckers. Branches slender, prostrate, rooting at nodes, not tapering, 4-angled, ca 6 mm wide, laterally furrowed. Leaves minute, ovate, glabrous, tip acute, arise on the tubercles of the angles. Inflorescence terminal, umbellate, 10-13-flowered. Flowers campanulate, pentagonal, apically flattened in bud. Bracts 2, minute, ca. 2.5 mm long, linear. Bracteoles inconspicuous. Pedicels ca. 17 mm long, green. Calyx divided up to the base, segments 5, alternating with corolla lobes, ca. 4 mm long, linear, acute, glabrous. Corolla ca. 2.5 cm across, corolla-tube ca. 6 x 6 mm, campanulate, segments 5, outside green mottled with purple, three distinct colouration on the tube inside, a deep purple ring at the middle with dark purple ring formed a rim of mouth and interior tubes light purple dotted white background with valvate limb, 5-fid, with pellucid glands at bottom. Corolla-lobes distinct, triangular, acute at tip, dark purple to brownish purple above, a few thin yellow transverse lines interrupted on the lobes, 3 or 4 golden yellow hairs on the margins at the base of corolla lobes. Corona ca. 4 mm in diameter, dark purple; outer corona 5-lobed, truncate tips, lobes prominently cuspidate on either side; inner lobes ligulate, elongate, ascending and appressed on dorsal surface of anthers; staminal column short, incumbent on the stigma; anthers light yellow, lobes broadly elliptic. Pollinia solitary, erect, yellowish red, compressed, oblong or obtuse, faintly transversely striped, attached laterally to the erect purple corpusculum, glabrous; stigma 5-angled. Follicles paired, erect, ca. 5 cm long, lanceolate, glabrous, light purplish streaks above, slightly beaked at the tips (Plate 6.7; Figure 6.9).

Distribution: INDIA (Karnataka-Tumkur, Tamil Nadu-Kuridimalai)

Abundance: A very few populations occur in small hill regions of Tumkur hills of Karnataka and Kuridimalai in Tamil Nadu.

Flowering and fruiting: November –March.

Etymology: The species have truncated (bifurcated) corona tip.

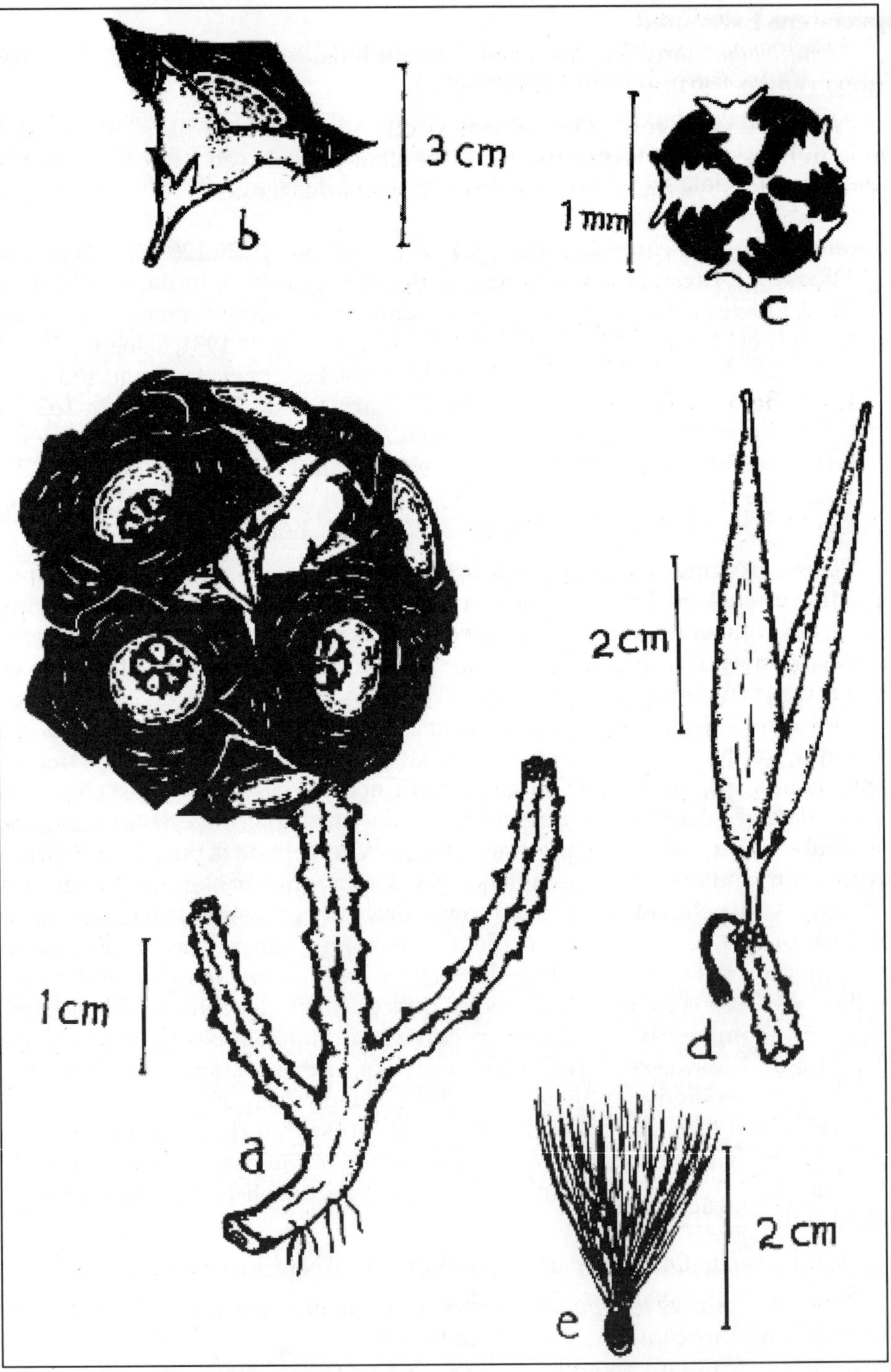

Figure 6.9: ***Boucerosia truncato-coronata*** **Sedgewick**
A: Habit; B: Flower; C: Corona; D: Fruit; E: Seed

Specimens Examined

Tamil Nadu: Coimbatore dt., Kuridimalai, Madhukarai, 10.5.2008, A. Ugraiah and S. Karuppusamy 31733 (SKU).

Karnataka: Tumkur dt., Pemmonalli temple opposite hills, 29.11.2008, A. Ugraiah and S. Karuppusamy 31767 and 31768 (SKU); CAL No. 296827 without collector name, collected date 18-5-1901 probably from Karnataka (P.V. Bruyns *det.*), specimen flowers destroyed completely (CAL).

Nomenclatural notes: *C. nilagiriana* (= *C. truncato-cronata*) was described by Kumari and Subba Rao (1976) from Nilgiri hills of Tamil Nadu.

Note: There are no herbarium specimens in any Indian herbaria except *B. nilagiriana* Kumari and Rao 39262 A (CAL), 39262, 39263, 38287 and 37329 (MH). The present collection made after a long gap of type collection approximately 400 km away from type locality. A fragmented population was observed in about 50 km surrounding areas of Tumkur district of Karnataka.

Boucerosia umbellata (Haw.) Wight et Arn., Contrib. Bot. Ind.: 34. 1834; Plowes in Haseltonia 3: 59. 1995; Hooker f. Fl. Brit. India 4: 77. 1883 (incl. var. *campanulata*); Meve and Liede in Plant Syst. Evol. 234: 200. 2002. *Caralluma umbellata* Haw., Syn. Pl. Succ.47, 1812; Type: from 'Eastern India', described from a plant cultivated in England, introduced 1804, ? no material preserved. Gamble, Fl. Pres. Mad. 2: 861. 1923; Gravely and Mayuranathan in Bull. Madr. Govt. Mus. n.s. N.H. 4(1): 13. 1931; S.R. Srinivasan in Henry *et al.* Fl. Tamil Nadu Analy. 2: 82. 1987; Sharma *et al.* Fl. Karnataka 165. 1984; Gilbert in Bradleya 8: 16.1990; Hanumanthappa in Pullaiah and Ali Moulali Fl.Andhra Pradesh 2: 584. 1997; Jagtap and Singh, Fasc. Fl. India 24: 209. 1999. *Stapelia umbellata* (Haw.) Roxb., Pl. Coast Corom. 3: 36. t. 241. 1819. *Desmidorchis umbellata* (Haw.) Decne in Sc. Mat. 9: 266. 1838. *Caralluma campanulata* (Wight) N. E. Br. in Gard. Chron. 12: 369. 1892; Gamble, Fl. Pres. Madras 2: 861. 1923. *Boucerosia campanulata* Wight. Icon. Pl. Ind. Orient. 4.2:1. 1848. Type: Tab.1287 in protologue based on plant from India, locality not known.

Stem fleshy, branched; branches erect, 60 cm tall, acute angled, not tapering, quadrangular. Leaves reduced, opposite decussate, sessile, deltoid, glabrous, leaf scars spine-like. Flowers terminal, many flowers in umbellate cymes, bracts ca 2–8 mm long, linear; pedicels terete, 1–2 cm long. Calyx 5-lobed, divided up to base, lobes linear, 5 mm long, apex acute, margin minutely hairy, glandular within, glabrous. Corolla campanulate, ca 1.5 cm long, lobes 5, apex acute, purplish transverse bands, velvety within, glabrous. Corona staminal, biseriate; outer 5-lobed, dark-purple, truncate, ca 9 mm across; inner 5-lobed, apex acute. Stamens 5, short, ca 1.6 mm long; pollinia 5, pollen masses solitary in each anther cell, yellow, waxy. Gynostegium ca 2.6 mm long. Follicles paired, 12-16 cm long, linear-lanceolate, tapering towards apex with blunt tip, glabrous. Seeds 4-8 mm, ovoid; coma 2.5 cm long (Plate 6.8; Figures 6.10 and 6.11).

Distribution: INDIA (Andhra Pradesh, Bihar, Karnataka, Kerala, Maharashtra, Orissa, Tamil Nadu)

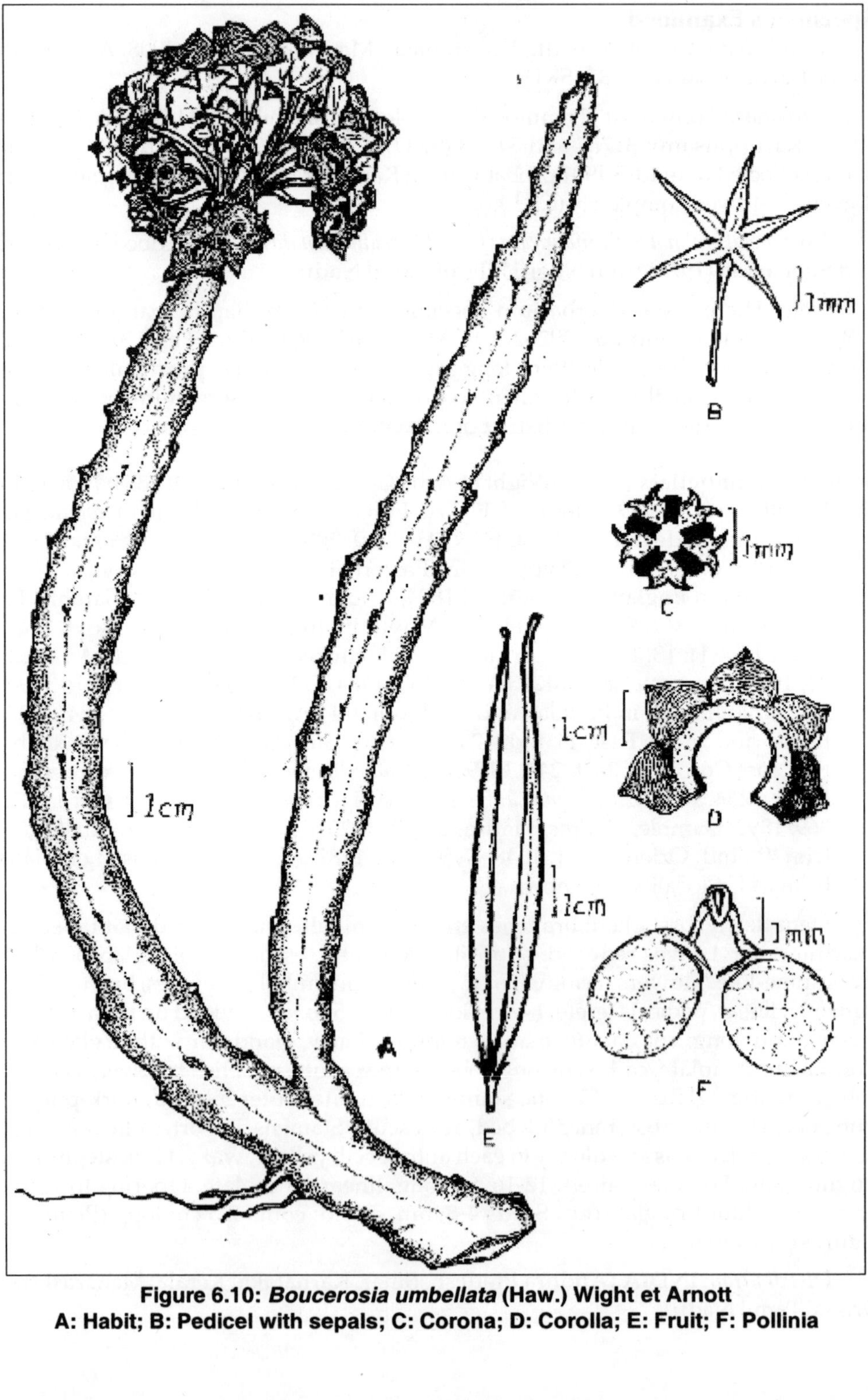

Figure 6.10: ***Boucerosia umbellata*** **(Haw.) Wight et Arnott**
A: Habit; B: Pedicel with sepals; C: Corona; D: Corolla; E: Fruit; F: Pollinia

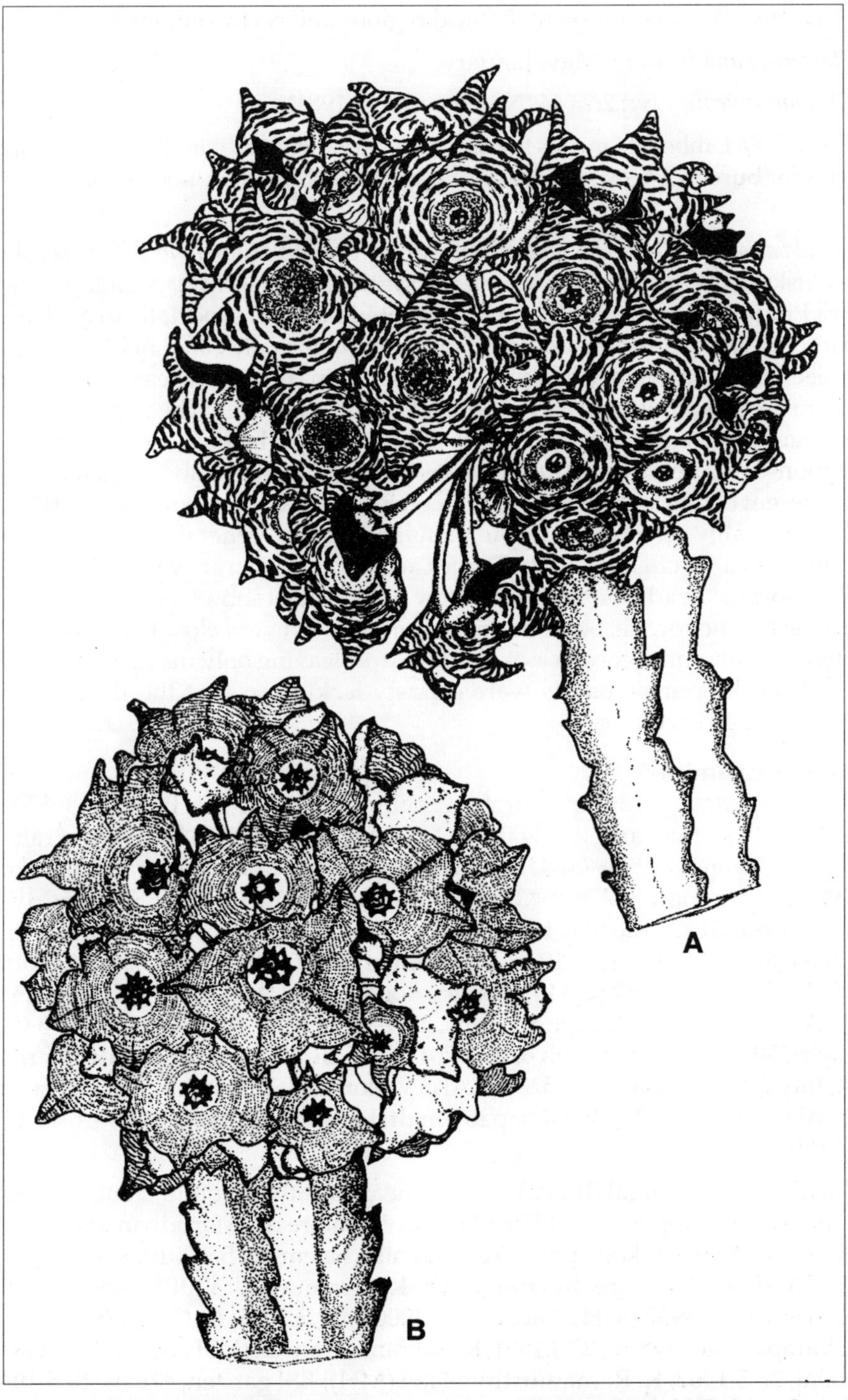

Figure 6.11: Floral Variations in *Boucerosia umbellata* (Haw.) Wight et Arnott
A: Striated flowers; B: Non-striated flowers

Abundance: Very common in dry arid regions and rocky regions.

Flowering and fruiting: May–January.

Chromosome number: 2n= 44 (Navaneetham, 1981).

Etymology: Umbellate means floral pedicels arise from the single point. The specific epithet is for bunch of flowers arise on the apical portion of the succulent stem of this plant.

Floral variations: During a recent field survey carried out *B. umbellata* was collected on the outskirts of the town Penukonda, beside the NH 7 highway Anantapur district, Andhra Pradesh. They occur in narrow isolated habitats especially in arid areas of scrub forests, rocky foot hills and dry lands among the cultivated fields. As a part of the project, frequent field visits were conducted in different areas during various seasons to observe flowering and fruiting nature of the genus. The populations show marked variations regarding the colour, striations and the hairs on the corolla. Previous publications have described *B. umbellata* as having purplish glabrous petals whereas three different colour patterns were noticed in the specimens collected in the above mentioned locality. Most of the populations showed the general characters - Corolla campanulate, ca 1.5 cm long, lobes-5, apex acute, purplish transverse bands, velvety within, glabrous. In addition to these a few populations showed different character with respect to the corolla. Some of the flowers showed very close bands of purple to the extent that the entire corolla looks deep purple leaving only the tip of the petals. In a few others the purple bands were entirely lacking so that the flowers appear yellowish orange in colour.

Specimens Examined

Andhra Pradesh: Anantapur dt, Batrepalli R.F. 17.10.1982, T. Pullaiah 852 (MH and SKU); Kalasamudram, 19.7.2008, A. Ugraiah 31749 (SKU); Kalasamudram R.F., 2.5.1986, E. Chennaiah 2948 (SKU), Cherukur, between Madakasira and Penukonda, 28.1.2009, A. Ugraiah 31778 (SKU); Nityapujakona, 23.10.1993, SRS Reddy 8739 (SKU); Chittoor dt, On the way to Japali from Tirupathi, 450 m, 26.6.1969, G.V. Subba Rao 32036 (MH); Nigidi, 18.3.1917, J.S. Gamble 14752 (MH); Palamaner,2200ft, 6-5-1923, C. E. C. Fischer 4789 (CAL); Horsley konda, 4000 ft, 26-5-1918, C. E. C. Fischer 4375 (CAL); Nellore dt., Veligonda hills, 28-7-1914, M. S. Ramaswami 1353 (CAL), Udayagiri, 30-7-1957, S.K.Wagh 6700, 6701, 6725 (BLAT); Cuddapah dt, Soambally, 2000 ft, July 1884, J. S. Gamble 15201 (CAL), Vekurkota, 2000 ft, July 1884, J.S. Gamble 15202 (MH, CAL and DD); Visakhapatnam dt, Lakshmipuram, 1.6.1900, C.A. Barber 1754 (MH).

Tamil Nadu: Dindigal dt., Palani hills, near Varathamanathi Dam, 9.5.2008, A. Ugraiah and S. Karuppusamy 31729 (SKU); Coimbatore dt., Marudhamalai, 21.5.1981, T. Pullaiah, 3 (SKU); Pakkoda point, Yercaud hills, Salem dt., 5.3.2010, S.Karuppusamy 24173 (Madura College herbarium); Kudirimalai, 3200ft, 29.7.1930, V. Narayanaswamy, 3937 (MH); Girmalam, 3000ft, 19.3.1931, K. C. Jacob, 433 and 434 (MH); Varapalayam, 666 m, 27.4.1951, K. Subramanyam 22 (MH and CAL); Nellimalai R.F, 400m, 26.5.1962, K. Ramamurthy 14135 (MH); BSI garden, 476 m, 19.5.1964, E. Vajravelu 17599 (MH); Anikatty, 785m, 17.3.1970, M.V. Viswanathan, 472 (MH);

Thekkumalai, 666 m, 2.4.1960, C. Gajapathy 9988 (MH); Adakkam, Pulnerp, 22.7.1897, J.S. Gamble *s.n.* (MH); Kalapatti-Attamalai slopes, Coimbatore, C. E. C. Fischer 296796 (CAL); Tholanpalaiyur-Coimbatore, 1600 ft, 24-4-1910, C. E. C. Fischer 1859 (CAL); Talamalai, 3000ft, 23-4-1906, C. E. C. Fischer 143 (CAL); North Arcot dt., Tippuradu R.F, 165 m, 28.6.1963, K. Ramamurthy 16603 (MH), 16603 (CAL); Nilgiri dt., Towards Ebanad, 950m, 16.3.1972, 40261 (MH), From Anaikatty towards Ebanad, 900 m, 23.11.1970, G.V. Subba rao, 37326 (MH); Salem dt., Hogainakal forest, 275 m, 12.7.1964, 20577 (MH), Channel near the road Hogainakal, 260m, 15.3.1965, E. Vajravelu, 23567 (MH); Pagoda point-Yecaud, ±1360 m, 5.5.1965, S. Karthikeyan 26826 (MH); Pachaimalai, Narippadi to Kumbakkal, 400 m, 27-7-1978, K. M. Mathew and N. Venugopal 15629 (CAL); Changalpattu dt., Kottakuppam near Athimangeripet, Pallipat (Tal), 60m, 20.4.1984, D. Narasimhan 472 (MH); Kanyakumari dt., Purathimalai, Kulasekaram range, ±200 m, 27.1.1978, A.N. Henry 53319 (MH and CAL); Dharmapuri dt., Thirthamalai, Vadakathikadu or Allizone, 360m, 18.6.1978, K.M. Mathew and N. Venugopal 14213 (MH); Hogainakkal and Vembanoormalai, K. M. Mathew and N. Venugopal 23074 (CAL); Madurai dt., Murugamalai, 333m, 20.9.1961, K.M. Sebastine 12993 (MH and CAL); lower Pulney, 1600 ft, Re. Rodriguez, K. M. Sebastine 1940 (CAL); South Arcot dt., Gingee R.F. 125m, 23.3.1961, K.M. Sebastine 12374 (MH); 3.3.1905, J.S. Gamble 753 (MH); Shanikulam, 11.9.1899, C.A. Barber 887 (MH); Krishnagiri jungle, 21.8.1930, V. Narayanaswamy 4089(MH); Pudukottai dt., Narthamalai forest, 125m, 25.6.1984, C. Arulappan 19 (MH); Madras dt., Chengan Javadis, 3400ft, May 1941, M. S. Raghavan 89075 and 76 (DD).

Orissa: Ganjam dt., Mohini hills, 1000ft, March 1884, J.S. Gamble, 13929 (MH); Similipal dt., Sitakund, Bahali and Agrawala 744 (CAL).

Kerala: Palghat dt, Walayer forest, 225m, 10.7.1963, J. Joseph 17052 (MH); Travancore dt., Travancore, J. S. Gamble 32877 (MH),

Karnataka: Tumkur dt., Pavagada taluk, Bhupoor, 24.2.2008, A. Ugraiah 31703 (SKU), Pavagada foot hills,18.6.2008, A. Ugraiah 31741 (SKU), Hirehalli hills, 29.11.2008, S. Karuppusamy and A. Ugraiah 31766 (SKU); Chitradurg dt., Lokadalal, 1.12.2008, A. Ugraiah 31771 (SKU), Chitradurg fort, 16.6.2008, A. Ugraiah 31740 and 31745 (SKU); Mysore dt., Maddur road, Bhimanbiri, 3.3.1905, C.A. Barber 6829 (MH); Chamundi hills, 975m, 12.3.1964, K.M. Sebastine 18737 (MH); road side Gundlapet, 675m, 27.4.1965, B.D. Naithani 23942 (MH); Maddur Road, 32870 (MH), Chamundi hills, J. S. Gamble 35660 (MH); Gundlapet, B. D. Naithani 46093 (MH), Mysore, Foot of Joti betta, 27-4-1962, R. V. Kammathy 80403 (CAL), Foot of Joti betta, A. S. Rao 80403 (BSI); Channarayapatnam-Holenarsipur road, 3-5-1971, C. Saldanha and T. P. Ramamurthy 1619 (CAL); Halebid, 3000ft, Oct 1908, A. Meebold 9412 (CAL); Shimoga dt., Shimoga, 3000ft, Oct 1908 A. Meebold 9413 (CAL); Bangalore dt, Doddabalapur, S. R. Ramesh 664 (CAL); Mandya dt., Adichenchanagiri, K. P. Sreeneth and K. R. Keshavamurthy 5037 (CAL); Kolar dt., Chickbalapur, Nandi-R.F, N. P. Singh 146925 (BSI).

Maharashtra: Ganeshkund Botanical Garden, 21-5-1908, P. Parayape 296814 (CAL).

Caralluma R. Brown in Mem. Wern. Soc.,i. 14. 1811.

= *Saurolluma* Plowes, Haseltonia 3: 54. 1995.

= *Somalluma* Plowes, Haseltonia 3: 57. 1995.

= *Spathulopetalum* Chiov., Ann.Bot. (Rome) 10: 392. 1912.

Type: *Stapelia adscendens* Roxburgh

Strongly succulent, perennial, branched, non-rhizomatous; stem-tips tapering, non-deciduous; branching epicutaneous. Leaves lanceolate, semi-persistent; stipular hairs tufted, glandilose. Flowers solitary or in pairs at the upper nodes. Sepals acute. Corolla broadly campanulate; lobes 5, narrow, valvate, usually brownish-purple with wibratile fusiform cilia. Corolla tube short, campanulate, apical half of corolla lobes replicate. Column very short; anthers short, retuse, incumbent on or confluent with stigma, tips inappendiculate: pollen-masses one in each cell, short, erect one margin pellucid. Gynostegium sessile or subsessile; corpuscular flange winged, ellipsoidal. Follicle pairs erect, v-shaped, slender, smooth, terete. Seeds comose.

Distribution: Southern tip of India, but two species extended via Arabia to Senegal and one variety occurs in NW Myanamar (Burma).

Key to the Species of Genus *Caralluma* (*sensu stricto*)

1. Corolla always dark-purplish throughout; hairs strongly spindle or club shaped, confined to margin of petals .... *C. stalagmifera*
1. Corolla with transverse striations, tip purplish or yellowish; hairs with or without 2
2. Flowers pendulous; corolla with long needle-shaped hairs along the margin or without 5
2. Flowers non-pendulous; corolla rotate 3
3. Stem grows above 50 cm tall, apically groved .... *C. moorei*
3. Stem grows less than 50 cm tall, not groved 4
4. Hairs only on distal half on margin of petals; corolla pale green .... *C. bhupinderiana*
4. Hairs without; corolla yellow green with darker-purplish transverse bands .... *C. sarkariae*
5. Angles of the branches round or acute; corolla with marginal hairs only .... *C. adscendens*
5. Angles of the branches sharply acute; corolla with geniculate hairs on the surface .... *C. geniculata*

Caralluma adscendens (Roxb.) R.Br. in Mem. Wern. Soc. 1: 14.1810.

Gravely and Mayuranathan (1931) classified this species into six varieties based on their stem and flower characters. The distribution of these varieties occupied different degree of frequency in Peninsular India. But most dominant and older varieties are var. *attenuata* and var. *fimbriata*, other varieties are evolved from degree of reduction in hairiness of flower and roundness of stem.

1. Key to the Varieties of *Caralluma adscendens* Based on Stem and Floral Morphology

1. Corolla-lobes hairy 2
1. Corolla-lobes glabrous .... var. *adscendens*
2. Stems rounded towards the base 3
2. Stems acute towards the base 5
3. Distal portion of the stem attenuate; 25–50 cm high .... var. *attenuata*
3. Distal portion of the stem not attenuate; 12–20 cm high 4
4. Flowers large, deep purple hairs along the margin; pedicel pendulous .... var. *fimbriata*
4. Flowers small, greenish purple; hairs not developed; pedicel erect .... var. *gracilis*
5. Pedicel semipendent; hairs on corolla completely absent; stems stout and not immediately attenuate .... var. *bicolor*
5. Pedicel never bent; hairs strongly developed; stems obviously attenuate .... var. *carinata*

2. Key to the Varieties of *C. adscendens* Based on Corolla Epidermal Morphology

1. Corolla epidermal cells homogeneous 2
1. Corolla epidermal cells heterogeneous 3
2. Epidermal cells with distinct apiculate or papillate growth on the top 4
2. Epidermal cells without apiculate process on the surface .... var. *fimbriata*
3. Papillary growth sharply mucronate, cells intermingled with long hairs .... var. *gracilis*
3. Papillary growth with blunt tip, cells without intermingled hairs 5
4. Apiculate process distinctly bottle-neck shaped .... var. *attenuata*
4. Apiculate process simply elongate, not constricted below the papilla .... var. *adscendens*
5. Papilla uniformly elongated, cells hexagonal .... var. *carinata*
5. Papilla differently elongated, cells polygonal .... var. *bicolor*

Caralluma adscendens (Roxb.) R. Brown in Mem. Wern. Soc. 1: 14.1810; Hooker f. Fl.Brit. India 4: 76. 1883; Gamble Fl. Pres. Madras 2: 861. 1923; Plowes in

Haseltonia 3: 52. 1995; Jagtap and Singh in Fasc. Fl. India 24: 193. 1999; Meve et Leide in Plant Syst. Evol. 234: 196. 2002. var. **adscendens**; Gravely et Mayuranathan in Bull. Madr. Govt. Mus. n.s. N.H. 4(1): 13. 1931; S.R. Srinivasan in A.N. Henry *et al.* Fl. Tamil Nadu Anal.2: 81.1987; Hanumanthappa in Pullaiah and Ali Moulali Fl. Andhra Pradesh 2: 583.1997. *Stapelia adscendens* Roxb. Pl. Coast Corom. 1: 28-29. 1795. Type: tab. 30 of protologue.

Stems fleshy, up to 1 m tall, quadrangular; internodes four-angled, 6–18 mm long and 2–6 mm across, slender above, glabrous. Latex watery. Leaves present only on young branches, reduced to scales, opposite, decussate, sessile, 1–2 mm long, subulate, tip acute, glabrous. Flowers terminal or subterminal, solitary or paired, axillary; pedicel terete, 3–5 mm long and ca 1 mm in diam., brown, glabrous. Calyx 5-lobed, divided up to base, lobes ca 2.5 x 1 mm, ovate, apex acuminate, margin thin, glabrous. Corolla campanulate, ca 8 mm long; corolla tube ca 1.5 mm long; lobes 5, 6–7 x 2.5 mm, lanceolate-oblong, apex apiculate, hairy or glabrous. Corona staminal, biseriate; outer annular, with two filiform filaments, ca 1.5 mm long, alternating with anther-lobes, glabrous; inner 5-lobed, flap-like, overlapping anther-lobes, ca 1 x 0.4 mm long, apex truncate or crenate. Stamens 5, ca 1.6 mm long; pollinia 5, pollen masses solitary in each anther cell, yellow, waxy, caudicles light brown, corpuscle dark brown. Follicles usually solitary, 5.5 × 2.3 cm long and 3.5–4.5 mm in diam., cylindrical, peaked with curved tip, base acute, glabrous; seeds many, ca 9.5 × 4.5 mm, oblong to obovate, base rounded, dark brown with light brown margin ca 1 mm wide; coma silky white, 2–3 mm long (Plate 6.9, Figure 6.12).

Distribution: Tamil Nadu, Karnataka, Andhra Pradesh, Maharashtra and Orissa.

Abundance: Discontinuous population in Peninsular India. Endemic.

Flowering and fruiting: Throughout the year.

Chromosome number: 2n = 22.

Etymology: From the Greek 'adscendens' means flowering branches upright or rising up. The variety is growing upright succulent stems with narrow flowering branches.

Specimens Examined

Andhra Pradesh: Medak dt., Pocharam tank,12.11.1992, T. Pullaiah and C. Prabhakar, 12048 (SKU); Medak tank, 25.8.1992, C. Prabhakar and B. Raviprasad Rao 11795 (SKU); Mahaboobnagar dt., Molachintapally forest, 25.1.1995, T. Dharmachandra Kumar,15320 (SKU); Kurnool dt., Kambagirikunta, 15.3.2000, S. Sunitha and A. Madhu 25867 (SKU); Sivapuram, 20.7.1994, Saiprasad Gowd 12954 (SKU); Cuddapah dt., Palakonda hills, 10.11.1988, C. Subbarayudu, 8203, (SKU); Gunjana River bed, J. L. Ellis, 29797 (MH), 14982 (CAL); Guntur dt., Vijayapuri south, 25.7.1988, V. Ramakrishnaiah 6826 (SKU); Srikakulam dt., Raivada R.F, 200 m, 13.5.1979, G. V. Subba Rao, 62398 (MH); Vishakapatnam dt, near Palagedda, 375 m, 11.10.1972, G.V. Subba Rao, 42543 (MH); West Godavari dt., Polavaram near Itikala kota, 21.9.1962, D. C. S. Raju 432 (CAL), 15 (CAL); Guntur dt., Nagarjunakonda valley, 17.7.1961, K. Thothathri 1937 (CAL).

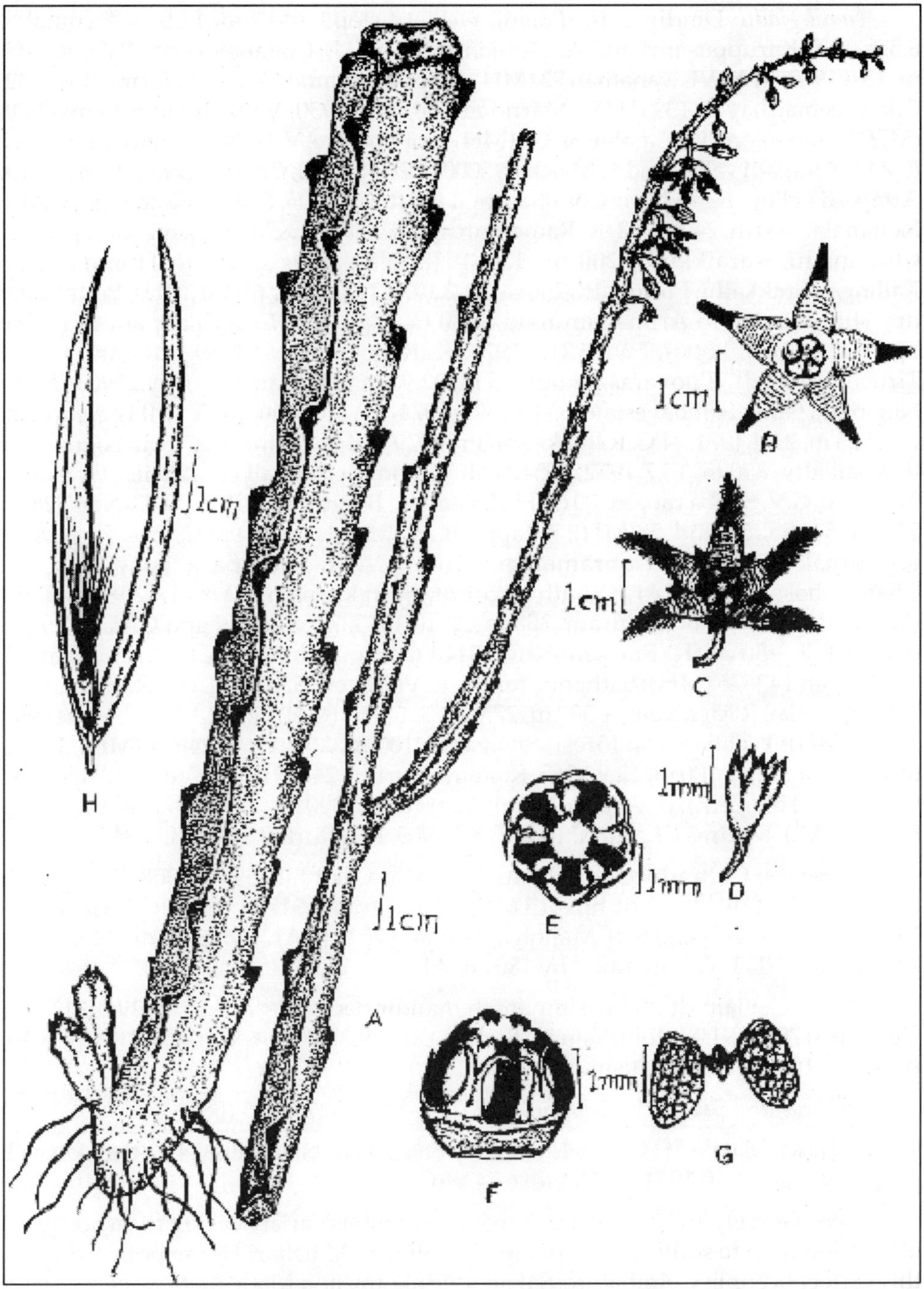

Figure 6.12. ***Caralluma adscendens*** **var.** ***adscendens***
A: Habit; B, C: Flowers; D: Sepals; E: Corona; F: Side view of corona; G: Pollinia; H: Fruit

Tamil Nadu: Dindigal dt., Palani, western slope and foot hills of Sirumalai, 8.5.2008, S. Karuppusamy and A. Ugraiah 31725 (SKU); Coimbatore dt., Palamai, 495 m, 13.8.1969, M.V. Viswanathan 72 (MH); Slope of Anamoolamalai, 650 m, 31.8.1962, C.P. Sreemadhavan 139 (MH); Marudamalai, 24.6.1930, V. Narayanaswamy 3238 (MH); Coimbatore, J.S.Gamble 32851 (MH); Coimbatore, V. N. Narayanaswamy 1017 (CAL); Attapadi valley and S. Malabar, 2000 ft, 26.10.1910, C.E.C. Fischer 2360 (CAL); Attapadi valley, Agali Near Coimbatore, 1400 ft, 2.7.1905, C.E. C. Fischer 50 (CAL); Nellimalai, 400 m, 24.8.1962, K. Ramamurthy 14803 (CAL&MH); Ramanathapur dt., Chettinadu, Karaikkudi, 200 m, 1.12.1977, N.C. Nair 53019 (MH and CAL); Kallingalparakkadu, Pudupatti, 250 m, 21.2.1979, N.C. Nair 61050 (MH); Pudukottai dt., Thirumayam to Arimanam road, ± 80 m, 14.7.1984, C. Arulappam 43 (MH); Kiranur to Pudukottai, 50 m, 21.9.1977, K. Ramamurthy 51359 (MH and CAL); Tiruchirapalli dt., Poovarasankudi, 75 m, 22.9.1965, K. Ramamurthy 25903 (MH); Nilgiri dt., Parali-Sambar estate, 650 m, 30.6.1974, E. Vajravelu, 15057 (MH); Avarihalli R.F, 925 m, 21.4.1971, N.C. Rathakrishnan 38029 (MH); On the way from Segur river to Anaikatty, 850 m, 15.7.1972, 40542 (MH); from Kedar halla to Anaikatty, 800 m, 22.8.1970, G.V. Subba rao, 36200 (MH); Salem dt., Bargur, 19.8.1918, N. C. Nair 32856, 52, 53, 54, 55, 57 and 58(MH); Edappadi, K. M. Mathew 19832, 296777 (CAL); Kamuthakudi, V. Balasubramaniam 2102 (CAL); Poomparai to Vilpati, M. Chandrabose 51362 (CAL); South Arcot dt, Marakkanam, 10 m, 17.2.1979, 60281 (MH and CAL), Sankarapuram, 300 m, 23.10.1983, 79681 (MH and CAL), Kurum barum R.F, ±50 m, K. Ramamurthy 90440 (MH); Tirumayam to Arimanam, C. Aralappan 143676 (MH); Sathanur forest, E. Vajravelu 52072 (CAL); Ramanad dt., Sanjeevimalai, Rajapalyam, ± 300 m, 27.9.1971, 38757 (MH), 26.12.1971, E. Vajravelu, 39550 (MH); Kalaiyer koil forest, Sivaganga,100 m, 20.8.1964, 24694 (MH), Ebani forest- Sivaganga, 100 m, 12.9.1965, K. Ramamurthy, 24694 (MH); Vellimalai R.F, N. C. Nair, 57414 (CAL); N. Arcot dt., Salbanur forest, 200 m, 25.11.1977, E. Vajravelu 52072 (CAL); Madras dt., Parlakinderi, 5.5.1909, I.H. Burkill 31862 (ISIM).

Karnataka: Chitradurga dt., Halumalleswara foot hills, 14.6.2008, A. Ugraiah 31735 (SKU); Lokadal foot hills,15.6.2008, A.Ugraiah,31738 (SKU); S. Melavalli-Kollegal, R. Ramesh and S. B. Manohar 3808 and 7532 (CAL); Mysore dt., Nagapuri, 790 m, 7.6.1971, T. P. Ramamurthy 1801 (CAL).

Orissa: Ganjam dt., Nhrusimhanath mandir back side, Sukinda, 29.8.2008, A. Ugraiah 31754 (SKU); Mohrikaluva, Berhampur, 29.8.2008, A. Ugraiah 31755 (SKU); Berkuda, 10.8.1919, N. Annandale 1233 (CAL).

Maharashtra: Satara dt., Bomnoli, I. D. Deshpande,166695 (BSI)

Sri Lanka: Matale dt., Ca 8 miles directly ESE of Damballa, hills above the Mahaveli project anicut, 11.10.1974, G. Davidse 7426 (CAL).

Notes: Gravely and Mayuranathan noted that this variety occurs from northeast of the Godavari to south end of Attapady valley of Malabar. Dense populations of this variety occur in Coimbatore, Salem, Pudukottai and Madurai districts of Tamil Nadu. In present study specimens were collected from Madurai and Pudukottai districts of Tamil Nadu, but a few populations have been observed in Nagamalai hills near Madurai, where they have flowers with short hairs on the margins of the petals and are prominently striped purple on the inner side of basal part. In the same district some populations do not have these hairs, and petals are glabrous with a greenish yellow background. All of these populations grow close to cultivated land and exposed dry scrub forests of the foothills. In dry areas they grow about 75 cm tall, but in fertile areas it can reach a height of 1 m.

Caralluma adscendens (Roxb.) R. Brown var. **attenuata** (Wight) Gravely et Mayuranathan in Bull. Madr. Govt. Mus. n.s. N.H. 4(1): 13. 1931; S.R. Srinivasan in A.N. Henry *et al.* Fl. Tamil Nadu Anal.2: 81. 1987; Gilbert in Bradleya 8: 11.1990; Plowes in Haseltonia 3: 52. 1995; Hanumanthappa in Pullaiah and Ali Moulali Fl. Andhra Pradesh 2: 583. 1997; Jagtap and Singh in Fasc. Fl. India 24: 194. 1999; Meve and Leide in Plant Syst. Evol. 234: 200. 2002. *Caralluma attenuata* Wight, Ic. Pl. Ind. Orient.4(1): 15. t. 1268. 1848. Type: tab. 1268 of protologue based on material from India; Hooker f. Fl. Brit. India 4: 76.1883; Gamble Fl. Pres. Madras 2: 861.1923.

Stems bushy growth, 75 cm tall, strongly attenuate, usually much branched distally, angles streaked reddish, rounded. Flowers hairy, pendulous, dark purple (Plate 6.10, Figure 6.13)

Distribution: Tamil Nadu, Karnataka, Andhra Pradesh, Maharashtra and Orissa.

Abundance: Common, distributed all over the Deccan Peninsula.

Flowering and fruiting: Throughout the year.

Chromosome number: 2n = 44 (Navaneetham, 1980, 1981).

Etymology: From the Greek 'attenuata' means thin or weak; the variety of the plant is having thin or weak stem apices.

Specimens Examined

Andhra Pradesh: Anantapur dt., Anantapur, T. Pullaiah,116995 (MH); Muchukota R.F, 300 m, 26.5.1981, T. Pullaiah and N. Yesoda 214 (SKU and MH); Chintakunta, 250 m, 9.10.1981, T. Pullaiah 462 (SKU and MH); Kalasamudram R.F, 13.10.1984, T. Pullaiah and E. Chennaiah 2823 (SKU); Kalasamudram, 19.7.2008, A. Ugraiah 31748 (SKU), Muchukotakanam, Tadipatri, 8.9.2008, A. Ugraiah 31756 (SKU), Between Kondapuram and Yarraguntapalli, 8.9.2008, A. Ugraiah 31758 (SKU), Mavatur road side towards Madakasira, 28.1.2009, A. Ugraiah 31777 (SKU); hills opposite, Gooty Rly station, 23.4.2008, S. Karuppusamy and A. Ugraiah 31711 (SKU); Kadiri, 2000 ft, 1884, J.S.Gamble 15204 (MH and CAL); Penakacherla 700 ft, 1889, J. S. Gamble, 21241 (MH); Kurnool dt., K. M. C. Campus,17.5.1984, Ameer Ahammad 2823 (SKU); Gulemullabad R.F, 30.5.1983, R. R. V. Raju 1452 (SKU); Gani R.F. 5.5.1984, R. R. V. Raju, 3113 (SKU); Kurnool, J. S. Gamble,16888 (BSI); Guntur dt., Guntur, K. M. Sebastine,32864 (MH); Nizamabad dt., Patharajampet, 9.3.1990, B.R.P. Rao 9702 (SKU); Ditchpally, 14.8.1988, B. R.P. Rao 6438 (SKU); Rangareddy dt., Kusuma samudram, 28.6.1990, M. Silar Mohammad, 10362 (SKU); Ramagundam, M. Silar Mohammad, 10317 (SKU); Cuddapah dt., On the way to Duggamakonda, Lankamalai R. F, 800m, 21.8.1958, K. Subramanyam, 6332 (MH) and (CAL); Palakonda hills, 10.2.1989, C. Subbarayudu 5548 (SKU); Nellore dt., Atmakur, 21.9.1937, K.C. Jacob, 380 (MH).

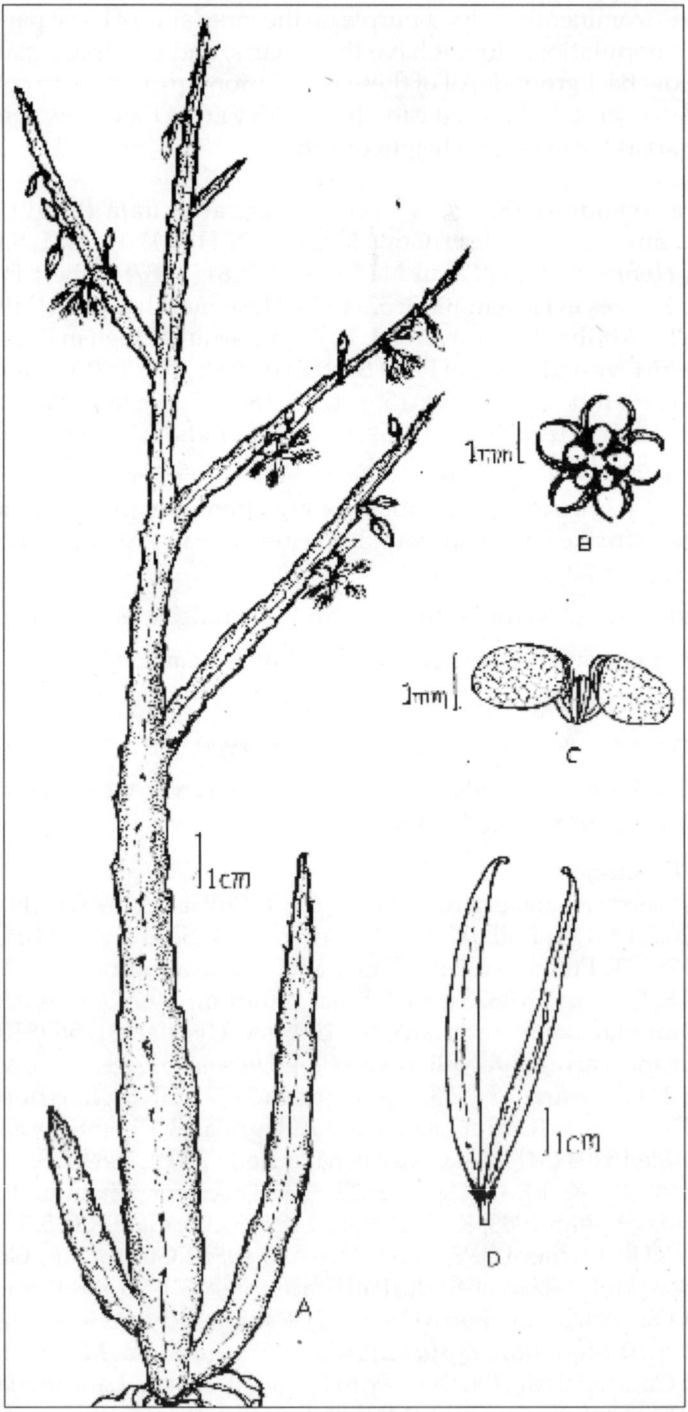

Figure 6.13: ***Caralluma adscendens*** **var.** ***attenuata*** **(Wight) Gravely et Mayuranathan A: Habit; B: Corona; C: Pollinia; D: Fruit**

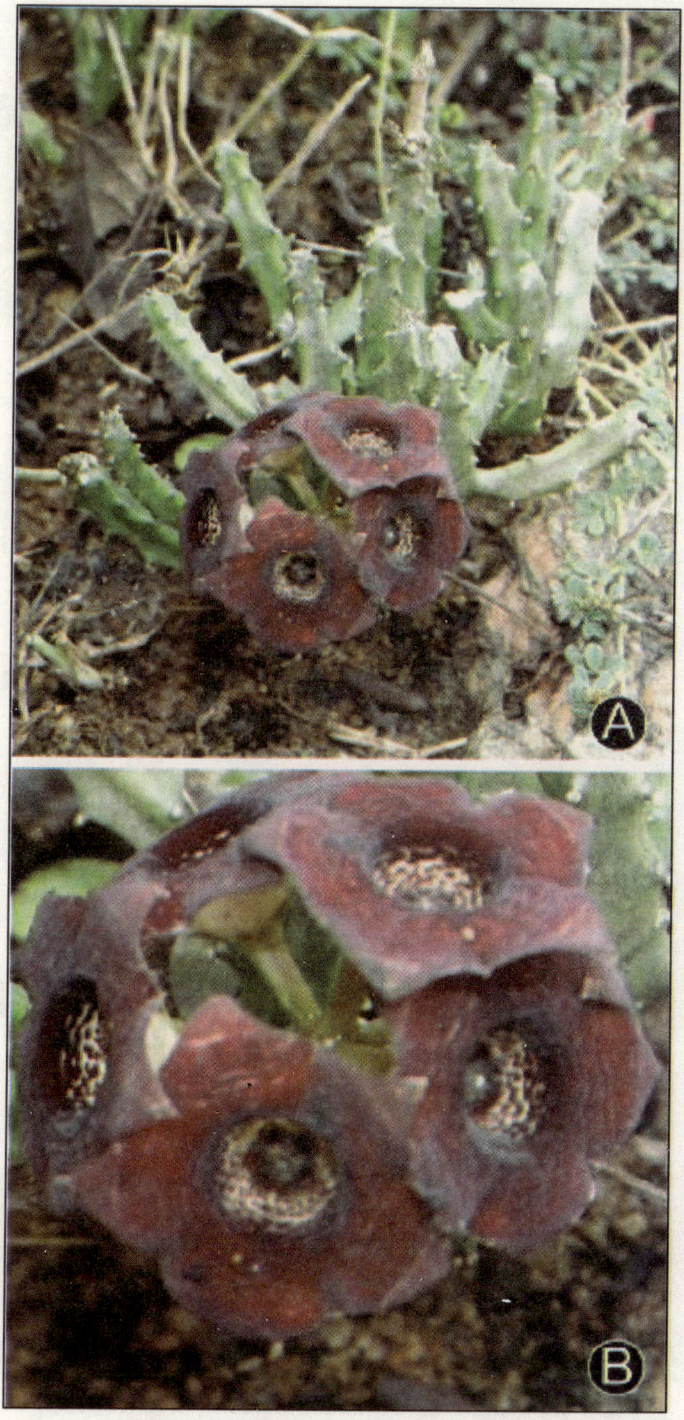

Plate 6.7. ***Boucerosia truncato-coronata*** **Sedgewick**
A: Natural habitat; B: Inflorescence

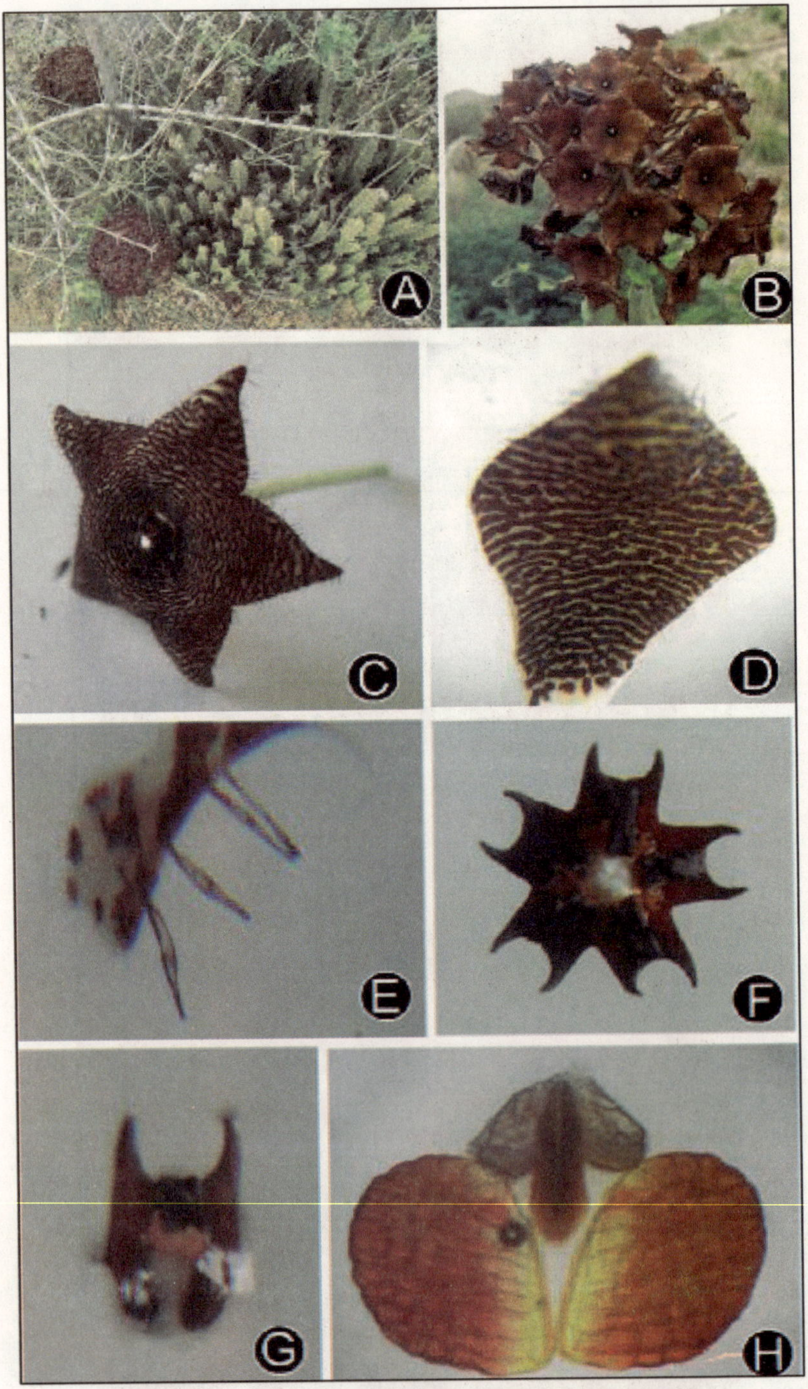

Plate 6.8. ***Boucerosia umbellata*** **(Haw.) Wight et Arn. A: Natural habitat; B: Inflorescence; C: Flower; D: Petal; E: Hairs; F: Corona; G: Outer corona; H: Pollinia.**

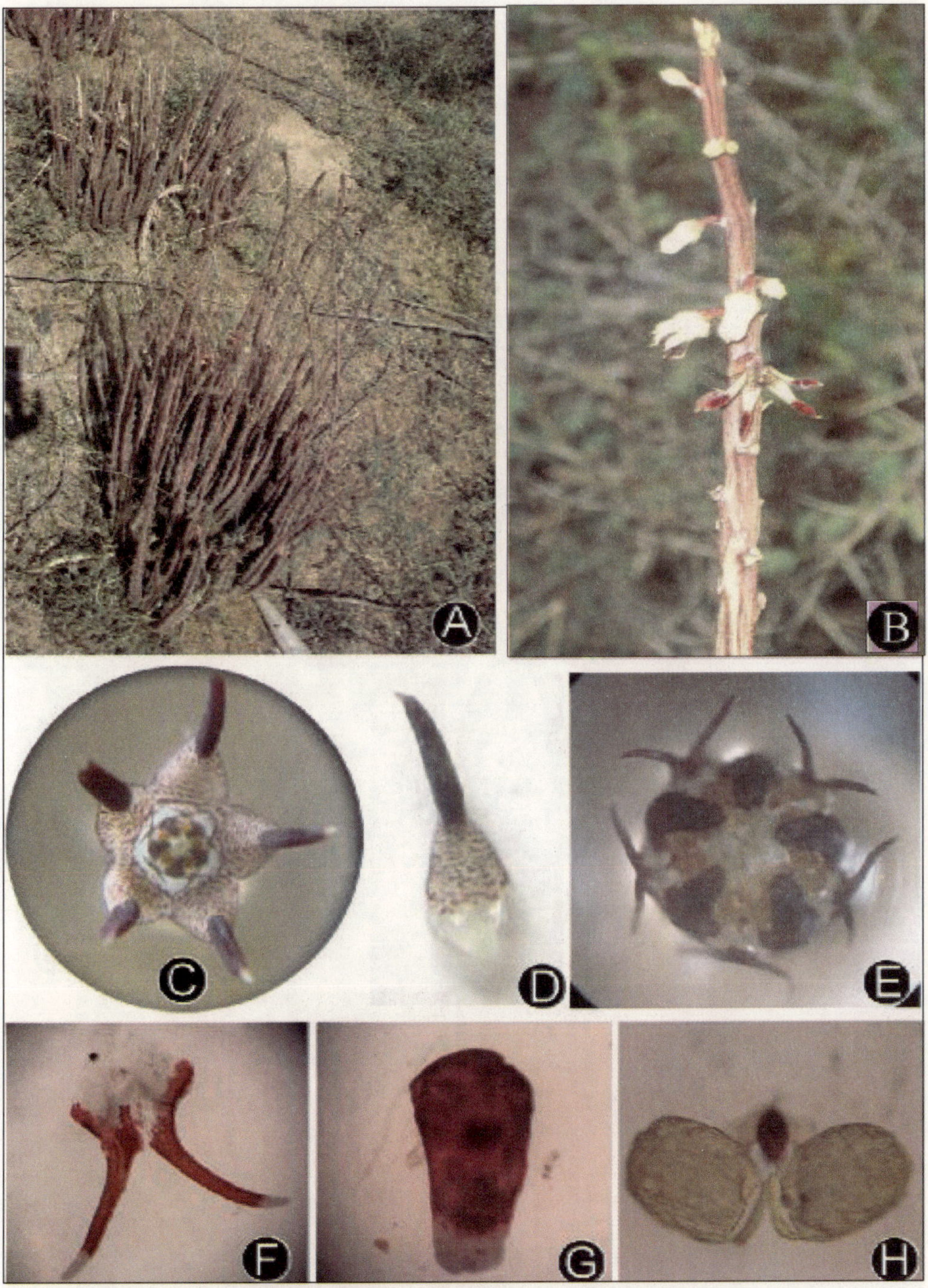

Plate 6.9. *Caralluma adscendens* (Roxb.) R.Br. var. *adscendens*
A: Natural habitat; B: Inflorescence; C: Flower; D: Petal; E: corona; F: Outer corona; G: Inner corona; H: Pollinia.

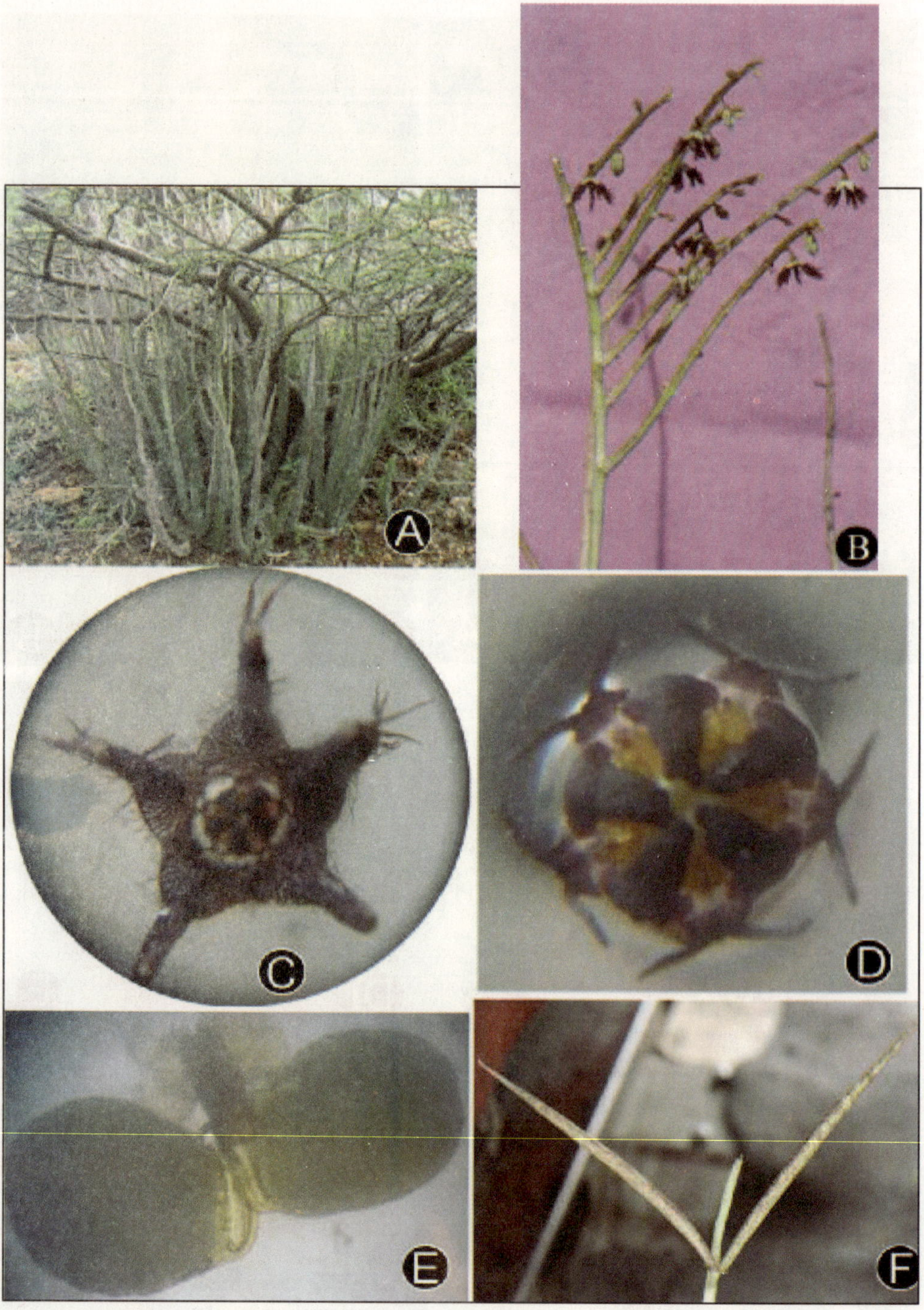

Plate 6.10. ***Caralluma adscendens*** **(Roxb.) R.Br. var.** ***attenuata*** **(Wight) Gravely et Mayuranathan**

A: Natural habitat; B: Inflorescence; C: Flower; D: Corona; E: Pollinia; F: Fruit.

Chittoor dt., Satyavedu to Ambakam, 125 m, 3.10.1974, M. Chandrabose, 45226 (MH); Panapakam-N.E of forest rest house, 375 m, 15.6.1062, 31857 (MH); on way to Amudalakona, 425 m, 27.9.1974, G.V. Subba Rao, 45833 (MH); Karimnagar dt., on the way from Kodimial, 400 m 19.7.1964, G. V. Subba Rao, 20148 (MH). Vishakhapatnam dt., Circuit house, 30 m, 4.10.1964, 21444 (MH); near Palagadda, 375 m, 11.10.1972, G.V. Subba rao, 42543 (MH); Godavari circars, G. V. S. Rao 296785 (CAL); Medak dt., ICRISAT site, 600 m, 28.5.1979, L. J. G. Van der Maesen 3793 (CAL); Hyderabad dt., Jubilee hills, 6500 ft, 26.6.1978, L. J. G. Van der Maesen 3205 (CAL); Srikakulam dt, Raivada R.F, 200 m, 13.5.1979, G. V. Subba rao, 62398 (CAL); Godavari dt., Rampachodavaram, 250 m, 20.8.1995, M. Mohan, 105069 (MH); Prakasam dt., Nandavanam hills, Velugundla R.F, 18.7.1984, R.K.Mohan 439 (CAL).

Tamil Nadu: Coimbatore dt., Madukarai-$CaCO_3$ mining area, 10.5.2008, S. Karuppusamy and A.Ugraiah 31731(SKU); Kuridimalai, Madukarai, 10.5.2008, S. Karuppusamy and A.Ugraiah 31732 (SKU); Marudhamalai, 21.5.1981, T. Pullaiah 2 (SKU); Hushia hills, J.S. Gamble 32863 (MH); Simasamudram, Kollegal, 18.2.1930, 20063 (MH); Mettur, 19.8.1929, V.Narayanaswamy 19049 (MH); Chinnathadagam (Thekkumalai), 653 m, 9.7.1956, 205 (MH and CAL), Aliyar submergible area, 350 m, 28.7.1962, K.M. Sebastine 14688 (MH); Coimbatore, A. N. Henry 83495 (MH); Nellimalai R.F, 400 m, 25.5.1962, K. Ramamurthy, 14112 and 14803 (MH); Lawbton's peak-Coimbatore, 2100 ft, 22.4.1911, C. E. C. Fischer, 2671 (CAL); Kuridimalai, 73 m, 13.8.1956, K. Subramanyam, 533 (MH and CAL); slope of Kuridimalai, 73 m, 10.7.1956, K. Subramanyam 246 (CAL); Chengleput dt., Vandalore R.F. ±100 m, 2.10.1974, A.N.Henry 45558(MH); Salem dt., Hogainakal forest, 275 m, 13.7.1964, E. Vajravelu 20607 (MH). Morappur, J.S. Gamble 32866 (MH); Kolli hills, Aruvithurai, 600 m, 5.7.1979, P. Perumal 23513 (CAL); Salem, K. Ramamurthy 38850 (MH); Edappadi, 250 m, 18.12.1978, K.M. Mathew 19832 (CAL); Shevaroy hills, Pallipatti slopes, 500 m, 7.11.1978, K. M. Mathew 19018 (CAL); Pachaimalai, Narippadu to Kummbakkal, 400 m, 27.7.1978, K. M. Mathew and N. Venugopal 15628 (CAL); Tirunelveley dt., above lower dam, Papanasam, 167 m, 7.7.1959, K.M. Sebastine 8364 (MH); Netrikal, 350 m, 10.3.1963, J. Joseph, 15893 (MH); Trichirapalli dt., Puliyamcholai, 233 m, 29.10.1958, K.M. Sebastine, 7049 (MH); Poovarasankudi, 75 m, 22. 9. 1965, K. Ramamurthy, 25892 (MH); S.Arcot dt., Kurumbarum R.F. near Marakkam,50 m, 14.3.1989, 90440 (CAL); Marakkanam, K. Ramamurthy 60281 (CAL); Kanyakumari dt., Maruthuvamalai, 200 m, 18.10.1985, A.N. Henry, 83375 (MH); Ramanathapuram dt., Pranmalai, Thirappathur, 250 m, 29.11.1977, N.C. Nair 52925 (MH and CAL), Vellimalai R.F, 175 m, 23.6.1978, N.C. Nair, 57414 (MH and CAL); Thavalazhapperumal kuttam, Periyar dam, 275 m, 16.2.1979, N. C. Nair 60840 (CAL); Karaikudi, N. C. Nair, 53019 (CAL); Visuvanoor, 30.10.1988, 1946 (MH); on the way to Mandapasalai, ±75 m, 15.11.1989, 2243 (MH), Kamuthakudi, ± 50 m, 15.1.1989, V. Balasubramanyam 2102 (MH); Palayampatti, 12.3.1953, G.H. Maduram, 21895 (MH); Vellimai, Sivaganga, 100 m, 12.8.1964, K. Ramamurthy, 20263 (MH); Marudhadi beat, Srivilliputtur R.F, 230, 16.7.1965, E. Vajravelu, 24707 and 39321(MH); North Arcot dt., way to Vaniampadi, 233 m, 14.12.1958, K. Subramanyam 7484 (MH and CAL); Vazhigur, 250 m, 26.3.1978, 54598 (MH), Salbanur forest, 200 m, 25.11.1977, E. Vajravelu 52072 (MH); Madurai dt, Bodirange, 500 m, 15.9.1961, K.M. Sebastine,

12907 (MH); Poomparai to Vilpatti, 500 m, 18.10.1977, M. Chandrabose, 51362 (MH and CAL); Vellore dt., Vellore, K.C. Jacob 83327 (MH); Ioukkuluru, P. Venkanna 140960 (MH); Tirunelvely dt., Palayamkottai, G. H. Maduram 86339 (MH); Netrikal, J. Joseph 15893 (MH); Narthamalai, C.Arulappan 141420 (MH); Tirumayam, C.Arulappan 143680 (MH); Dultalur, S. India, C. E. C. Fischer 296784 (CAL); Dharmapuri dt., Urigam R.F, 700 m, 6.9.1978, K. M. Mathew and N. Venugopal 16912 (CAL); Thanjavur dt., Sibhal to Velamkanni, 25 m, 17.9.1977, K. Ramamurthy, 51292 (MH); Dhai thoppu, 25 m, 29.10.1989, S. Ragupathy 1115 (CAL). Nilgiri dt., way to Thengumaruda, 525 m, 6.11.1970, E. Vajravelu, 36730 (MH); Pudukottai dt, Narthamalai, ± 130 m, 30.3.198, 403 (MH), Tiramayam, ± 80 m, 14.7.1984, C. Arulappan, 47 (MH); Dindigul dt., Sirumalais, 13-8-1959, P.Pallithanan 4865 (BLAT).

Karnataka: Tumkur dt., Pavagada taluk, Bhupoor, 24.2.2008, A. Ugraiah 31701 (SKU); Sira -Madugiri road, 18 km, Madugiri, N. P. Singh, 146920 (BSI); Chitradurg dt., Halumalleswar foot hills, 14.6.2008, A. Ugraiah 31734 (SKU); Lokadal foot hills, 15.6.2008, A. Ugraiah 31739 (SKU); Chitradurg foot hills, 16.6.2008, A. Ugraiah 31744 (SKU); Devaragudda R.F. Holalkere, N. P. Singh, 143300 (BSI); Alospet, Hospet J. S. Gamble 328959 (MH); Bellary dt., J. Joseph 83126 (MH); Virampuram, J.S. Gamble 296786 (CAL); Virampuram, 5.5.1909, I.H. Burkill 31861 (ISIM); Bellary- Hospet road, T. S. Puri 41548 (BSI); Kolar dt., Sonnipalli, 24.6.1978,T. M. Ramakrishna 1168 (MH); Bijapur dt., Kamatagi R.F, Hugund, N. P. Singh, 142603 (BSI); Huliyal R.F. Jamkhand, N. P. Singh 142955 (BSI).

Orissa: Ganjam dt., Mohri hills, 1000ft, 1884, J.S.Gamble, 13915 (MH); Ruke konda, 24.8.1931, V. Narayanasamy 82968 (MH); Barkuda, N. Annandale 296776 (CAL).

Maharashtra: Poona, Law college, A. S. Rao 87164 (CAL); Poona, College garden, Seshagiri Rao Rolla 296779 (CAL); 8 km from Songamner, Seshagiri Rao Rolla 83629 (BSI); Along Diveghat, Seshagiri Rao Rolla, 86509 (BSI).

Notes: This is the most widely distributed of the varieties of C. *adscendens*. The present study found it at Coimbatore, Dindigul, Madurai, Salem and Pudukottai districts of Tamil Nadu; Anantapur, Kadapa, Nellore, Chittoor districts of Andhra Pradesh and Chitradurga, Tumkur districts of Karnataka. It was first described from the foothills of Nilgiris, and Hooker quotes Cochin as another locality, but at that time *Caralluma stalagmifera* unknown and seems often to have been confused with *C. attenuata*. This variety has more hybridizable potency with neighboring *Caralluma* varieties, hybridized forms having been recorded by Gravely and Mayuranathan (1931) from Madurai and Pudukottai districts of Tamil Nadu.

Caralluma adscendens (Roxb.) R. Brown var. **bicolor** (Ramachandran *et al.)* Karuppusamy, Ugraiah and Pullaiah, *Stat. nov*. Basionym: *Caralluma bicolor* Ramachandran *et al*. in Nordic J. Bot. 29: 447-450. 2011. Type: Siljo Joseph 1501 (CAL) (holo).

Succulent herb. Vegetative stem fleshy, 45-120 cm high, slightly branched from the base, slender. Branches quadrangular, angles acute, uniformly green at the base, paler at the top with reddish-brown tinge along ribs, fertile apical portion very slender, internodes 20 – 45mm long. Leaves triangular (sagittate), 2-4 mm long, almost sessile, decussate, acute at apex, glabrous, deciduous. Flowers 5-merous, axillary, in pairs along the attenuated apical portion of stem, opening in succession. Bracts and bracteoles 3, minute, glabrous. Pedicel terete, ca 3-5 mm long, glabrous. Calyx divided to base, ca 1.5- 1.0 mm, triangular, acuminate at apex, fleshy, glabrous, with imbricate aestivation. Corolla bud ca 1.0-1.4 cm long, with valvate aestivation. Corolla ca 2.0-2.8 cm across, glabrous throughout; tube ca 2 mm long, pale greenish yellow with a few reddish brown striations; lobes ca 1.2 - 0.3 cm, rotate, lanceolate-oblong, with the base similar in colour to the tube, distal two thirds strongly revolute, slightly geniculate at junction with the dark reddish brown proximal portion, cuspidate at apex. Corona staminal, biseriate; outer corona deeply forked with linear, slightly curved lobes, ca 1 mm in long, with a small projection between the lobes, broad at base, margin concave; inner corona, 0.8 mm long, incumbent on anthers, not meeting, slightly keeled near base, keel rounded, apex forked with short rounded lobes, with a small projection between the lobes, basally united with the outer corona, reddish brown. Anther 0.5 mm long, yellowish, basally united with inner surface of the middle corona, swollen; Pollen masses ca 1 mm long, solitary in each anther cell, yellow, round, waxy, attached by reddish brown caudicles, widened to dark brown corpuscle to form five pollinia. Gynostegium ca 1 mm long; stigma cap star shaped pentagonal, with a small depression at the centre; ovary apocarpous, ovules on marginal placenta. Follicles creamy white with pale purplish streaks, 13 -14 cm long, tapering towards the apex, glabrous. Seeds oblong-obovoid, ca 9-4 mm; coma silky white, ca 2.8 cm long.

Distribution: Tamil Nadu (endemic).

Abundance: Common in base of Maruthamalai hills, Coimbatore; Nagamalai hills and Alagar hills in Madurai and Sirumalai hills at Dindigul distirct.

Flowering and fruiting: Throughout the year.

Etymology: The variety is possessing two colors on the corolla lobes.

Specimens Examined

Base of Maruthuvamalai hills, behind the Bharathiar University play ground, 19.7.2010, S. Karuppusamy 846, 852 (Madura college herbarium).

Notes: This newly described taxon is more closely related to *Caralluma adscendens* and *Caralluma stalagmifera*. Only the differences mentioned by the authors are size of the plant, nature of stem angle and size of the corolla lobes. But the variations are very common in all succulent stapeliads. During our field investigation we observed many *Caralluma adscendens* populations in Nagamalai hills and Alagar hills of Madurai district, and Sirumalai hills in Dindigul district showed great variations in height, very stout and angled stems, variously banded corolla lobes, great degree of variations in hairs on the corolla margin without to densely fringed, and purple streaks on stems. It may be due to polyploidy in the population as mentioned many earlier workers. This variety is more alike with Roxburgh illustration in his Plants of the Coast Coramandal in 1795. In this ground the new taxon *Caralluma bicolor* is considered under the variety of *Caralluma adscendens*.

Caralluma adscendens (Roxb.) R. Brown var. **carinata** Gravely et Mayuranathan in Bull. Madr. Govt. Mus. n.s. N.H. 4(1): 16. 1931. Type: Plate II. 6 in protologue collections from Nagamalai and Alagar hills, Madurai district, Tamil Nadu, India; Gilbert in Bradleya 8: 16.1990; Plowes in Haseltonia 3: 52. 1995; Jagtap and Singh in Fasc. Fl. India 24: 195. 1999; Meve and Liede in Plant. Syst. Evol. 234: 200. 2002.

Plants ca.35 cm tall. Stems acute angled, green, distally strongly attenuate, rarely branched. Flowers purplish, hairy, usually pendulous and campanulate but sometimes semi-erect and rotate; pedicels not bent (Plate 6.11, Figure 6.14).

Distribution: This variety is distributed on road side and waste lands near MKU and Sirumalai foot hills of Tamil Nadu (endemic).

Abundance: Very small populations.

Flowering and fruiting: July- December.

Etymology: From the Greek 'carinata' means keeled; the flower petals of the variety is having keeled or bands.

Specimens Examined

Tamil Nadu: Madurai dt., Near MKU road side, 4.5.2008, S. Karuppusamy and A. Ugraiah 31717 (SKU); Dindigul dt., Sirumalai western slope of foot hills, 8.5.2008, S. Karuppusamy and A. Ugraiah 31727 (SKU).

Notes: Very few populations known in Tamil Nadu (endemic). This variety has been observed only in the Nagamalai and Azhargar hills of the Madurai district and Sirumalai hills of Dindigul district of Tamil Nadu. This variety is threatened due to habitat modification.

Caralluma adscendens (Roxb.) R. Brown var. **fimbriata** (Wall.) Gravely et Mayuranathan in Bull. Madr. Govt. Mus. n. s. 4(1): 13. 1931; Santapau and Irani in Univ. Bombay Bot. Mem. 4: 21. 1962; Sharma *et al*. Fl. Karnataka 165. 1984; Gilbert in Bradleya 8: 16.1990; Jagtap and Singh in Fasc. Fl. India 24: 195. 1999; Plowes in Haseltonia 3: 52. 1995; Meve and Liede in Plant Syst. Evol. 234: 200. 2002. *Caralluma fimbriata* Wall., Pl. As. Rar. 1: 7. 1830. Type: tab. 8 of protologue based on material collected Burma, Yenangeum or Pagamew, and cultivated in Calcutta; Hooker f. Fl. Brit. India 4: 77.1883; Cooke, Fl. Pres. Bombay 2: 244. 1905.

Stems up to 45 cm tall, not definitely attenuate, equal thickness throughout, creamy reddish distally, not streaked, angles rounded. Flowers dark purple, usually pendulous, petals densely hairy along the margins (Plate 6.12, Figure 6.15).

Distribution: This variety is distributed in road sides, waste lands along with thorny bushes in Andhra Pradesh, Karnataka, Tamil Nadu and Maharashtra.

Abundance: Very common

Flowering and fruiting: Throughout the year.

Etymology: From the Greek 'fimbria' means fringes; the hairy fringes on the corolla margins.

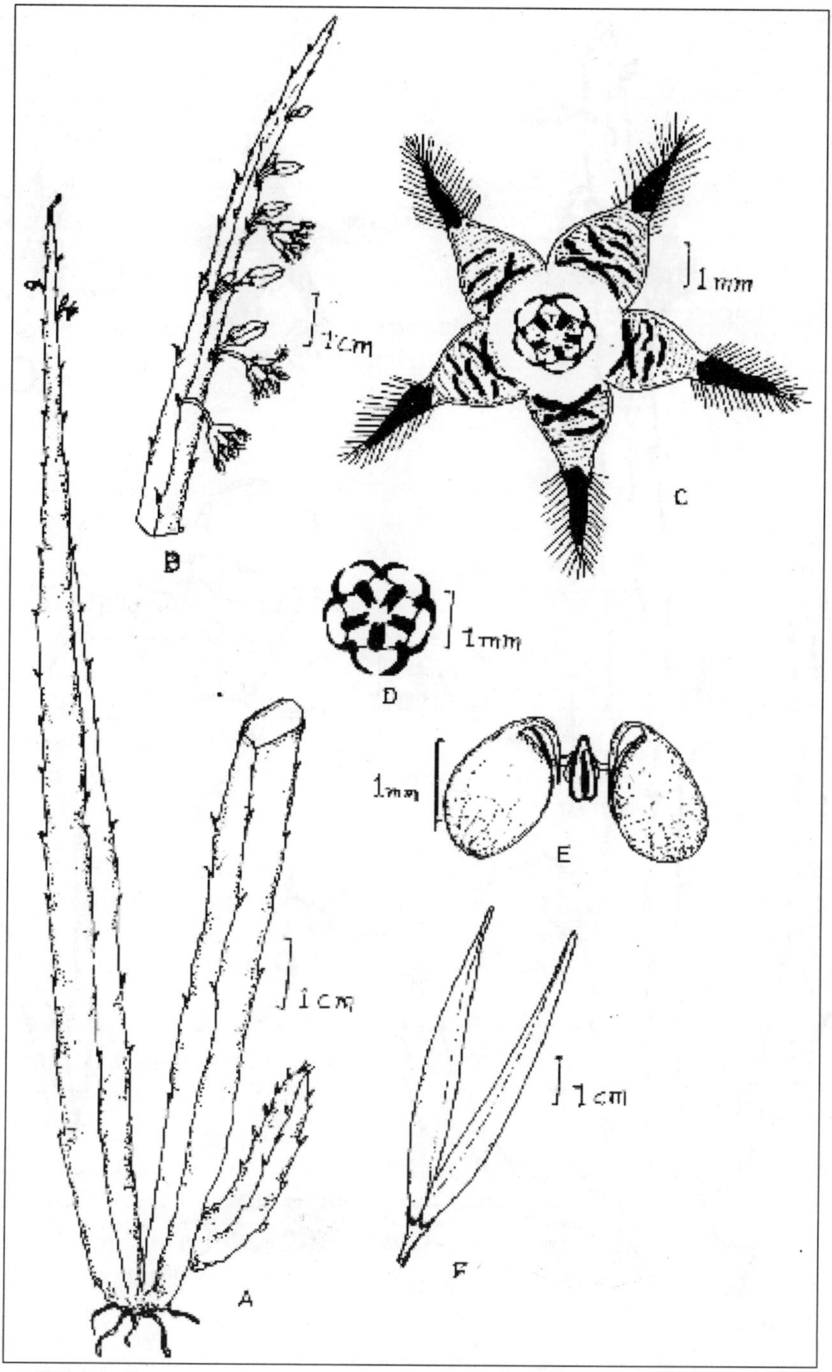

Figure 6.14: ***Caralluma adscendens*** **var.** ***carinata*** **Gravely et Mayuranathan**
A: Habit; B: Inflorescence; C: Flower; D: Corona; E: Pollinia; F: Fruit

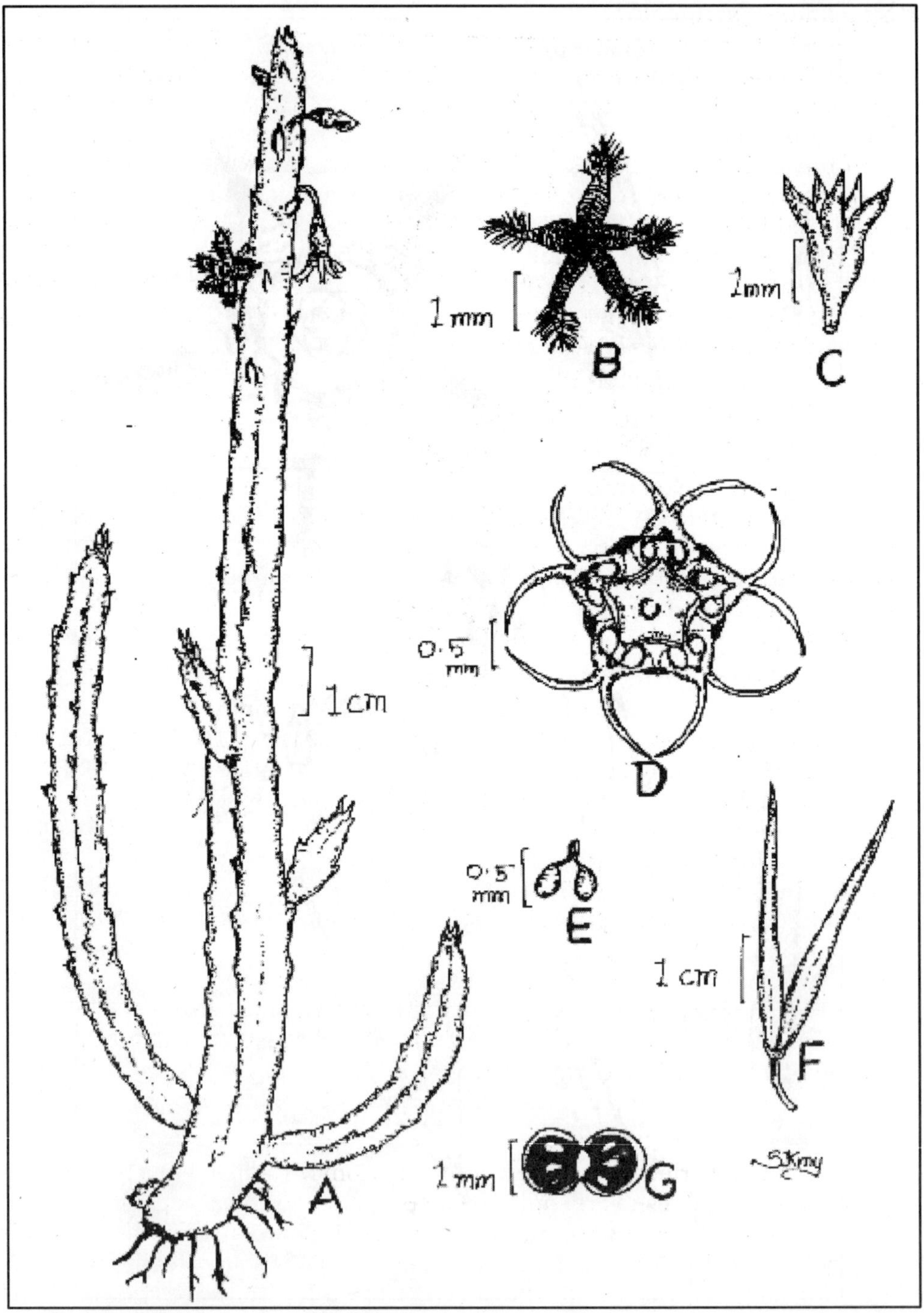

Figure 6.15: ***Caralluma adscendens*** **var.** ***fimbriata*** **(Wall.) Gravely et Mayuranathan**
A: Habit; B: Flower; C: Sepals; D: Corona; E: Pollinia; F: Fruit; G: T.S. of ovary

Specimens Examined

AndhraPradesh: Anantapur dt., Kalasamudram, 19.7.2008, A. Ugraiah 31750 (SKU), Bugga, Tadipatri, 8.9.2008, A.Ugraiah and S.Sandhyarani 31759 (SKU), Gooty foot hills, 23.4.2008, S. Karuppusamy and A. Ugraiah, 31707 and 31708 (SKU), Gooty hills, 1600 ft, July 1884, J. S. Gamble 16485 (CAL), Penakacherla, 700 ft, July 1884, J.S. Gamble 15261 and 21242 (DD); Kurnool dt., Srisailam 5 km towards Sundipenta,10.9.2008, A.Ugraiah and S. Sandhyarani 31761 (SKU); Guntur dt., Kondaveddu, 7-9-1956, SKW 3732 (BLAT); Mahaboobnagar dt., Mallelathertham, 10.9.2008, A.Ugraiah and S.Sandhyarani 31762 (SKU); Nellore dt., Sangan, 23.7.1914, M. S. Ramaswami 1158 (CAL), Cuddapah dt., Cuddapah, 19.10.1938, E.K.Krishnan 79302 (DD), Gaverkota, 1000 ft, July 1884, J.S. Gamble 15039 (DD); Visakhapatnam dt., Madgol, 15-7-1958, SKW 8442 (BLAT).

Tamil Nadu: Nerinjipat, C.E.C. Fischer 296805 (CAL); Anamalais, Thirumurti-Palar valley, 296782 (CAL); Shembaganur, Rev. L. Anglade, 296792 (CAL). Salem dt., Moratopur, 16.3.1915, *s.n.* 11649 (MH)

Karnataka: Tumkur dt, Bhupoor, 24.2.2008, A.Ugraiah 31702 (SKU), Tumkur hills, 18.6.2008, A.Ugraiah 31747 (SKU); Pavagada foot hills, 18.6.2008, A.Ugraiah 31743 (SKU); Dharwar dt., Hubli taluk, Soudatti, 26.3.2008, A.Ugraiah 31704 (SKU), Dharwar dt., 22.4.1909, W. Burns 296794 (CAL); Chitradurga dt., Halumalleswar foot hills,14.6.2008, A.Ugraiah 31736 (SKU); Molakalmuru – Bellary road, N. P. Singh, 141455 (BSI); Belgaum dt., Yallapur, Potchapur 26.7.2009, A.Ugraiah 31781 (SKU);

Maharashtra: Sangli dt., Gurhathwadi hills, 27.7.2009, A. Ugraiah 31783 (SKU), Bahabuli foot hills, 27.7.2009, A. Ugraiah 31785 (SKU), Shalupuri towards Bahubuli, 27.7.2009, A. Ugraiah 31782 (SKU), Lakshmi hills, Athrige, 27.7.2009, A. Ugraiah 31784 (SKU), Saganeswar forest, Tasgaov taluk, A. N. Landhe 170120 (BSI), Valva taluk, Islampur A. N. Landhe,170212 (BSI); Sindewadi area, Malegao range, P. L. Narasimhan 165288 (BSI); Poona dt., Diveghat, between Swarghat and Saswad, A. Ugraiah 31780 (SKU); Poona law college, 12.7.1962, A.S. Rao 87614 (CAL), Law College hill, Poona, Razi 5155 A (BLAT), Pashan 8 miles from Poona, N.Irani 178, 179, 1021 (BLAT), Bopudi 3 miles north of Poona, June 1888, s.l. 107, 21996 (BLAT), Chattarshingu hill, Poona, 17-5-1917, s.l. 30449; Nasik dt., Nayaydangri, 166305 (BSI); Ahamadnagar dt., Kargighat on the way from Ahamadnagar to Pathardi, K. P. Janardhanan 98971 (BSI); Kuruli, Khed Taluk, K. P. Janardhanan 72296 (BSI); East slopes of Bhuthinath jungle, K. P. Janardhanan 100393 (BSI); Khandgaon, Dec. 1986, R.D.Shinde 913 (BLAT); Katraj Ghat, 14-8-1955, N.Irani 1063; Mumbai, St. Xavier College terrace Garden, 4-5-1955, G.L.Shah 4537 (BLAT); Kolhapur dt., Kolhapur Aug, 1920, ACK 704 (BLAT).

Notes: This variety is described originally from Myanmar, but it has since been recorded from India and Sri Lanka. It exists in discontinuous populations in drier regions of peninsular India. Large numbers of natural populations have suddenly declined due to the increased demand in pharmaceutical market for its glycosides. It is not currently cultivated for this purpose, markets relying on wild collected material. *Caralluma* extracts have also been found to be appetite suppressant, a property which is well known to Indian tribals and hunters. Indian folklore records its use as a potent appetite suppressant and weightloss promoter. *Caralluma adscendens* var. *fimbriata* is used in the treatment of obesity. The extract of *Caralluma adscendens* var. *fimbriata* in the form of capsules has been released under trade name GENASLIM for body weight control (Lawrence and Choudary, 2004).

Caralluma adscendens (Roxb.) R. Brown var. **gracilis** Gravely et Mayuranathan in Bull. Madr. Govt. Mus. n. s. 4(1): 14. 1931. Type: Plate II.5 in protologue; Gilbert in Bradleya 8: 16.1990; Plowes in Haseltonia 3: 52. 1995; Jagtap and Singh in Fasc. Fl. India 24: 198. 1999; Meve and Liede in Plant Syst. Evol. 234: 200. 2002.

Stems greenish ca. 70 cm in height, acute angled, slightly attenuate at distal portion. Flowers slightly hairy, axillary paired below the distal apex, pedicel 1.5 cm; corolla chestnut brown (Plate 6.13, Figure 6.16)

Distribution: Distributed from Pudukottai forest area to southern districts of Tamil Nadu (endemic).

Abundance: Dense population.

Flowering and fruiting: Throughout the year.

Etymology: From the Greek 'gracile' means graceful and slender; graceful and slender pedicel of the flower is a character of this variety.

Specimens Examined

Tamil Nadu: Dindigul dt., Palani hills, near Varadhamanathi dam, 9.5.2008, S. Karuppusamy and A. Ugraiah, 31730 (SKU).

Notes: Gravely and Mayuranathan (1931) originally collected and described this variety from the of Pudukottai forests of Tamil Nadu. It is distributed throughout Tamil Nadu and occurs in dense populations in Pudukottai forests. In the present investigation specimens were collected from the forests of Palani hills. This variety also hybridizes with *C. stalagmifera* and other neighboring varieties presenting intermediate forms (Gravely and Mayuranathan, 1931).

Caralluma bhupinderiana Sarkaria Nat. Cact. Succ. J. 35 (3): 68-72, 1978. Type: India Sarkaria J93-78 (PAN); S.R. Srinivasan in A.N. Henry *et al.* Fl. Tamil Nadu Anal.: 81.1987; Gilbert in Bradleya 8: 16.1990; Plowes in Haseltonia 3: 52. 1995; Jagtap Singh, Fasc. Fl. India 24: 195. 1999; Meve and Leide in Plant Syst. Evol. 234: 200. 2002.

Stem fleshy, up to 70 cm high, quadrangular; internodes ca 1.5 cm thick, tapering towards apex with acute tips, glabrous. Latex watery. Leaves rudimentary, opposite decussate, sessile, ca 3 × 1 mm, lanceolate, broad at base, usually present on young branches, deciduous, glabrous. Flowers axillary, from thin apical portion of the stems, paired; bracts three, thin, ca 0.5 mm; pedicels semi-erect or at right angle to the stem, terete, 6–8 mm long, pale yellow, glabrous. Calyx five-lobed, divided up to base, pale green, lobe ca 1.5 × 0.5 mm, lanceolate, apex acute, glabrous. Corolla rotate, slightly reflexed; lobes 5, ca 5 × 3 mm, ovate-oblong, apex acute, margin densely hairy in distal part, outer surface of corolla-tube slightly concave, glabrous, occasionally few cilia on midline on inner surface; corolla-tube ca 0.5 mm high, finely ciliate at the mouth within. Corona staminal, biseriate, ca 2 mm in diam., outer deeply bifid

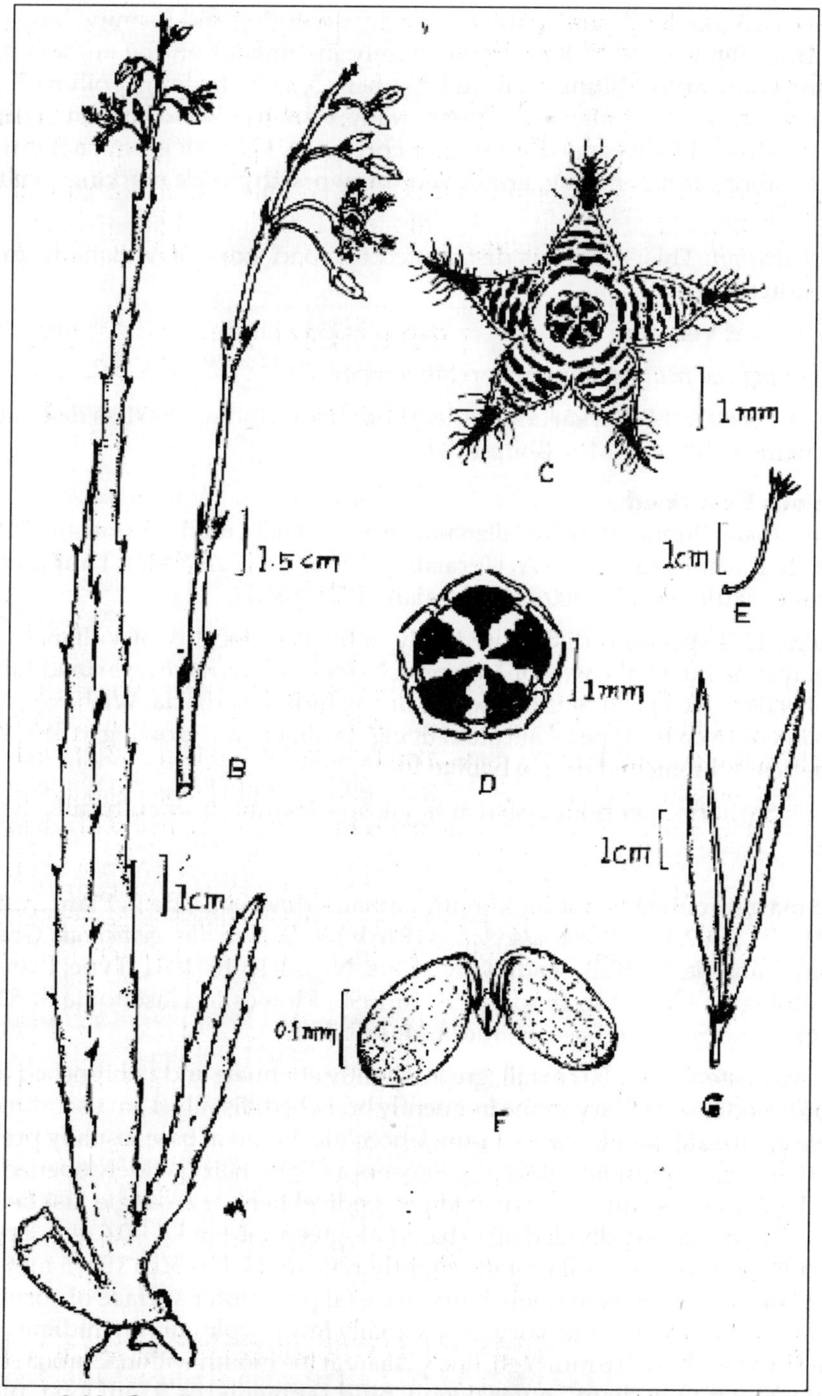

Figure 6.16: ***Caralluma adscendens var. gracilis*** **Gravely et Mayuranathan**
A: Habit; B: Inflorescence; C: Flower; D: Corona;
E: Pedicel with sepals; F: Pollinia; G: Fruit

segments, ca 3 mm long, transparent, laterally diverging and forming loops; inner arising from the base of outer corona, closely incumbent on the anthers but not exceeding them, apices blunt, recurved. Stamens 5, ca 2 mm long; pollinia 5, pollen masses solitary in each anther cell, yellow, waxy, brown pellucid layer attached with a light-brown caudicles and dark-brown corpuscle. Gynostegium ca 2 mm long. Follicle fusiform, ca 8.5 cm long, linear, deep brown with purple markings (Plate 6.14, Figure 6.17).

Distribution: This species is distributed on road sides of Vallanadu forest in Tamil Nadu (endemic).

Abundance: Very rare

Flowering and fruiting: September–November.

Etymology: Dr. J.S. Sarkaria succulent collector in India, who has dedicated the species name to his wife Mrs. Bhupinder.

Specimens Examined

Tamil Nadu: Pudukottai dt., Vallanadu forest foot hills, road side toward Tuticorin, 5.5.2008, S. Karuppusamy and A. Ugraiah, 31720 and 31721 (SKU); Thuthukudi dt., Veerapandipattinam, 17.1.2009, A. Ugraiah 31775 (SKU).

Notes: This species is distributed only in the type locality of Vallanadu forest near Palayamkottai on the way of Tuticorin. No collections have been made since the type collection. No specimens deposited in any Indian herbaria. We have collected the specimens from the type locality and living specimens are growing in SKU garden. This species is threatened due to habitat loss.

Uses: Sarkaria mentioned that it is an ornamental, horticulturally desirable species.

Caralluma geniculata (Grav. et Mayuranathan) Meve et Liede in Plant Syst. Evol. 234: 200. 2002. *Caralluma adscendens* (Roxb.) R. Brown var. *geniculata* Gravely et Mayuranathan in Bull. Madr. Govt. Mus. N. S. 4(1): 16. 1931. Type: Plate II. 7 in protologue; Gilbert in Bradleya 8: 16.1990; Plowes in Haseltonia 3: 52. 1995; Jagtap and Singh in Fasc. Fl. India 24: 195. 1999.

Stems acute angled, 50 cm tall, green, slightly attenuate and unbranched distally, but more slender secondary stems frequently branched distally. Leaves rudimentary, opposite decussate, sessile, ca 3 × 1 mm, lanceolate, broad at base, usually present on young branches, deciduous, glabrous. Flowers axillary, hairy, widely opened, facing upwards, dark chestnut brown markings, pedicel bent at an angle just below the flower. Calyx five-lobed, divided up to base, pale green, lobe ca 1.4 × 0.6 mm, lanceolate, apex acute, glabrous. Corolla rotate, slightly reflexed; lobes 5, ca 10 × 5 mm, ovate-oblong, apex acute, margin finely hairy in distal part, outer surface of corolla-tube slightly concave, short white hairy, occasionally few purple cilia on midline on inner surface; corolla-tube ca 0.6 mm high, finely ciliate at the mouth within. Corona staminal, biseriate, ca 3 mm in diam., outer deeply bifid segments, ca 5 mm long, purplish, laterally diverging and forming loops; inner arising from the base of outer corona,

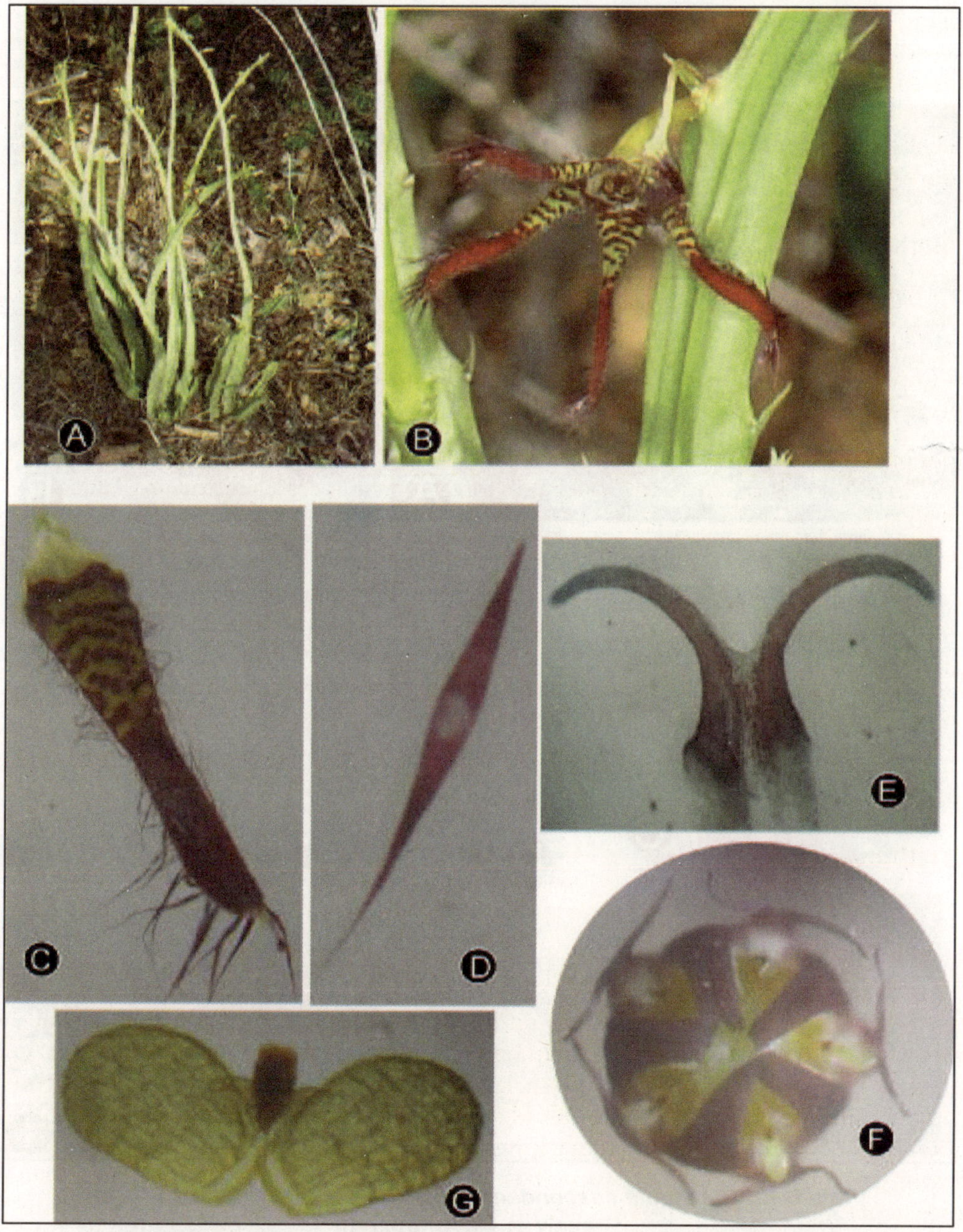

Plate 6.11. *Caralluma adscendens* (Roxb.) R.Br. var. *carinata* Gravely et Mayuranathan
A: Natural habitat; B: Flower; C: Petal; D: Hair; E: Outer corona; F: Corona; G: Pollinia.

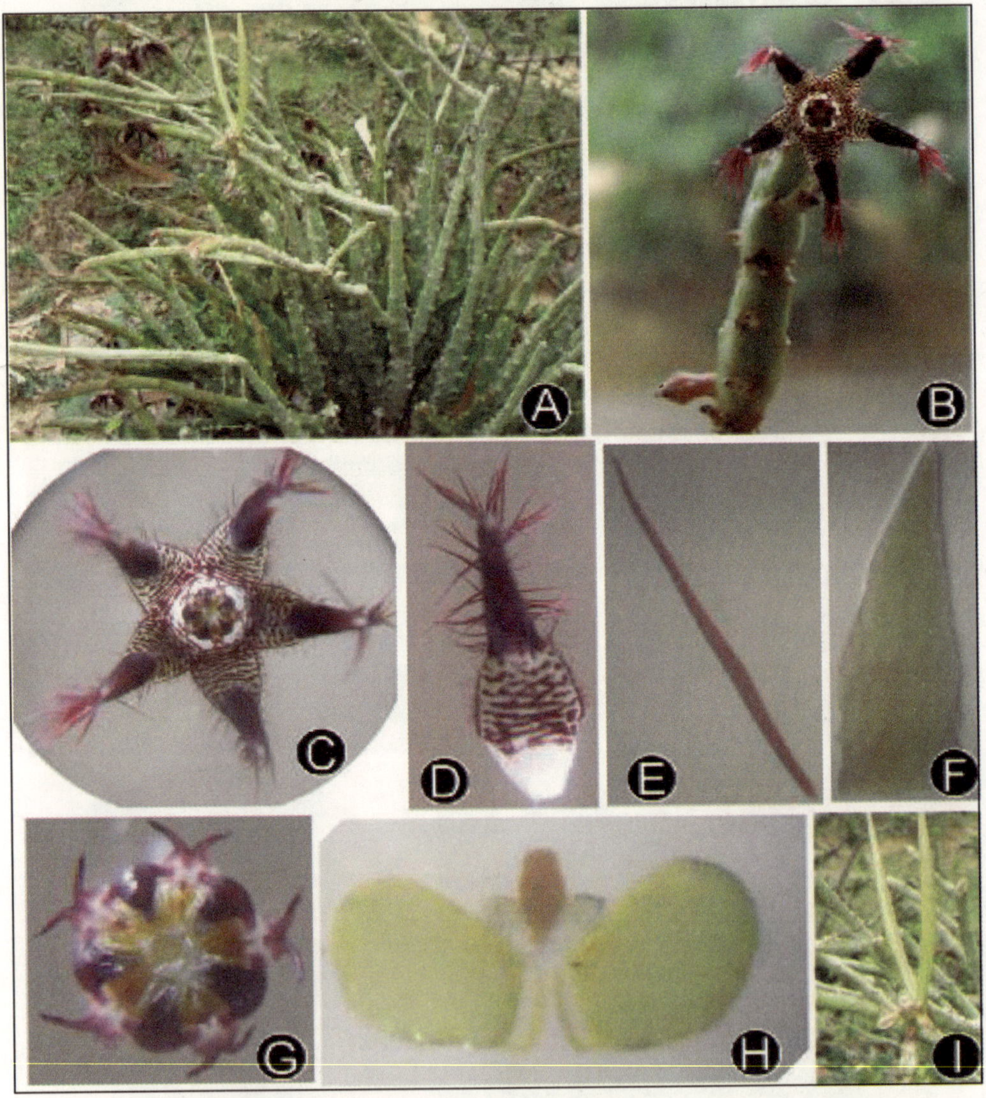

Plate 6.12. *Caralluma adscendens* (Roxb.) R.Br. var. *fimbriata* (Wall.) Gravely et Mayuranathan
A: Natural habitat; B: Inflorescence; C: Flower; D: Petal; E: Hair; F: Sepal; G: Corona; H: Pollinia; I: Fruit.

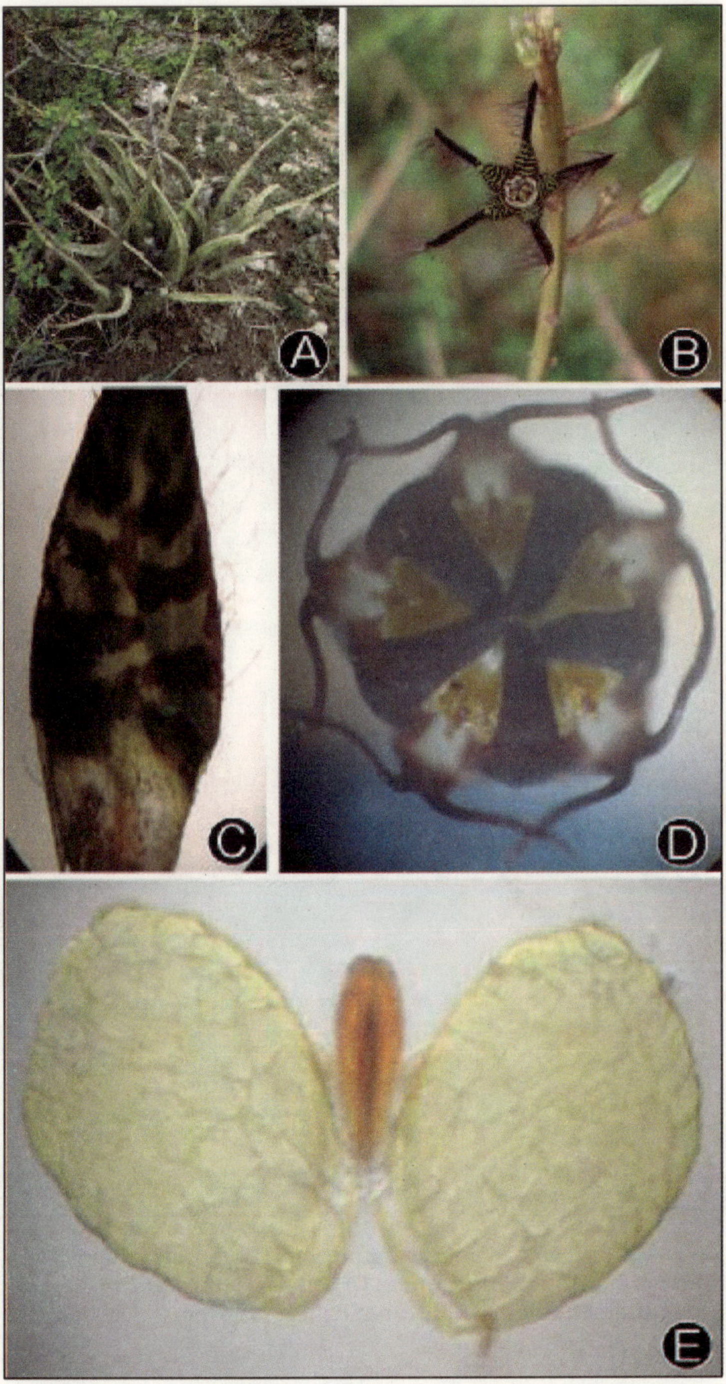

Plate 6.13. ***Caralluma adscendens*** **(Roxb.) R.Br. var.** ***gracilis*** **Gravely et Mayuranathan**
A: Natural habitat; B: Flower; C: Petal; D: Corona; E: Pollinia

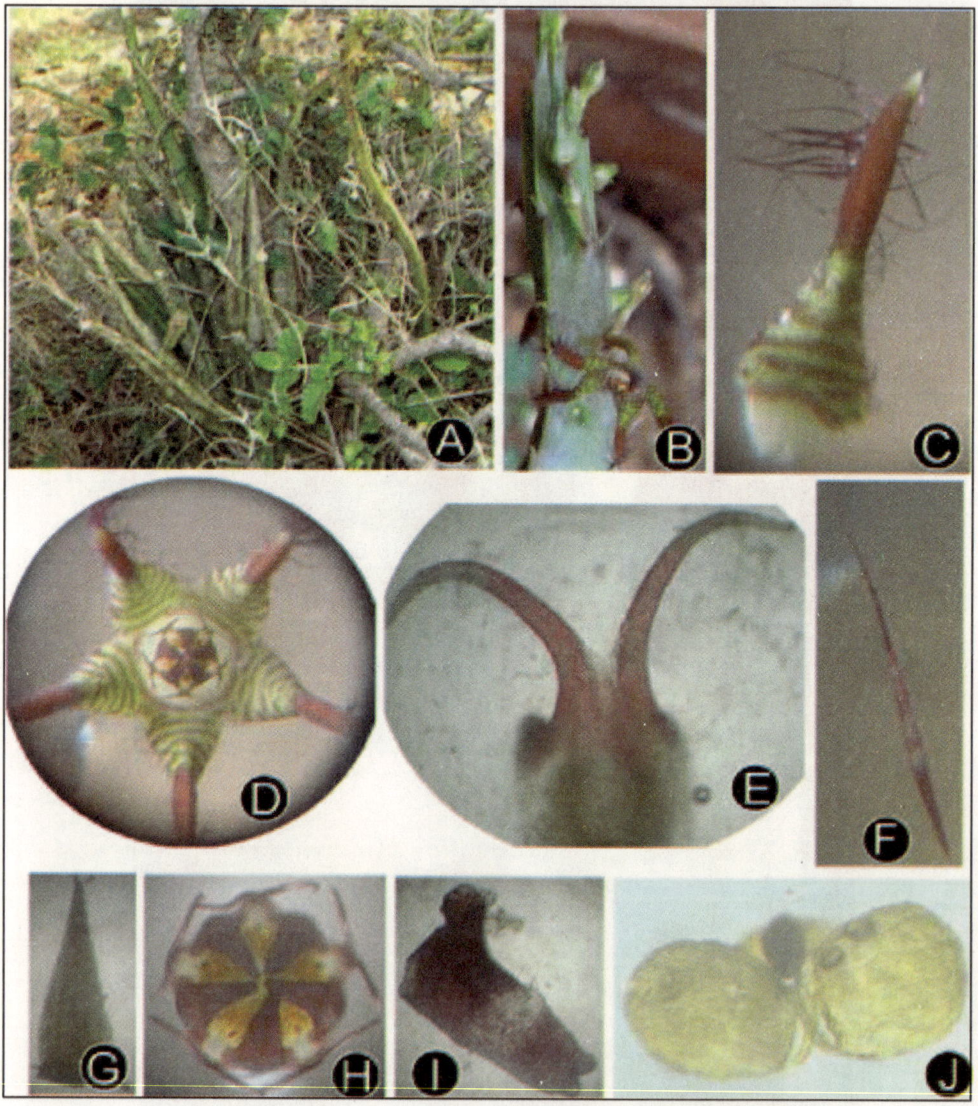

Plate 6.14. ***Caralluma bhupinderiana*** **Sarkaria**
A: Natural habitat; B: Inflorescence; C: Petal; D: Flower; E: Outer corona; F: Hair; G: Sepal; H: Corona; I: Inner corona; J: Pollinia

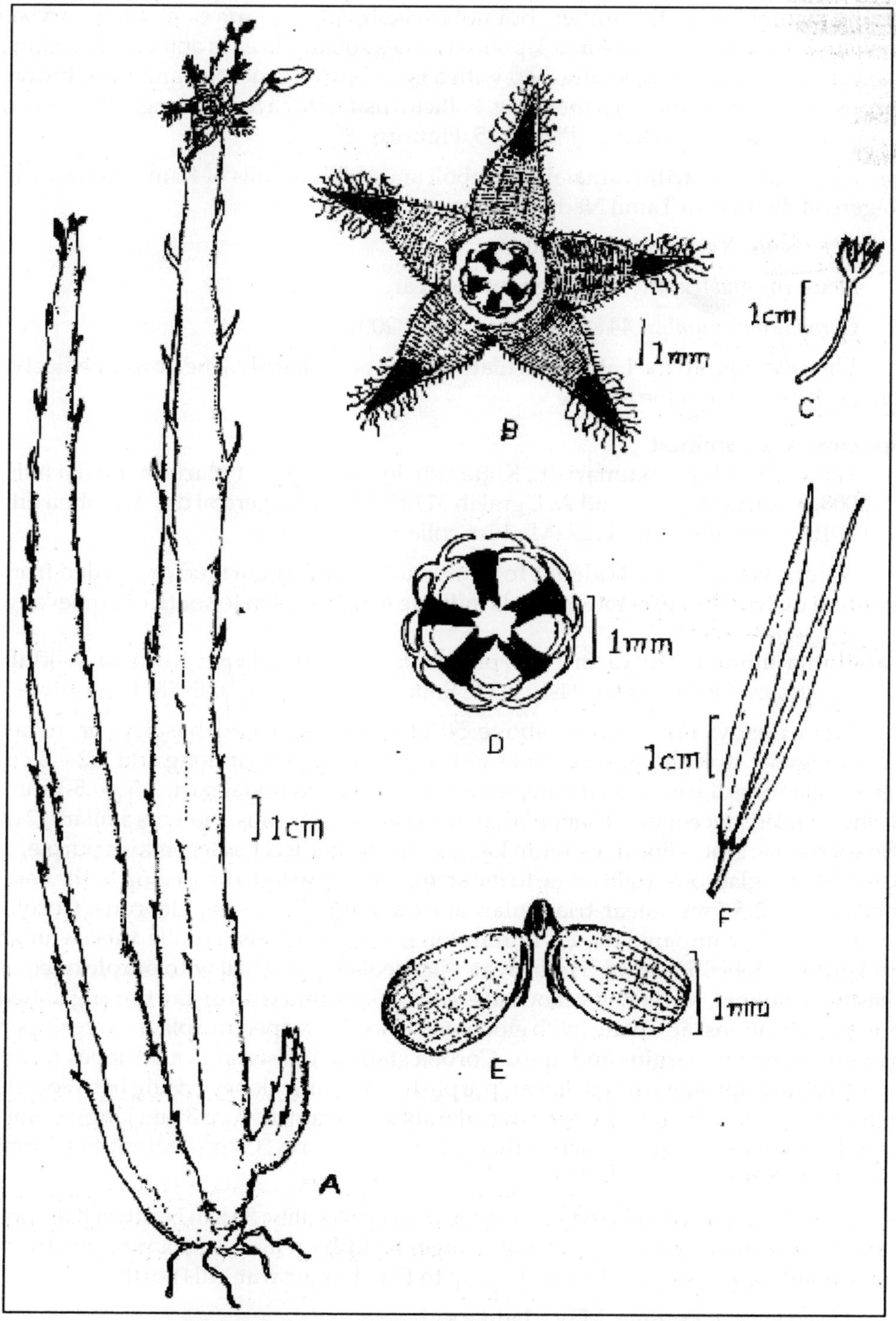

Figure 6.17: ***Caralluma bhupinderiana*** **Sarkaria**
A: Habit; B: Flower; C: Pedicel with sepals; D: Corona; E: Pollinia; F: Fruit

closely incumbent on the anthers but not exceeding them, apices blunt, recurved. Stamens 5, ca 3 mm long; pollinia 5, pollen masses solitary in each anther cell, yellow, waxy, brown pellucid layer attached with a light-brown caudicles and dark-brown corpuscle. Gynostegium ca 3 mm long. Follicle fusiform, ca 8.5 cm long, linear, deep brown with purple markings (Plate 6.15, Figure 6.18).

Distribution: Marthuvamalai, Aramboli and Valliyur hills of Kanyakumari and Nagercoil districts in Tamil Nadu (endemic).

Abundance: Very few populations.

Flowering and fruiting: Throughout the year.

Chromosome number: 44 (Albers and Meve, 2002).

Etymology: From the Latin geniculate means; bent sharply. The flower pedicel of the species bent from the middle.

Specimens Examined

Tamil Nadu: Kanyakumari dt., Kottaram, lower slopes of Maruthuamalai hills, 7.5.2008, S. Karuppusamy and A. Ugraiah 31722 (SKU); Nagercoil dt., Aramboli hill, 10.9.2010, S. Karuppusmy 1127 (Madura college herbarium).

Notes: This variety is endemic to Tamilnadu. The present study recorded from Madurai district, but previous records indicate a distribution to south of Tinnevally.

Caralluma moorei Aditya in Asklepios 110: 3-10-2011. Type: Kuldiha Wildlife Sanctuary, Orissa, India. 24-10-2009, Soumen Aditya SA-30-095M (Khosotype).

Stem fleshy, erect, grow above 50 cm tall, branched basally; branches quadrangular, apically groved, internodes elongated, 1-3 cm long and 1.2 – 2 cm across, glabrous. Leaves decussate, sessile on protruded nodal part, 3-5 x 0.5-1 mm, fleshy, elliptic-lanceolate – triangular, pointed at tip, glabrous. Flowers axillary, 2 or 3 in each axile; bracts linear, ca 1 mm long, subulate; pedicel terete, pinkish purple, 1-3.8 mm long, glabrous, right angle to the stem. Calyx 5-lobed, divided up to the base, lobes ca 5 x 2.5 mm, linear-triangular, apex acuminate, fleshy, glabrous. Corolla rotate, basally campanulate, ca 12 mm long, 1.3 cm across; corolla tube whitish background; lobes 5, ca 8 x 1.5 mm, ovate – lanceolate, disal half with purplish red or chestnut coloured, lower half yellowish green background with distinct strong dotted purplish striations, apiculate, with elongated – needle shaped purplish white tipped hairs hanging on margins and apex. Corona staminal, biseriate; outer lobes forms two erect and apically curved, linear, purplish lobes; inner lobes arising between the outer lobes at their base; incumbent over the anthers. Stamens 5, ca 3 mm long; pollinia 5, pollen masses solitary in each anther cell, yellow, waxy. Gynostegium ca 1.5 mm long (Plate 6.16).

Distribution: Southeastern India (endemic). Type locality: 35 Km North of Balasore, Orissa, eastern part of Eastern Ghats range, Kuldiha wild life sanctury, northern entry point, upper slopes, distribution up to Panchlingeswar hills north.

Flowering and Fruiting: May – January.

Etymology: The species name is commemorated to Gwen Moore, who is one of the foremost experts on rock gardening in the United States.

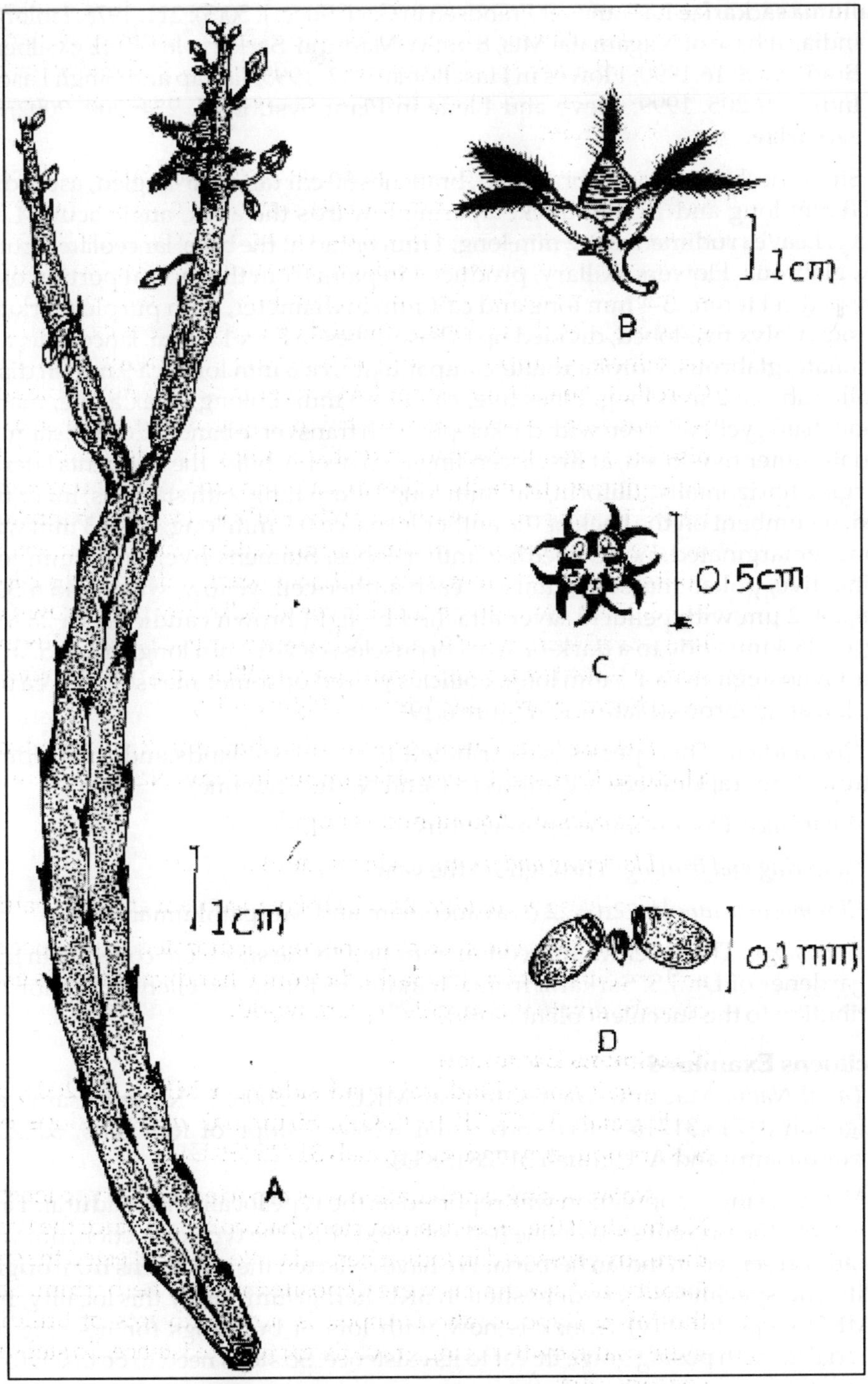

Figure 6.18: ***Caralluma geniculata*** **Meve et Liede**
A: Twig; B: Flower; C: Corona; D: Pollinia

Caralluma sarkariae Lavranos et Frandsen in Cact. Succ. J. 50(5): 211. 1978. Holotype: India, at base of Nagamalai Mts, 8 km W Madurai, Sarkaria J64-77 (E); Gilbert in Bradleya 8: 16.1990; Plowes in Haseltonia 3: 52. 1995; Jagtap and Singh Fasc. Fl. India 24: 205. 1999; Meve and Liede in Plant Syst. Evol. 234: 200. 2002; *var.* **sarkariae**.

Stems fleshy, profusely branched, branches 50 cm tall, four-angled, ascending, to 300 mm long and 15 mm thick, tapering towards the apex, angle acute. Latex watery. Leaves rudimentary, 2 mm long, 1 mm broad at the base, lanceolate, acute at apex, glabrous. Flowers axillary, produced in pairs from thin apical portion of the stem; pedicel terete, 3-4 mm long and ca 1 mm in diameter, with purple markings, glabrous. Calyx five-lobed, divided up to base, lobes ca 2.5 x 1.5 mm, lanceolate, apex acuminate, glabrous. Corolla rotate-campanulate, ca 6 mm long, ca 9 mm in diam.; Corolla tube ca 2 mm long; lobes five, ca 4 x 1.5 mm, oblong, apex acute, margin without hairs, yellow-green with darker-purplish transverse bands. Corona staminal, biseriate; outer five-lobed, at first ascending then deeply bifid, the segments laterally diverging horizontally, filiform, ca 1 mm long, alternating with stamens, inner five-lobed, incumbent on the back of the anther lobes, ca 0.5 mm long, 0.2-0.3 mm wide, oblong, emarginated, not exceeding anther-lobes. Stamens five, ca 1.5 mm long; pollinia five, pollen masses solitary in each anther-cell, yellow, waxy, 345.6-360 x 244.8-259.2 µm with pellucid layer attached by light brown caudicles, ca 28.8 µm long, ca 86.4 µm wide to a dark-brown corpuscles, ca 201.6µm long and ca 57.6 µm wide. Gynostegium ca 1.5 mm long. Follicles paired or sometimes solitary, ca 6 cm long, linear, glabrous (Plate 6.17, Figure 6.19).

Distribution: This species is distributed in the waste lands and road sides at Madurai Kamaraj University campus in Tamil Nadu (endemic)

Abundance: Discontinuous populations

Flowering and fruiting: Throughout the year.

Chromosome number: 2n = 22 (Navaneetham and Sampathkumar, 1984).

Etymology: The species name commemorated to the succulent collector in India and gardener of Dr. J.S. Sarkaria from Chandigarh for his excellent collection and contribution to the succulent plant world.

Specimens Examined

Tamil Nadu: Madurai, road side near MKU, 4.5.2008, S. Karuppusamy and A. Ugraiah 31713,31716 (SKU), Sirumalai western slope of foot hills, 8.5.2008, S. Karuppusamy and A. Ugraiah 31728 (SKU).

Notes: A single population was reported as the type locality in Madurai, Tamil Nadu. Until the present study none had collected since the type collection, nor were there any preserved in Indian herbaria. We have collected the specimens from original locality and specimens were deposited in SKU herbarium. Sadly this locality, near the MKU (type locality) Annex is now with lots of buildings for housing and industrial growth posing grave threat to its existence. So steps need to be taken for its conservation.

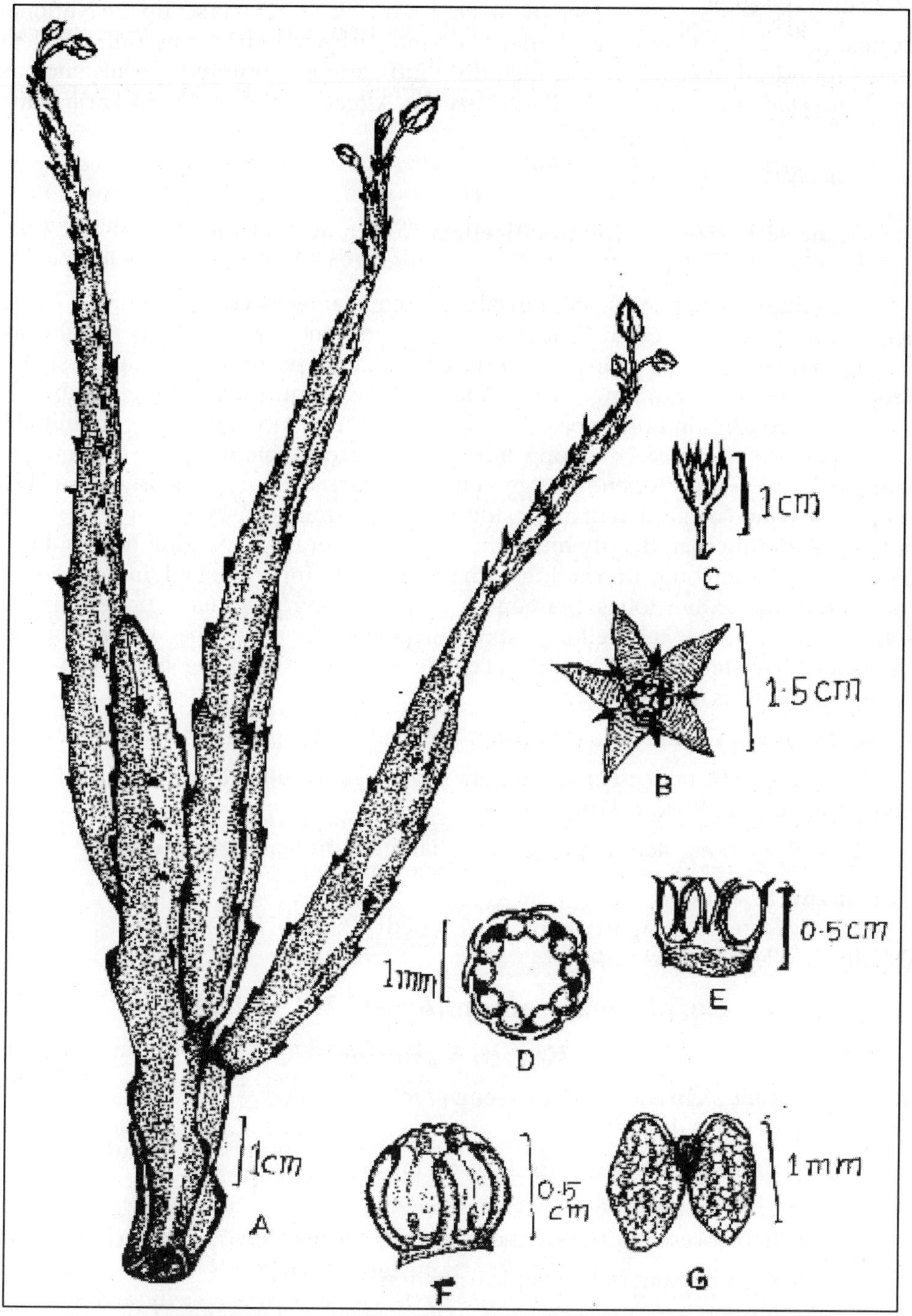

Figure 6.19: ***Caralluma sarkariae*** **Lavranos et Frandsen** ***var. sarkariae***
A: Twig; B: Flower; C: Sepals; D: Upper view of corona;
E: Side view of outer corona; F: Side view of coronal series; G: Pollinia

This species is a good garden plant. Dr. J. Sarkaria (1987) has set up the National Cactus and Succulent Botanical Garden at Chandigarh and he has grown all succulent plants found all over the world including indigenous attractive species such as *Caralluma bhupinderiana* and *Caralluma sarkariae.* After death of Dr. J.S. Sarkaria many of these succulents are neglected.

Tamil Nadu (endemic).

Caralluma sarkariae var. **longipedicellata** Aditya in Asklepios 110: 18-24. 2011. Type: Madurai, India, 10-5-2010, Soumen Aditya SA 50-126M (K. holotype).

Stem fleshy, squarish angled, 1 m tall, ca 15 cm diameter across, tapering towards apex, angles acute. Leaves small, apetiolate, 3 x 1 mm, lanceolate, acute apex, glabrous. Flowers axillary, produced in pairs or thrice, on lateral position of the apical stems. Pedicel terete, 6 – 7 mm long, ca 1 mm in diam., with purple markings, glabrous. Calyx 5-lobed, divided up to base, lobes ca 3 x 2 mm, lanceolate, apex acuminate, glabrous. Corolla tube ca 4 mm long, lobes 5, ca 6 x 2 mm, oblong, apex acute, margin without hairs, widely open, orange yellow to dark brown, sometimes purplish transverse bands on basal half inner side. Corona staminal, biseriate, outer 5-lobed, at first ascending then deeply bifid, the segment laterally diverging horizontally, filiform ca 1.5 mm long, alternating with the stamens; inner 5-lobed, incumbent on the back of the anther lobes. Stamens 5, ca 2 mm long, pollinia 5, pollen masses solitary in each anther cell, yellow, waxy with pellucid layer attached by dark brown caudicles. Gynostegium ca 2 mm long. Follicles paired, ca 8 cm long, linear, brownish streaked, glabrous (Plate 6.18).

Distribution: Tamil Nadu (Madurai, Theni and Dindigul district; endemic).

Flowering and Fruiting: Throughout the year. In cultivation flowered only in March and September (Aditya, 2011b).

Etymology: Long slender pedicel is a characteristic feature of this species.

Specimens Examined

Tamil Nadu: Usilampatty kanavai, Theni dt., 20.8.2011, S. Karuppusamy 1026 (Madura College herbarium).

Caralluma stalagmifera C.E.C. Fisch.

Key to Varieties

1. Angles of the stem acute; pedicel semi-erect, greenish; flowers <1 cm in diameter .... var. *intermedia*
1. Angles of the stem terete; pedicel erect, pink or purple; flowers >1 cm in diameter 2
2. Spindle hairs present all along the margin of corolla lobes .... var. *longipetala*
2. Spindle hairs present only on apical portion of corolla lobes or absent .... var. *stalagmifera*

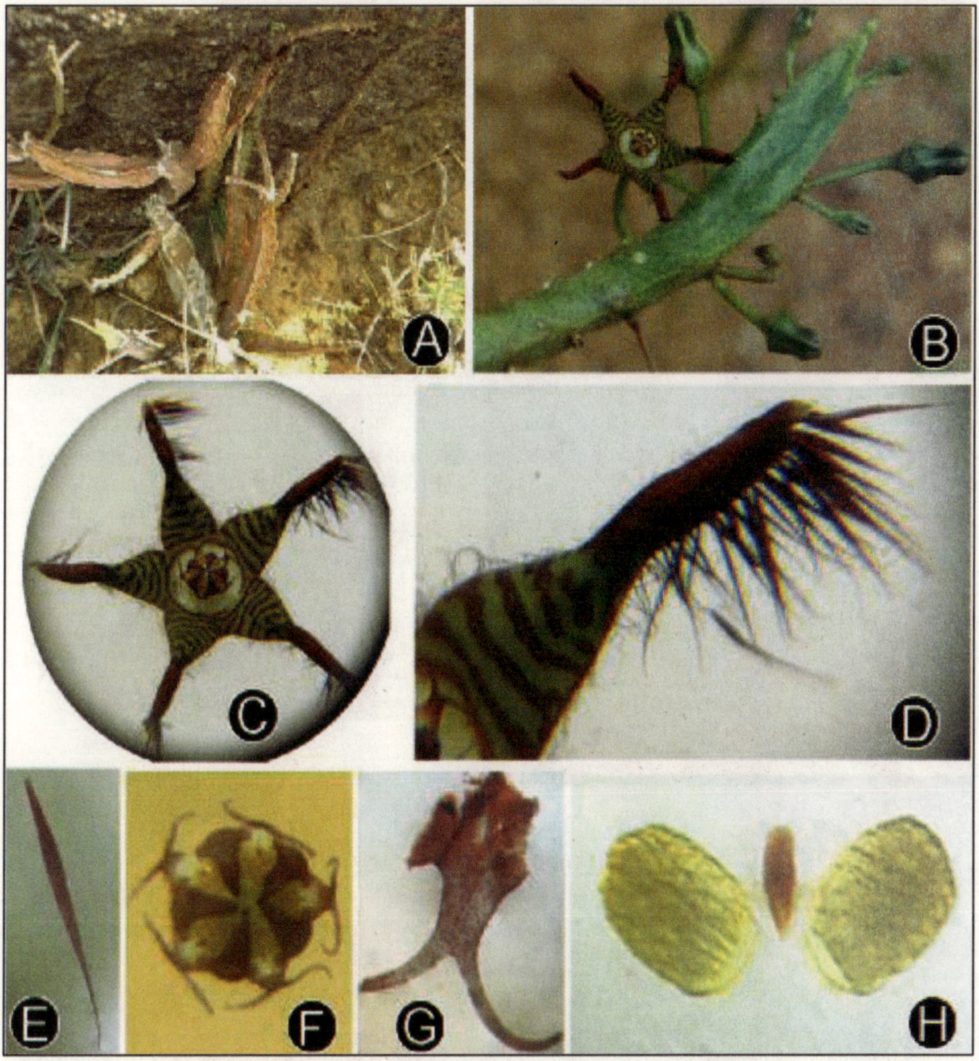

Plate 6.15. ***Caralluma geniculata*** **(Gravely et Mayuranathan) Meve et Liede**
A: Natural habitat; B: Inflorescence; C: Flower; D: Petal; E: Hair; F: Corona; G: Outer corona; H: Pollinia

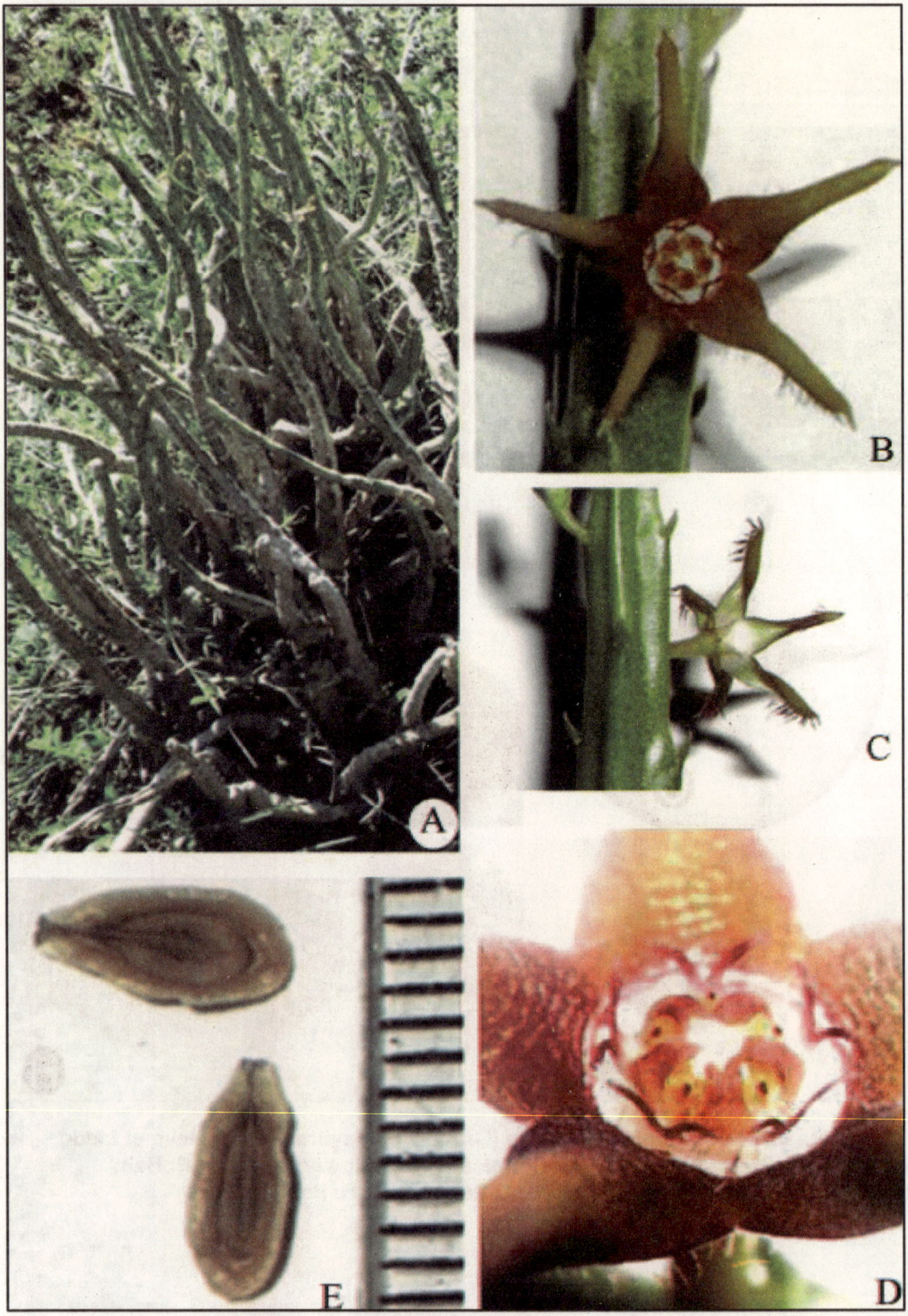

Plate: 6.16. *Caralluma moorei* Aditya
A: Natural habitat; B: Flower front side; C: Flower backside; D: Corona; E: Seeds
(Courtesy: Aditya)

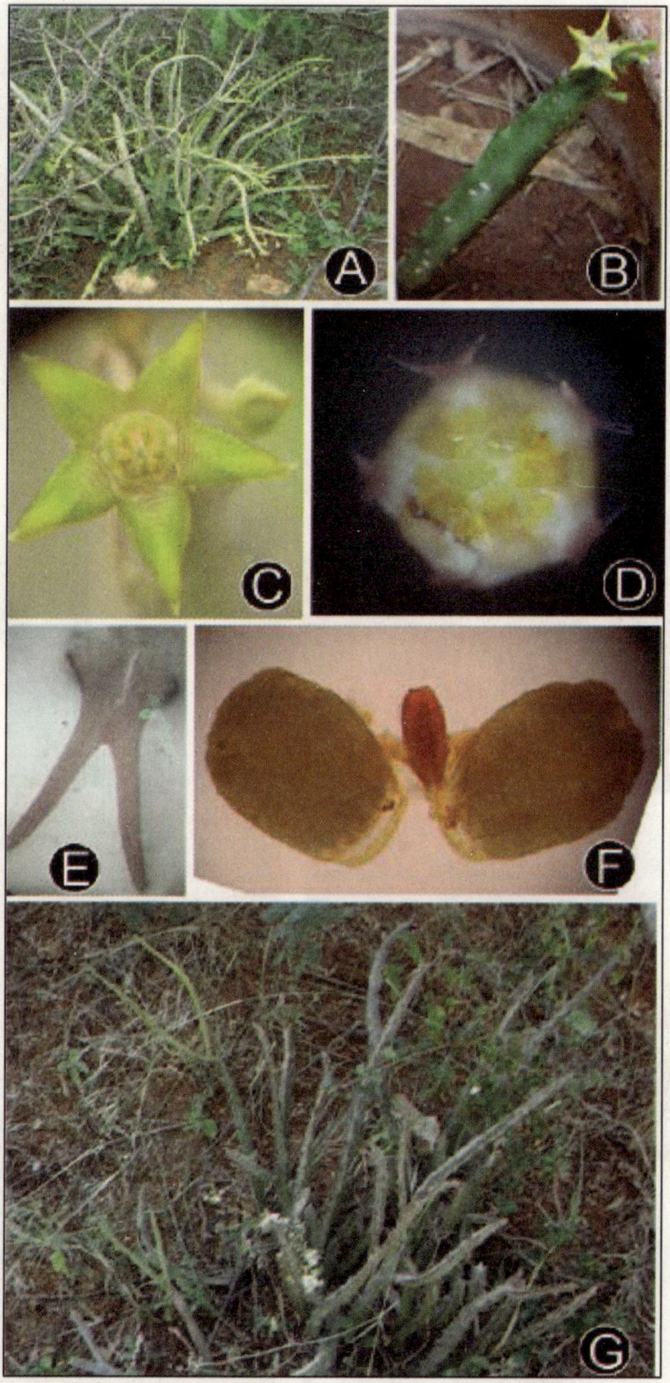

Plate 6.17: ***Caralluma sarkarieae*** **Lavranos et Frandsen var.** ***sarkariae***
A: Natural habitat; B: Inflorescence; C: Flower; D: Corona; E: Outer corona; F: Pollinia; G: Fruit

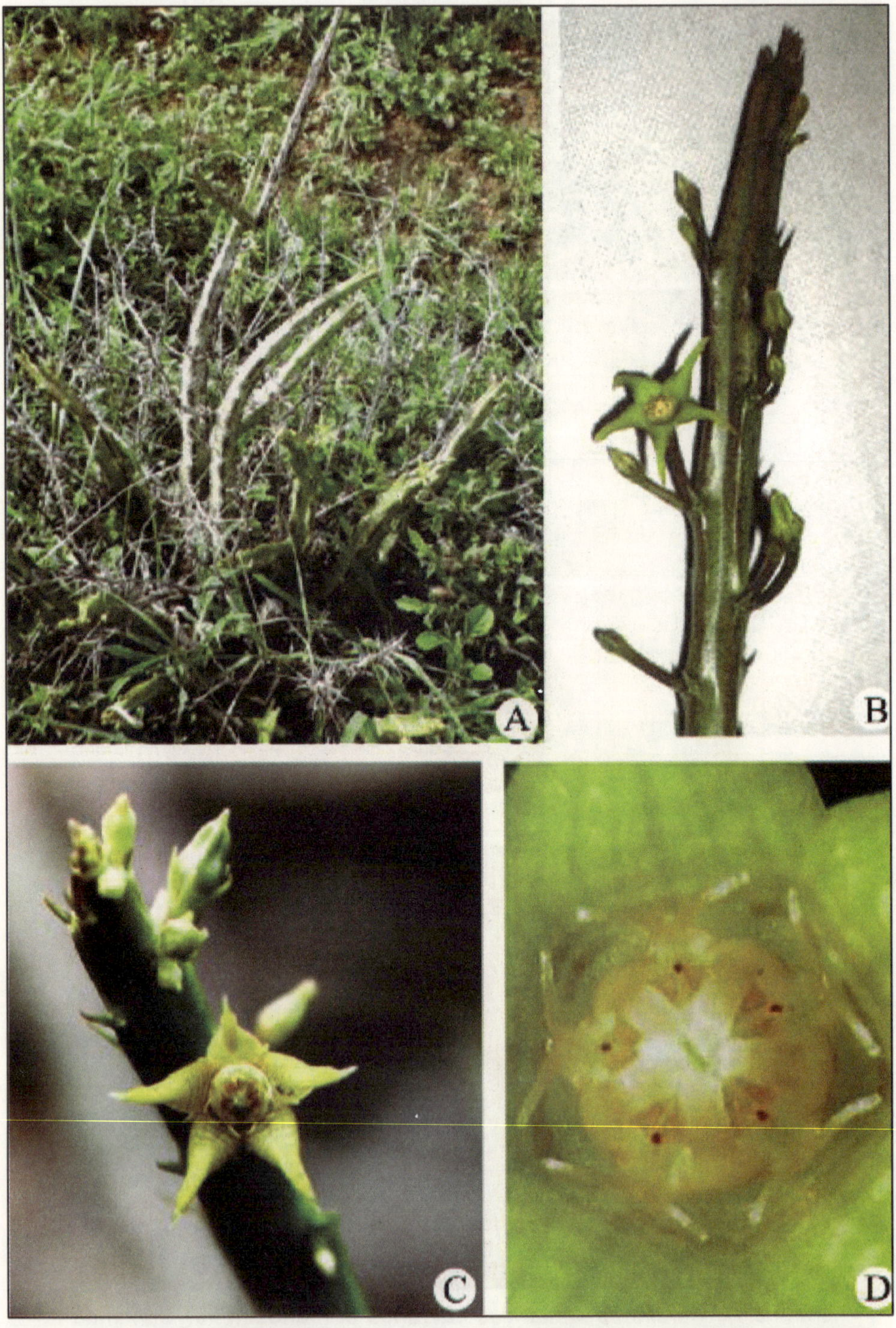

Plate 6.18. ***Caralluma sarkarieae*** **Lavranos et Frandsen var.** ***longipedicellata*** **Aditya**
A: Natural habitat; B: Inflorescence; C: Flower; D: Corona
(Courtesy: Aditya)

Caralluma stalagmifera C. E. C. Fisch. in Bull. Misc. Inform. Kew 1925: 431.1925. Type: India, Madras (*Mayuranathan s.n.* (K); Sharma *et al.*, Fl. Karnataka 165. 1984; S.R. Srinivasan in A.N. Henry *et al.* Fl. Tamil Nadu Anal. 2: 82. 1987; Gilbert in Bradleya 8: 16.1990; Plowes in Haseltonia 3: 52. 1995; Jagtap and Singh Fasc. Fl. India. 24: 206.1999.Type: S. India, Vandalur, near Madras, Mayuranathan (comm. F.H. Gravely, May, 1925); Meve and Liede in Plant Syst. Evol. 234: 200. 2002. var. **stalagmifera**; Karuppusamy and Pullaiah in Rheedea 17: 41. 2007.

Shrubs; stems fleshy, branched; branches 70 cm tall, quadrangular; internodes small, 6-11 mm long, 2.5-8 mm across, distally terete, glabrous. Leaves decussate, sessile, 3-4 x 0.5-1 mm, triangular, pointed at tip, fleshy, glabrous. Flowers axillary, solitary; bracts minute, triangular; pedicel terete, erect, up to 6 mm long, ca. 1 mm in diameter, glabrous; calyx five-lobed, divided up to base, lobes ca 2.5 x 1.5 mm, triangular, apex acuminate, fleshy, glabrous; corolla campanulate, ca. 8 mm long; corolla tube ca. 2 mm long; lobes five, ca. 6 x 1.5 mm, ovate-lanceolate, deeply purplish red inside, apiculate with spindle shaped, easily detachable hairs hanging all along the distal margin and apex; corona staminal, biseriate; outer lobes of two erect, linear-lanceolate slightly curved segments, ca. 1.5 mm long; inner lobes arising between the outer corona lobes at their base, incumbent over the anthers; stamens five, ca. 2 mm long; pollinia five, pollen masses solitary in each anther cell, yellow, waxy, attached by light brown caudicles; gynostegium ca. 1.5 mm long. Follicles paired, creamy white in young, light purplish streaked, ca. 6-11 x 0.5-1 cm, tapering towards apex, glabrous (Plate 6.19; Figure 6.20).

Distribution: INDIA (Andhra Pradesh, Tamil Nadu, Karnataka), endemic.

Abundance: Very common.

Flowering and Fruiting: June-July.

Chromosome number: 2n = 22 (Navaneetham 1980, 1981).

Etymology: Stalagmite crystal-like hairs on the corolla tip and margins of the flower of this species.

Specimens Examined

Andhra Pradesh: Chittoor dt., Horsley hills, S. Karuppusamy 27931 (SKU); Cuddapah dt., Gunjana river bed, J.L. Ellis 29797 (MH).

Karanataka: Dharwad dt., Soundatti hills, 26.3.2008, A. Ugraiah 31705 (SKU), Tumkur dt., Basti betta, 29.4.2008, S. Karuppusamy and A. Ugraiah 31769 (SKU); Mysore dt., Hirisave, 27.10.1969, C. J. Saldanha 15346 (CAL); Mandya dt., Malavalli-Kollegal road, 14.5.1978, S.B. Manohar and S.R. Ramesh 7531 (CAL).

Tamil Nadu: Madurai dt., Nagamalai hills, S. Karuppusamy 27910 (SKU); Dindigal dt., Sirumalai hills, S. Karuppusamy 27812 (SKU).

Caralluma stalagmifera C. E. C. Fisch. var. **intermedia** Karuppusamy et Pullaiah in Rheedea 17: 45. 2007. Type: INDIA, Andhra Pradesh, Anantapur district, Hillocks opposite to Gooty Railway station, 19 August 2005, S. Karuppusamy 26991 (Holotype, SKU; Isotypes, MH).

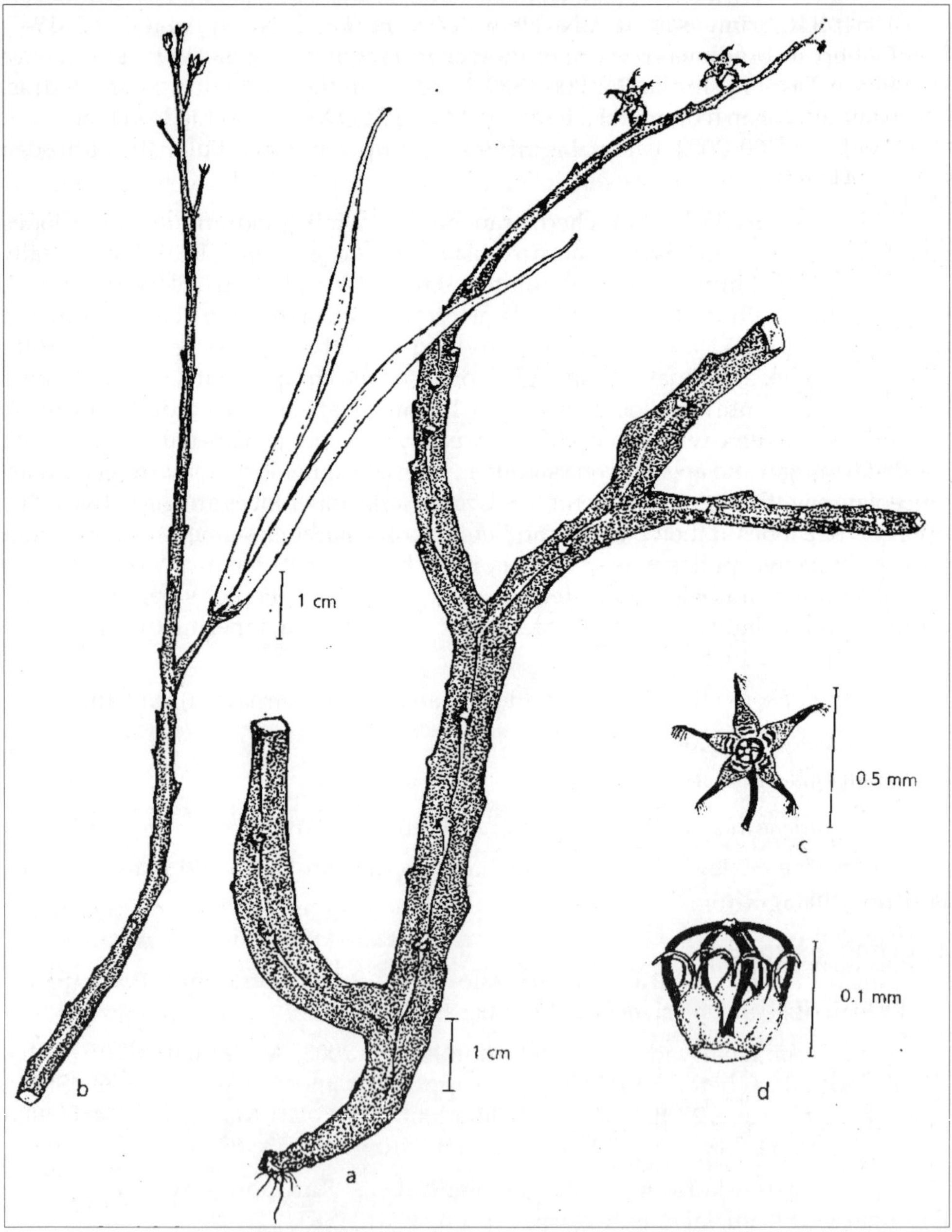

Figure 6.20: *Caralluma stalagmifera* C.E.C. Fisch. var. *intermedia* Karuppusamy et Pullaiah
A: Flowering twig; B: Fruiting twig; C: Flower; D: Corona

Shrubs; stems fleshy, branched; branches 1 m tall, quadrangular; internodes 10-15 mm long and 2.5-10 mm across, quadrangular, glabrous. Leaves decussate, sessile, 3.5 x 0.5-1 mm, triangular, pointed at apex, fleshy, glabrous. Flowers axillary, solitary; bracts minute, triangular; pedicel terete, semi-erect, up to 5 mm long, ca. 1 mm in diameter, pinkish, glabrous. Calyx five-lobed, divided up to base, lobes ca. 2 x 0.5 mm, triangular, apex acuminate, fleshy, glabrous. Corolla rotate or campanulate, ca. 6 mm long, ca. 1 mm across; corolla- tube ca. 1.5 mm long; lobes five, ca. 5 x 1.2 mm, ovate-lanceolate streak at base, tip yellowish brown, spindle hairs a very few at tip or absent; corona staminal, biseriate; outer lobes formed of two semi-erect, linear-lanceolate curved segments, ca. 1 mm long; inner lobes arising from between the outer corona lobes at their base, incumbent over the anthers; stamens five, ca. 1 mm long; pollinia five, pollen masses solitary in each anther cell, yellow, waxy, attached by dark brown caudicles; gynostegium ca. 2.5 mm long. Follicles paired, creamy white with light purplish streaks, ca. 5-8 x 0.5-0.8 cm, tapering towards apex, glabrous (Plate 6.20; Figure 6.21).

Note: This variety is allied to *C.stalagmifera* var. *stalagmifera* and *C. stalagmifera* var. *longipetala* but differs in having distally attenuating, acute angled stem, small flowers, a few or no spindle hairs at tip of the corolla lobe, chestnut brown corolla, sometimes with a very few yellow streaks at basal portion and short pendulous pedicel.

Distribution: India: Andhra Pradesh and Tamil Nadu, endemic.

Abundance: Not very common.

Flowering and fruiting: July-August.

Etymology: Flowe size is medium between other two varieties of the species.

Specimens Examined

Andhra Pradesh: Anantapur dt., Hills opposite Gooty Rly station, 23.4.2008, S. Karuppusamy and A. Ugraiah, 31710 (SKU, MH).

Caralluma stalagmifera C. E. C. Fisch. var. **longipetala** Karuppusamy et Pullaiah in Rheedea 17. 45. 2007. Type: INDIA, Tamil Nadu, Madurai district, waste lands near airport, 28 July 2005, S. Karuppusamy 27968 (Holotype, SKU; Isotype, MH).

Shrubs, stems fleshy, branched; branches slender, 1 m tall, deeply green, quadrangular at base, terete towards apex; internodes 10-30 mm long, 3-15 mm across, glabrous. Leaves decussate, sessile, 4-6 x 0.5-1.5 mm, lanceolate, pointed at apex, fleshy, glabrous. Flowers axillary, solitary; bracts large, 0.2 mm long, triangular; pedicels terete, erect, up to 15 mm long and ca. 1 mm in diameter, glabrous. Calyx five-lobed, divided up to base, lobes ca. 3.5 x 1.5 mm, lanceolate, apex acuminate, fleshy, glabrous. Corolla campanullate, ca. 13 mm long, ca. 1 mm across; corolla tube ca. 2.2 mm long; lobes 5, ca. 8.5 x 1.5 mm, linear-lanceolate, dark purple or dark brown inside, apiculate with spindle shaped hairs along the margin and apex; corona staminal, biseriate; outer lobes formed of two semi-erect, linear lanceolate curved segments, ca. 2 mm long; inner lobes arising from between the outer corona lobes at

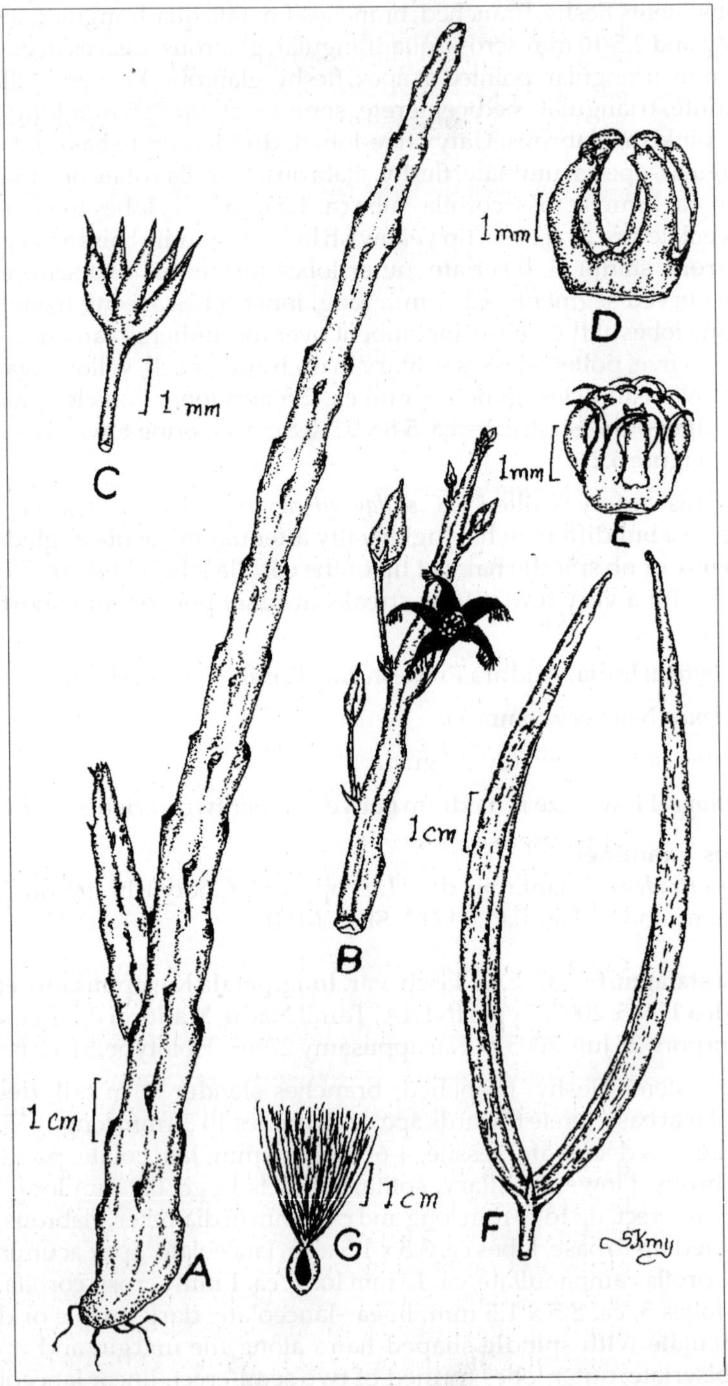

Figure 6.21: *Caralluma stalagmifera* C.E.C.Fisch. var. *stalagmifera*
A: Twig; B: Inflorescence; C: Pedicel with petals; D: Corona; F: Fruit, G: Seed

their base, incumbent over the anthers; stamens 5, ca. 2.5 mm long; pollinia 5, pollen masses solitary in each anther cell, yellow, waxy, attached by dark brown caudicles; gynostegium ca. 2.5 mm long. Follicles paired, terete, purplish streaked, ca. 11-15 x 0.5-1 cm, tapering towards apex, glabrous (Plate 6.21; Figure 6.22).

Distribution: India (Tamil Nadu- Madurai district), endemic.

Abundance: Very few populations in waste lands.

Flowering and fruiting: February-August.

Etymology: Elongated petals in the variety.

Specimens Examined

Tamil Nadu: Tamil Nadu: Madurai dt., waste lands near Airport, 28.7.2005, S. Karuppusamy 27968 (Holotype, SKU; Isotype, MH). Madurai dt., near MKU road side, 4.5.2008, S. Karuppusamy and A. Ugraiah, 31715 (SKU).

Notes: This variety is allied to *C. stalagmifera* var. *stalagmifera,* but differs in having the stem distally attenuating in varying degrees, large flowers and spindle hairs along the margin of corolla lobes.

***Caudanthera* Plowes in Haseltonia 3: 58-59.1995**

= *Cryptolluma* Plowes, Haseltonia 3: 57. 1995.

= *Spiralluma* Plowes, Haseltonia 3: 53. 1995.

Type: *Cryptolluma edulis* Plowes

Plants with a rhizomatous habit and slender tapering sub-cylindrical, purple-streaked, edible stems; branching infrequent, epicutaneous, basal. Flowers on the undifferentiated stem-apex, apical flowering portion of stem ultimately deciduous; occasional subsequent pedunculate branches from apical axils. Leaves lanceolate, stipular glands terete, lacking hairs; corolla tube globose, glabrous. Gynostegium stipitate: corpusculum flange-winged, clavate.

Distribution: NW India and Pakistan via SW Arabian and northern Somali coast to red sea coast of Sudan.

Caudanthera edulis (Edgew.) Meve et Liede. in Plant Syst. Evol. 234: 201. 2002. *Boucerosia edulis* Edgew. in J. Linn. Soc. 6: 205. 1862. Type: India, Multan, Edgeworth 6035 (K, holo.). *Cryptolluma edulis* (Edgew.) Plowes in Haseltonia 3: 57.1995. *Caralluma edulis* Benth. et Hook. f. Gen. Pl. 2: 782. 1876; Hooker f. Fl. Brit. India 4: 76. 1883; Cooke, Fl. Pres. Bombay 2: 244.1905; Gravely and Mayuranathan in Bull. Madr. Govt. Mus. N. S. 4(1): 16. 1931; Bhandari Fl. Indian Desert. 220. 1978; Gilbert, in Bradleya 8: 14. 1990; Jagtap and Singh in Fasc. Fl. India 24: 202. 1999. *Spiralluma longidens* Plowes in Haseltonia: 53.1995. *Caralluma vittata* N. E. Br., Th.-Dyer, Fl. Trop.Afr. 4(1): 483 1904. *Boucerosia stocksiana* Boiss. Fl. Orient. 4: 63.1879. *Desmidorchis stocksiana* Kuntze, Rev. Gen.: 418. 1891.

Succulent, branched, perennial herb, stems erect, 15-60 cm high with viscous watery sap, stolons whitish; erect branches green or with longitudinal grey blotches

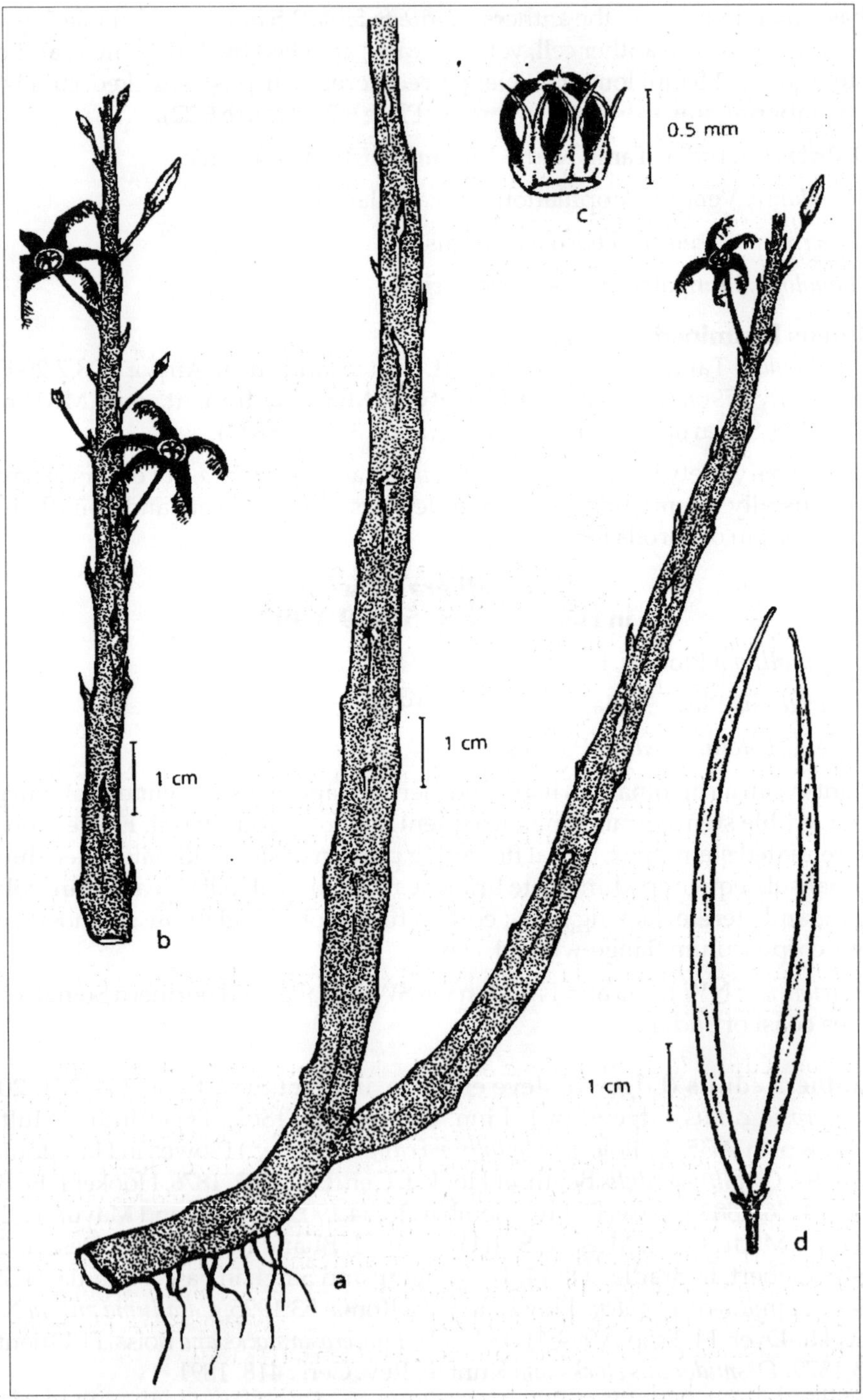

Figure 6.22: *Caralluma stalagmifera* var. *longipetala* Karuppusamy et Pullaiah
A: Habit; B: Inflorescence; C: Corona; D: Fruit

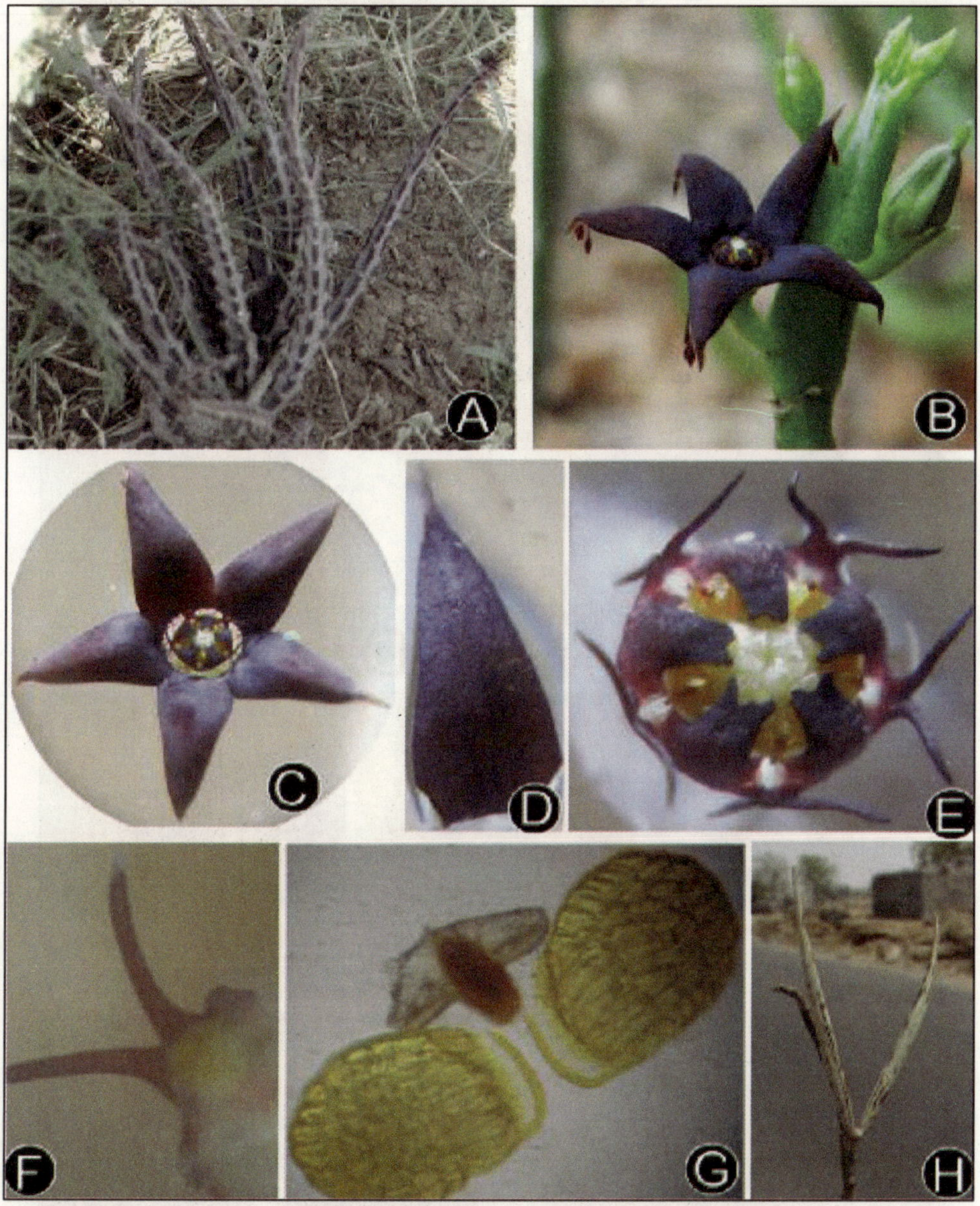

Plate 6.19. ***Caralluma stalagmifera*** **C.E.C.Fischer var.** ***stalagmifera***
A: Natural habitat; B: Inflorescence; C: Flower; D: Petal; E: Corona; F: Outer corona; G: Pollinia; H: Fruit.

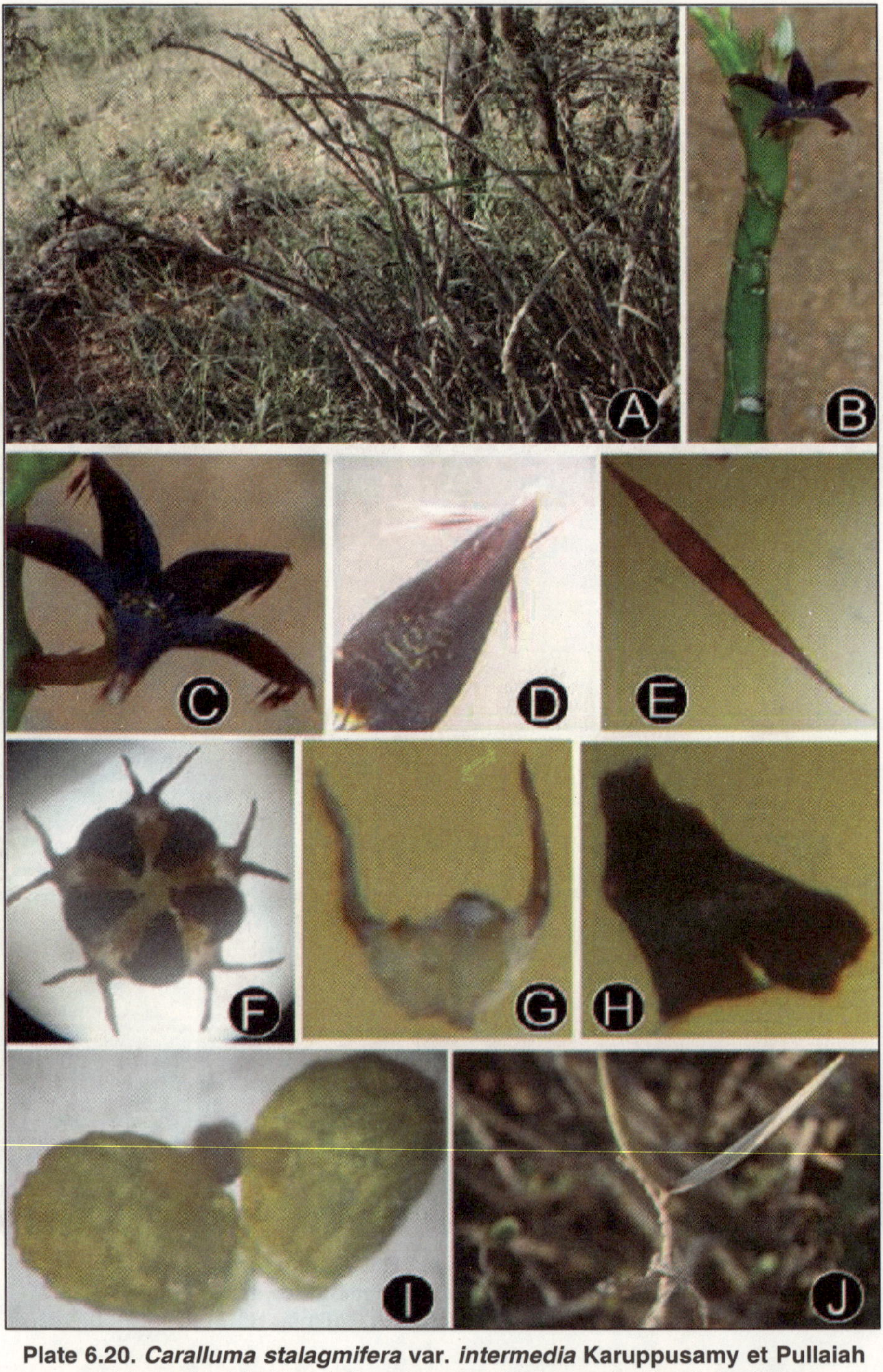

Plate 6.20. ***Caralluma stalagmifera*** **var.** ***intermedia*** **Karuppusamy et Pullaiah**
A: Natural habitat; B: Inflorescence; C: Flower; D: Petal; E: Hair; F: Corona; G: Outer corona; H: Inner corona; I: Pollinia; J: Fruit

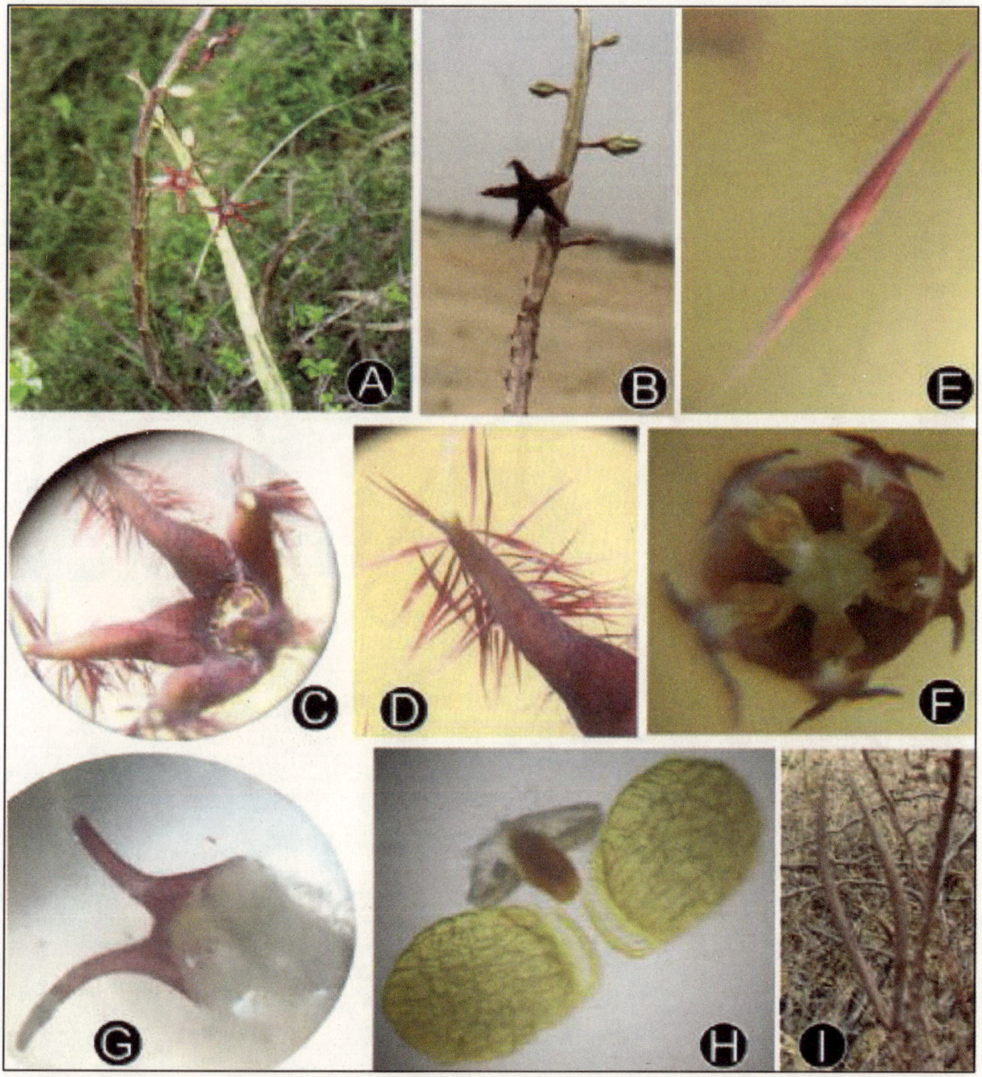

Plate 6.21. ***Caralluma stalagmifera*** **var.** ***longipetala*** **Karuppusamy et Pullaiah**
A: Natural habitat; B: Inflorescence; C: Flower; D: Petal; E: Hair; F: Corona; G: Outer corona; H: Pollinia; I: Fruit

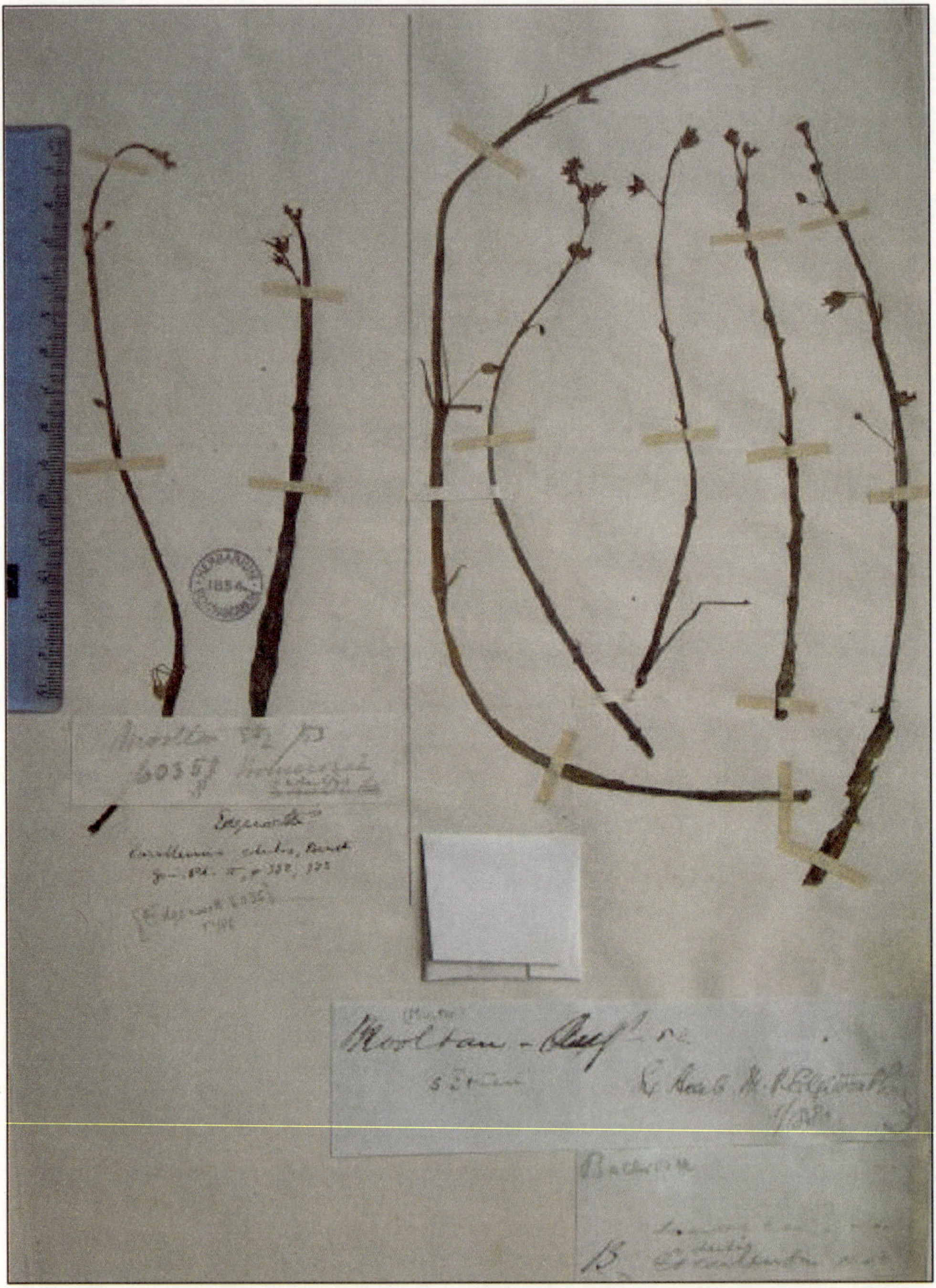

Figure 6.23: Type Specimen of *Boucerosia edulis* Edgew. (=*Caudanthera edulis* Edgew. Plowes) in J. Linn. Soc. 6: 205. 1962. Type: India, Multan, Edgeworth 6035 (K, holo)

throughout, distinctly tapering distally, 4-angled; angles rounded and toothed with scars of the fallen leaves. Leaves 6-8 x 2 mm, ovate-lanceolate, sessile, acute, soon caduceus, leaving upwardly directed protuberances on the stem. Flowers paired from the axils of the leaves on tender portions; pedicel slender, 2 cm long, sub pendulous then erect, with 2 minute subulate bracts. Calyx lobes 3 x 1 mm, divided to the base, ovate-lanceolate, acute, margins membranous. Corolla glabrous on both sides, with longitudinal purplish lines inside, divided half-way down, glabrous, lobes 5, 3-4 mm long, ovate-lanceolate, acute, margins slightly recurved. Corona in two rows, the outer 5-lobed, cupular, each lobe produced into 2 distinct, subulate teeth; inner corona 1 mm long, linear, subacute. Staminal column short, arising from the bottom of the corolla; pollen masses subhorizontal. Follicles in pair, 12-17 x 0.8-0.9 cm, slender, smooth, terete, lanceolate, tapering to a sharp point. Seeds to 9 x 3 mm, brown, margin winged; coma 2.5 cm long (Plate 6.22; Figures 6.23, 6.24).

Distribution: *INDIA*: This species is distributed in waste lands of sandy soil near Jaisalmer and Jodhpur districts of Rajasthan.

WORLD: *Caudanthera edulis* has been reported from Mauritania, Sudan, Eritrea, Somalia, Saudi Arabia, United Arab Emirates, Pakistan, India and possibly Iran and Afghanistan.

Abundance: Not very common

Flowering and fruiting: September –December.

Chromosome number: 2n= 22, 44.

Etymology: From the Latin 'edule' means edible; this species is used for edible purposes in Northern India.

Specimens Examined

Rajasthan: Jaisalmer dt., Kuyyala surroundings, 14.11.2008, A. Ugraiah 31764 (SKU);

Jodhpur dt., Bilad, 10.11.2009, A. Ugraiah 37716 (SKU); Mohangharh, 28.8.1964, B.M. Wadhwa 5071 (CAL).

Nomenclatural notes: *Desmidorchis stocksiana* and *Caralluma mouretii,* both species were placed as synonyms of *Caralluma edulis* by Bruyns (Bradleya 7/1989) and this position also was adopted by Gilbert (1990), this is not accepted here. It is hard to understand why Bruyns placed *Spiralluma longidens* under *Caralluma edulis*, as he indicated that he had examined the type specimen –this sheet has a set of three very clear drawings by N. E. Brown showing the unusual circinate inner corona lobes, the short erect extension at the apex of the anther, and the obtriangular pollinium, all of which represent major divergences from those of *Caudanthera edulis*; in addition, the color of the corolla lobes of *Spiralluma longidens* is also different, as was noted by Brown in his description.

Similarly, the protologue of *Spiralluma mouretii* states that it also possesses circinate inner corona lobes, and the type sheet shows that there are significant differences in the corolla compared with *Caudanthera edulis* (twice as large and campanulate-urceolate with shorter lobes). In addition, the type sheet of *Spiralluma*

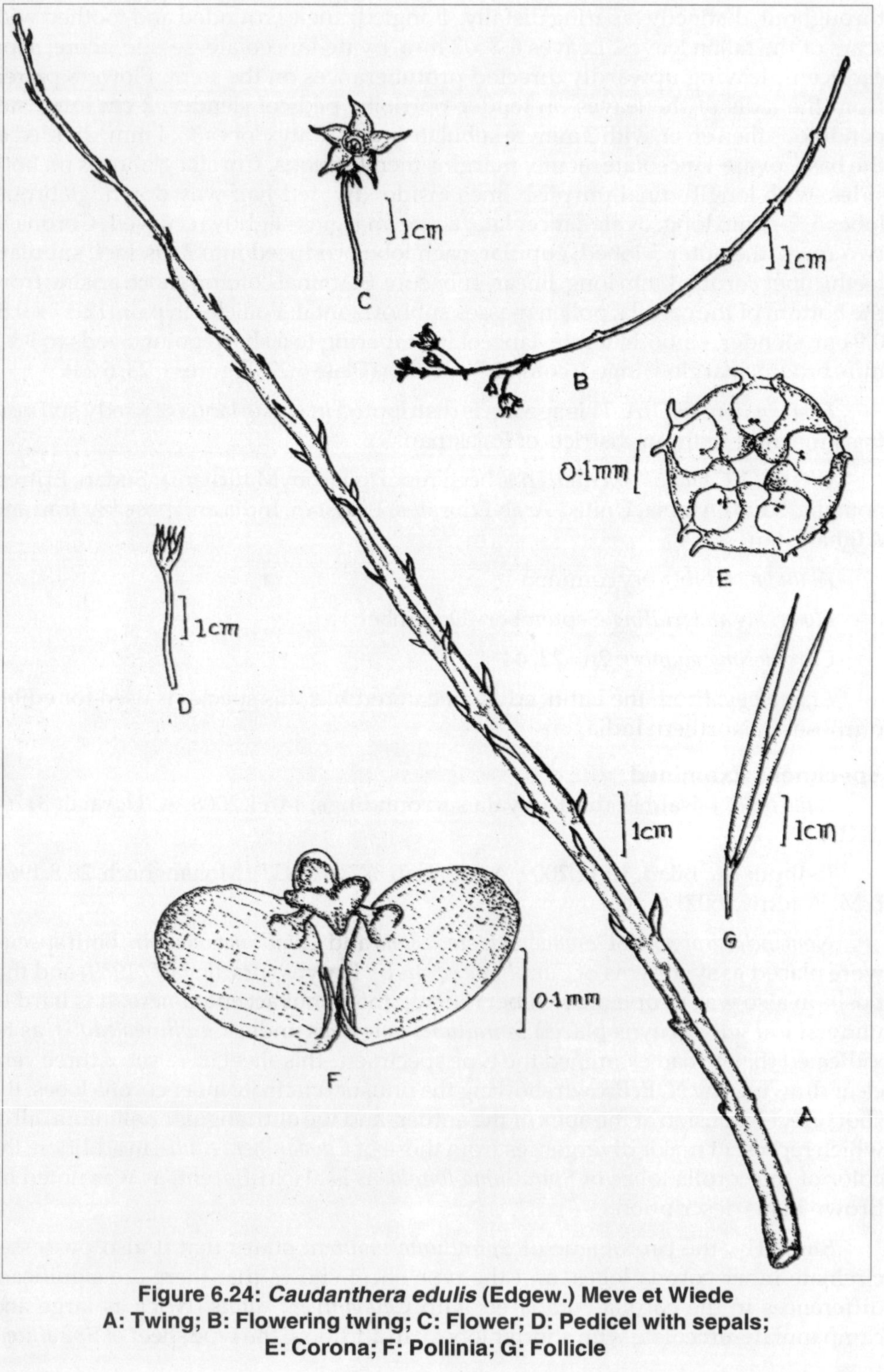

Figure 6.24: ***Caudanthera edulis*** **(Edgew.) Meve et Wiede**
A: Twing; B: Flowering twing; C: Flower; D: Pedicel with sepals;
E: Corona; F: Pollinia; G: Follicle

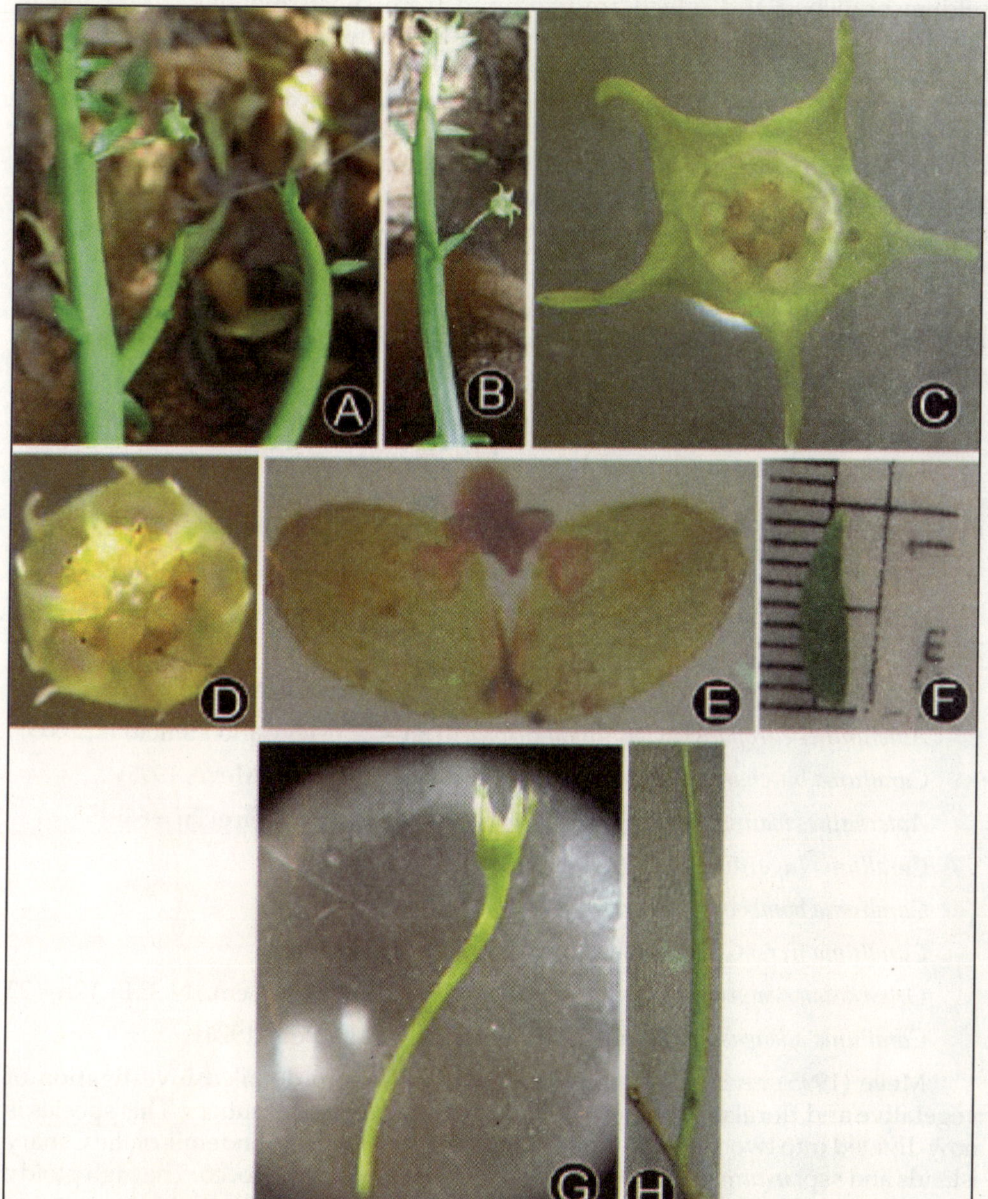

Plate 6.22. ***Caudanthera edulis*** **(Edgew.) Meve et Liede**
A: Natural habitat; B: Inflorescence; C: Flower;
D: Corona; E: Pollinia; F: Leaf; G: Pedicel; H: Fruit

mouretii shows that it is a shrubby much branched monopodial plant with linear stems, whereas *Caudanthera edulis* has slender erect tapering 35 cm tall stems that are seldom branched and which are produced from short rhizomes. The habit of *Spiralluma longidens* is not known: however, the material on Schweinfurth's type sheet suggests that were broken off from a shrubby plant because they are thicker at the base. If the habit of *S. longidens* was also rhizomatous as in *Caudanthera edulis*, then the stems would be narrowed basally. *Spiralluma longidens* and *Spiralluma mouretii* do not appear to be conspecific (the flowers of *S. longidens* are smaller and closer to those of *Caudanthera edulis* in size, and there are other differences) despite both Gilbert and Raynal arriving at this determination in notes on the type sheet of *Spiralluma mouretii* (Paris).

Uses: Fresh stems of *Caudanthera edulis* are edible and are sold as a vegetable in local vegetable shops ('situn') at Jaisalmer in India. As a succulent herb it has ornamental value.

Chromosome Numbers of Other *Caralluma* Species

The basic chromosome number in the genus *Caralluma (sensu lato)* n = 11 is constant in all the genera segregated from *Caralluma* and diploid number 2n = 22 is the more frequent. Six tetraploids and five hexaploids are known.

Caudanthera sinaica (Decne) Plowes 2n = 22 (Loewenstern and Garbari, 2004)

Borealluma plicatiloba (Lavranos) Plowes 2n = 22 (Loewenstern and Garbari, 2004)

Apteranthes negevensis (Zohary) Plowes 2n = 22 (Loewenstern and Garbari, 2004)

Apteranthes europaea (=*Caralluma europaea*) 2n = 22 (Meve and Heneidak, 2005)

Caralluma burchardii ssp. *maura* Meve et F.Albers 2n = 66 (Meve, 1995)

Apteranthes joannis (Maire) Plowes (=*Caralluma joannis* Meire) 2n = 66

Caralluma lugardi 2n = 22 (Albers, 1976)

Caralluma bomboensis Verd. 2n = 44 (Albers, 1976)

Caralluma frerei G.D.Rowley 2n = 44 (Albers, 1981)

Orbea decaisneana (Lem.) Bruyns (= *Caralluma decaisneana* (Lem.) N,.E.Br.) 2n = 22

Caralluma adenensis (M.Deflers) A.Berger 2n = 22 (Albers, 1976)

Meve (1995) revised *Caralluma burchardii* based on detailed investigation of vegetative and floral morphology as well as chromosome numbers. This species is now divided into two taxa, the dodecaploid ssp. *burchardii*, an endemic of the Canary islands and ssp. *maura*, a hexaploid from the West coast of Morocco. The high ploidy levels involved, the highest known in the Asclepiadaceae, are discussed in conjunction with biogeographical aspects.

Caralluma Websites

http://www.asclepiad-exhibition.org/Notes_Caralluma.htm

http://caralluma.tv/caralluma-explained.php

http://www.absoluteastronomy.com/topics/Caralluma

http://carallumafimbriatamfg.com/Caralluma_Fimbriata_information.html

http://www.fda.gov/ohrms/dockets/dockets/95s0316/95s-0316-rpt0252-08-Exhibit-02-vol184.pdf

http://www.livestrong.com/article/189005-what-is-caralluma/

http://en.wikipedia.org/wiki/Caralluma

http://caralluma.ash.com/caralluma.html

http://en.wikipedia.org/wiki/Caralluma_fimbriata

http://carallumareviewswarning.com/

http://carallumafimbriata.ash.com/

https://www.dragonherbs.com/prodinfo.asp?number=529

http://www.shopping.com/caralluma/products

http://thyroid.about.com/od/loseweightsuccessfully/a/caralluma.htm

http://www.webmd.com/vitamins-supplements/ingredientmono-1160-CARALLUMA.aspx?activeIngredientId=1160&activeIngredientName=CARALLUMA

http://carallumafimbriatamfg.com/

http://carallumasafe.in/caralluma/

http://www.carallumafimbriata-extremeweightloss.com/

http://caralluma.us/

http://www.shopping.com/caralluma/products~NS-1~linkin_id-8011124~cid-5405835109

http://www.thyroid-info.com/articles/caralluma.htm

http://www.carallumaburn.us/

http://www.carallumafimbriata.net/

http://www.ehow.com/about_5127416_caralluma.html

www.aggressivehealthshop.com/caralluma.htm

http://carallumareview.org/

http://www.caralluma-actives.net/

http://www.succulent-plant.com/families/asclepiadaceae/caralluma.html

http://carallumareviewswarnings.com/

http://www.mynaturalslimming.webs.com/caralluma.htm

http://www.dietsinreview.com/diets/Caralluma_Burn/

http://carallumafimbriata1.wetpaint.com/

http://caralluma.com.au/

http://www.nextag.com/caralluma/products-html

http://carallumaactivereviews.com/caralluma-review

http://carallumaactivereviews.com/

http://www.carallumaburnreviews.com/

http://www.facebook.com/pages/Caralluma/140827409276993?v=stream

http://ezinearticles.com/?Caralluma—The-Next-Hoodia?&id=239654

http://www.flowersofindia.in/catalog/slides/Caralluma.html

http://www.tradeavail.com/caralluma.html

http://caralluma.thepowerof30.com/

http://natural-appetitesuppressants.com/Caralluma.html

http://www.lifenatural.com/caralluma.htm

http://www.ehow.com/about_5729379_caralluma-fimbriata-side-effects.html

http://www.facebook.com/pages/Caralluma-fimbriata/127318780645235

http://getdietsolutions.com/caralluma/

http://www.fitnesstipsforlife.com/caralluma-appetite-suppressant.html

http://carallumafimbriataextract.org/

http://carallumafimbriatatrial.com/

http://www.maxoutbody.com/proxylean.php

http://carallumaactivesinfo.com/

http://store.naturalnews.com/index.php?main_page=product_info&cPath=100370&products_id=1003975

http://www.dietspotlight.com/caralluma-review/

http://www.carallumaburn.org/

http://www.carallumaburnfat.com/

http://www.slimaluma.com/caralluma.htm

http://caralluma.org.uk/

http://www.carallumaburnfat.com/caralluma-fimbriata.html

http://www.tucson-gardener.com/graphics/succulent/Caralluma.html

http://www.slimmingpillsreview.com/caralluma/

http://carallumaburnreview.org/

http://carallumaextract.wetpaint.com/

http://www.caralluma.tv/

http://caralluma.wikispaces.com/

http://www.carallumaactiveswebsite.com/

http://www.botany.com/caralluma.html

http://where-to-buy-caralluma-fimbriata.blogspot.com/

http://caralluma-weight-loss.blogspot.com/

http://www.buycarallumaburn.com/

http://www.carallumaburn.co.uk/

http://www.carallumaburn.us/caralluma-user-reviews.html

http://www.vitaminoptions.com/remedies/caralluma

http://www.iflorist.co.uk/p-1336-caralluma.aspx

http://www.absoluteastronomy.com/topics/Caralluma_fimbriata

http://au.shopping.com/caralluma/products

http://carallumafimbriataextract.ash.com/

http://www.carallumaactivestest.com/

http://hereshowtoloseweightfast.com/caralluma-actives

http://caralluma-fimbriata-advice.com/

http://carallumaactive.com/

http://fimbriatacaralluma.com/

http://www.longevitywarehouse.com/Caralluma-p/carallumadragonherbs.htm

http://www.cactus-mall.com/stapeliad/picture2.html

http://en.goldenmap.com/Caralluma

http://carallumaextract.net/caralluma-burn/

http://vitanetonline.com/description/66054/vitamins/Caralluma-Extract/

http://www.nextag.com/Of-Caralluma/shop-html

http://www.gardening.eu/plants/Succulent-Plants/Caralluma-joannis/2909/

http://www.carallumareviewer.com/buy-caralluma/

http://www.amazon.com/s?ie=UTF8&rh=i per cent 3Aaps per cent 2Ck per cent 3Acaralluma&page=1

http://www.rxlist.com/caralluma/supplements.htm

http://carallumafimbriatamfg.com/Caralluma_Fimbriata_uses.html

http://carallumafimbriata11.blogspot.com/

http://caralluma-fimbriata-diet.com/

http://carallumaforyou.com/

http://www.slideshare.net/Margarettrem/caralluma

http://pediaview.com/openpedia/Caralluma

http://www.raysahelian.com/caralluma.html

http://doescarallumawork.com/caralluma-actives/

http://carallumaactive.org/cgi-sys/suspendedpage.cgi

http://www.physicianformulas.com/store/scripts/prodview.asp?idproduct=327&name=Caralluma

http://www.carallumaburn.biz/does-caralluma-work.html

http://carallumaactivesreview.com/tag/fimbriata/

http://www.ebay.com/sch/i.html?_nkw=caralluma

http://caralluma.edublogs.org/

http://www.iherb.com/Slimaluma-Caralluma

http://review.350.com/caralluma-actives/

http://www.carallumaburnreviews.com/ingredients-of-caralluma-burn.html

http://carallumaactivesreport.com/

http://doescarallumawork.com/privacy-policy/

http://www.carallumaactives.com/.php

http://www.trendsnnews.com/caralluma

http://www.ideamarketers.com/?What_is_Caralluma_Fimbriata&articleid=737686

http://www.carallumaactivesreview.net/

http://classifiedsforlouisiana.com/caralluma-actives/

http://www.carallumafimbriataonline.com/

http://neutral-izer.blogspot.com/2009/02/caralluma-fimbriata-weight-loss.html

http://www.gencorpacific.com/caralluma.htm

http://www.carallumafimbriatareview.org/

http://www.vitalhealthpartners.com/caralluma-fimbriata-review/

http://www.righthealth.com/topic/Caralluma

http://wheretobuycarallumafimbriata.net/

http://www.theplantlist.org/browse/A/Apocynaceae/Caralluma/

http://www.buycaralluma.biz/category/caralluma-fimbriata

http://carallumaextract.net/buy-caralluma/

http://www.arkive.org/caralluma/caralluma-flava/

http://honestreview4u.com/caralluma-fimbriata

http://bensbins.com/product/dh529.html

http://www.freepatentsonline.com/7390516.html

http://www.carallumaburnreview.net/

http://www.multiherbal.com/caralluma.html

http://www.buzzle.com/articles/caralluma-fimbriata-plant.html

http://naturamedhealth.com/caralluma_fimbriata.html

http://carallumareviewswarning.com/about

http://www.federalabs.com/analyses/Saftey per cent 20of per cent 20Caralluma.pdf

http://www.livamed.com/products/Solaray-Caralluma-500mg- per cent 252d-30-Vegetarian-Capsules.html

http://carallumafimbriataguide.org/

http://www.commentarypage.com/caralluma-burn-reviews-and-side-effects/

http://caralluma.onlinewebshop.net/

http://plants.usda.gov/java/profile?symbol=CARAL

http://sites.google.com/site/carallumafimbriata12/caralluma-fimbriata—try-it-for-free

http://caralluma-fimbriata-diet.com/caralluma/

http://www.ebay.co.uk/sch/i.html?_nkw=caralluma

http://www.carallumafimbriatareview.org/page/7/

http://www.prnewswire.com/news-releases/caralluma-fimbriata—all-natural-appetite-suppressant-58049817.html

http://www.lithops.net/caralluma_socotrana_detail.htm

http://carallumafimbriata.biz/?tag=caralluma-fimbriata-cactus

http://species.wikimedia.org/wiki/Caralluma

http://www.liquida.com/caralluma/

http://www.curvesparis.com/caralluma-actives/

http://al-hudaz.blogspot.com/

http://www.thefreelibrary.com/Caralluma+Fimbriata+-+A+Natural+Appetite+Burner-a01073872525

http://www.plantcare.com/encyclopedia/caralluma-1508.aspx

http://www.carallumaburnbonus.com/reducta/

http://www.desert-tropicals.com/Plants/Asclepiadaceae/Caralluma_socotrana.html

http://shop.qbased.com/Caralluma-Actives-Weight-Loss-s/91.htm

http://www.succulents.co.za/Asclepiadaceae/caralluma/caralluma.htm

http://www.succulents.co.za/Asclepiadaceae/caralluma/caralluma_speciosa.htm

http://www.f-lohmueller.de/botanic/Asclepiadaceae/Caralluma/Caralluma011.htm

http://www.meemelink.com/prints per cent 20pages/18464.Asclepiadaceae per cent 20- per cent 20Caralluma per cent 20fimbriata.htm

http://www.f-lohmueller.de/botanic/Asclepiadaceae/Caralluma/Caralluma01.htm

http://zipcodezoo.com/Plants/C/Caralluma_arabica/

http://jean-andre.audissou.pagesperso-orange.fr/ASCLEPIADACEAE.htm

http://www.thecactusking.com/category/plants/succulent-families/asclepiadaceae

http://www.labome.org/topics/plants/plant/angiosperms/asclepiadaceae-3673.html

http://diptera.myspecies.info/category/citation-keywords/pollinating-caralluma-sp-asclepiadaceae

http://www.labome.org/topics/organisms/plants/plant/angiosperms/asclepiadaceae-3673.html

http://www.plantthis.com.au/plant-information.asp?gardener=10727&plantSpot=3

http://www.jardin-botanique-lyon.com/jbot/sections/en/the_gardens_plants/collec/zoom/asclepiadacees/

http://www.picsearch.com/pictures/plants/garden per cent 20plants/Caralluma.html

http://www.flickr.com/photos/joeysplanting/2189059985/

http://toptropicals.com/catalog/uid/Caralluma_speciosa.htm

http://onlinelibrary.wiley.com/doi/10.1111/j.1756-1051.1995.tb00178.x/abstract

http://davesgarden.com/guides/pf/b/Asclepiadaceae/Caralluma/quadrangula/cultivar/0/

http://s902.photobucket.com/albums/ac229/slimacaifan/?action=view&current=Asclepiadaceae_Caralluma_fimbria-1.jpg&newest=1

http://carallumafimbriatas.com/caralluma-fimbriata-common-names/

http://www.wikigenes.org/e/mesh/e/20255.html

http://www.cactus-art.biz/schede/CARALLUMA/Caralluma_meintjesiana/Caralluma_meintjesiana/Angolluma_meintjesiana.htm

http://www.asianflora.com/Apocynaceae/Caralluma-judaica.htm

http://www.galanthus.cat/Flora/Asclepiadaceae/Asclepiadaceae.htm

http://www.ars-grin.gov/cgi-bin/npgs/html/genus.pl?2064

http://www.junglekey.com/wiki/definition.php?terme=Caralluma_burchardii

http://www.plantthis.com.au/plant-information.asp?gardener=10727&tabview=photos&plantSpot=3

http://www.crac-grn.com/Carallumadalzielii.html

http://www.absoluteastronomy.com/topics/Asclepiadaceae

http://www.efloras.org/florataxon.aspx?flora_id=5&taxon_id=250077198

http://www.hear.org/starr/images/family/?q=asclepiadaceae&o=plants

http://www.gardenology.org/wiki/Caralluma

http://www.photomazza.com/?Asclepiadaceae-archivio

http://luirig.altervista.org/famiglie/asclepiadaceae.htm

http://www.hort.purdue.edu/newcrop/FamineFoods/ff_families/ASCLEPIADACEAE.html

http://www.ngkenya.com/flora/caralluma-01.html

http://www.specks-exotica.com/en/photo/15036/caralluma/

http://public.fotki.com/PanosS/asclepiadaceae—apo/caralluma-/caralluma-burchardi/carallumaburchardii-2.html

http://swbiodiversity.org/seinet/taxa/index.php?taxon=Caralluma

http://www.thefreelibrary.com/Antitrypanosomal+activity+of+some+pregnane+glycosides+isolated+from...-a0226382359

http://en.goldenmap.com/Frerea

http://en.goldenmap.com/Caralluma_fimbriata

http://www.gardentia.net/asclepia_004.htm

http://www.quicksales.com.au/buy/auction_arc.aspx?itemid=10647438

http://www.israbat.ac.ma/html/PublicationsIS/BIS_SV_31_1/11-Bensusan.pdf

http://pooranee.com/~botanicg/herbarium/index.php?option=com_sobi2&catid=434&Itemid=90

http://toptropicals.com/cgi-bin/garden_catalog/cat.cgi?family=Asclepiadaceae

http://plants.usda.gov/java/profile?symbol=CARU23

http://lib.bioinfo.pl/meid:231933

http://luirig.altervista.org/famiglienam/asclepiadaceae.htm

http://www.trueknowledge.com/q/example_of_an_asclepiadoideae

http://species.wikimedia.org/wiki/Caralluma_priogonium

http://arctos.database.museum/TaxonomyResults.cfm?full_taxon_name=Caralluma+quadrangula

http://arctos.database.museum/TaxonomyResults.cfm?full_taxon_name=Caralluma+quadrangula

http://www.succulent-plant.com/families/asclepiadaceae/aclass.html

http://www.cactusmania.it/en/the-collection-details.php?f=3

http://www.ars-grin.gov/cgi-bin/npgs/html/taxon.pl?312273

http://opendata.keystone-foundation.org/category/asclepiadaceae

http://www.uni-muenster.de/Biologie.Botanik/agalbers/publ.htm

http://www.body-detox-info.com/caralluma-fimbriata.html

http://www.mendeley.com/research/antinociceptive-antiinflammatory-activity-carumbellosidei-isolated-caralluma-umbellata/

http://chestofbooks.com/gardening-horticulture/Cyclopedia-2/Camphora-Caralluma.html

http://www.flowersofindia.in/catalog/slides/Indian per cent 20Frerea.html

http://www.kew.org/science/directory/people/Gilbert_Mike.html

http://lib.bioinfo.pl/auid:4716225

http://wn.com/Caralluma

http://www.tiuli.com/flower_info.asp?lng=eng&flower_id=714

http://cacti.fr/Asclep/Asclepiadaceae.html

http://florawww.eeb.uconn.edu/200202428.html

http://home-and-garden.webshots.com/photo/1122343863048225527PoDuzi

http://www.golatofski.de/Pflanzenreich/gattung/c/caralluma.htm

http://maharashtradirectory.com/catalog/digvijaypharma/herbal-extracts.html

http://www.asclepiad-international.org/asclep87.html

http://www.succulent.com.ua/succulents.htm

http://www.cssainc.org/index.php?option=com_content&task=view&id=244&Itemid=212

http://www.ccss-online.org/pdf/Jan08-CCSS-POI.pdf

http://www.evri.com/news/for?query=caralluma

http://www.freepatentsonline.com/y2005/0202103.html

http://apocynaceae.blogspot.com/

http://www.marengowalks.com/new_fams.html

http://www.bennyskaktus.dk/Asclepiadaceae/apteranthes.htm

http://www.succulent-plant.com/families/asclepiadaceae/frerea.html

http://www.bgci.org/index.php?option=com_article&id=0091&print=1

http://www.succulentguide.com/cactus/?genus=Boucerosia

http://www.ingentaconnect.com/content/tandf/ganp/2008/00000010/00000011/art00003?crawler=true

http://de.wikipedia.org/wiki/Boucerosia

http://www.succulentguide.com/synonyms/?initial=B

http://www.astrokaktus.com/CactusBase/cactusbase/c/rod_caralluma_seznam.html

http://www.grabsomehealth.com/product/overview/Caralluma_Burn_Weight_Loss/

http://database.prota.org/PROTAhtml/Caralluma per cent 20adscendens_En.htm

http://www2.arnes.si/~sspimule/plants.html

http://www.stapeliads.info/serv/core.s3

http://www.theplantlist.org/tpl/record/kew-2358335

http://www.ars-grin.gov/cgi-bin/npgs/html/genus.pl?19726

http://www.treebase.org/treebase-web/search/study/taxa.html?id=892&treeid=5717

http://www.zuerich-herbarien.unizh.ch/datenbanken/list.php?l=d&spTaxFlg=&spTypFlg=&spCouCod=&spColFlg=&spFam=Asclepiadaceae&spHer=ZSS

http://les-cactus.com/caralluma.php

http://carolajuhasz.girlshopes.com/carallumaex/

http://www.bolus.uct.ac.za/research.html

http://www.plantzafrica.com/plantnop/orbea.htm

http://www.homolaicus.com/scienza/erbario/utility/botanica_sistematica/hypertext/1453.htm

http://www.cactus-art.biz/schede/WHITESLOANEA/Withesloanea_crassa/Withesloanea_crassa/Whitesloanea_crassa.htm

Pioneer Workers and Contributors for Stapeliad Taxonomy

The first collectors and also the first people to recognise these fascinating flowers will undoubtedly be the indigenous tribes that crisscrossed the countryside before the advent of the scientific man. They usually depended upon these plants for food and sustenance during periods of drought, which surely often occurs, especially in Africa and India. The history of stapeliads started earlier from 17th century.

Justus Heurnius (1624–1639)

Justus Heurnius (1624-1639), the Dutch missionary from Leyden, who sailed for the Dutch East Indies in 1624 full of enthusiasm and returned 15 years later 1639, a sadder and wiser man. He was the first collector of Cape plants and his inclusion in his little collection of *Stapelia variegata* (*Orbea variegata*) gives this species the distinction of having been among the very first South African plants to become known in Europe.

Johannes Bodaeus Stapelius (1602–1636)

Johannes Bodaeus Stapelius (Latinized form of 'van Stapel') was born in 1602 in Amsterdam, The Netherlands. Stapelius had a deep interest in botany, having been trained under Adolphus Vorstius while studying for his medical degree. His life's ambition was to publish an annotated edition of the botanical works of Theophrastus (370-287 BC). However, he died in 1636, a short time before the book was finished, and it was edited and published in 1644 by his father, Egbert Bodaeus Stapelius as 'Theophrasti Eresii de Historia Plantarum'. Included in the 1644 book were plants drawn by Justus Heurnius (1587-1653) from his brief stay at the Cape in South Africa in April 1624, one plant of which was *Fritillaria crassa* (*Stapelia variegata*, now known as *Orbea variegata*). Stapelius was commemorated with the genus *Stapelia* that was described in 1753 by Carolus Linnaeus in his 'Species Plantarum.

The description of *Stapelia variegata*, refers to a *"tuberous root, that is most likely the reason for calling it Fritillaria, a sort of lily. Or the similarity of the flower to the flower of Fritillaria meleagris. The corolla (annulus), has a cavity within, in which another sort of floret is seated (corona)"*.

From Fritillaria to Stapelia (1678–1753)

After the publication of van Stapel's book, the inconsistency of the name *Fritillaria crassa* for *Stapelia variegata* began to manifest, but what else to call it was the problem (not so for our modern day taxonomers).

Botanical nomenclature in the second half of the 17th century was in some confusion and at times was hard to follow the methods adopted by the different botanists to name and describe their plants (today 300 years later they still can't agree and taxonomy is alive and well). Generic names were defined by French botanist Joseph Pitton de Tournefort (1656-1708) based on the forms and emphasize of the plant, but our modern specific names were little more than adjectival differentiations and were often extended to form a long sequence of words, and so virtually defined the species. Kaspar Bauhin in the beginning of the 17th century foreshadowed the binary nomenclature, but no such system was adopted before Linnaeus.

Pre-Linnaean period, different botanists were building up different botanical classifications, based on differences in plant structure, and not taking into account the whole plant. Then Tournefort and the German "Rivinus" (Augustus Quirinus Bachmann, 1652-1725) concentrated on the form of the corolla in each species.

Robert Morrison (1620-1683), a Scottish botanist in 1680 published a system based on external form of plant, fruits, which he called seeds. Paul Herman, a follower of Morrison, in his "Catalogue of Plants" in the Leyden Gardens, 1687 called *Stapelia variegata* as *"Apocynum humile aizoides siliquis erectus"*. Other botanists followed suit.

John Ray (1627-1705), theological student, scientist, zoologist, and botanist realised the importance of the inner structure of seeds, and observed the difference between embryos with two cotyledons, and those with one or none. 1696 Leonard Plunket (1641-1706) botanist to Queen Mary II, also noted this difference.

R. Bradley (1716-1727), professor of botany at the University of Cambridge, wrote the first work wholly devoted to succulents. the History of Succulent Plants, he explains why the stapeliads were referred to *Apocynum* by saying *"When the blossom is past there succeed long Cods, which contain seeds resembling those of an Apocynum, or Dogbane, of a chestnut colour, being pointed with a down or cotton-like substance"*.

The Stapelids were transferred to the genus *Asclepias*, by Robert Morrison himself in the last volume of his History of Plants, published after his death, 1699. Tournefort in 1703 and Caspar Commelin in 1715 continued with this arrangement.

Heinrich Bernhard Ruppius (1688-1719), was first to place Stapeliads in a distinct Genus in the Flora Ienensis, Jena, 1718. He established Genus *Crassa* and called

Stapelia variegata and *Stapelia hirsuta* by the names of *Crassa rivini* and *Crassa minor*, respectively, Crassa meaning "succulent", and Rivini was in honour of A.Q. Bachmann.

Laurens Heister (1683-1758) termed an interesting early generic name *Stisseria*, he was Professor of Anatomy and Botany at the Academy in Helmstedt, Germany. He was also in charge of the Botanical Gardens of the Academy. In 1730 Heister printed a catalogue of the rare and medicinal plants grown by him, which included *Stapelia variegata*, *Stapelia hirsuta* and a rare cristate plant of *Stapelia variegata*. He split the two species from Genus *Asclepias*, because he wrote *"their leafless, angled, succulent stems"* seemed completely distinct, and he established a new genus to provide for them, which he called *Stisseria*, in honour of Andre Stisser the founder of the Botanic Gardens.

Carl Linnaeus (1707-1778), the great Swedish botanist, finally established the genus *Stapelia* in his Critica Botanica, 1737. It is worth noting two tears previously, in the first edition of the Systema Naturae, Regnum Vegetabile, Leyden, 1735, Linnaeus had adapted Heister's name *Stisseria*. He now made the change to *Stapelia* as stated. Dr Marloth wrote that Otto Kuntze, of reforming fame, described this action as one of the numerous instances of abuse to which the great Linnaeus subjected his contemporaries if they dared not to accept his system of plants, and tried to reintroduce an original name (Revisio generum 1891). It is amazing that today in the 21st century we still have Linnaeus's in the taxonomy field.

Pre-Linnaeian Stapeliads (1696–1738)

The pre-Linnaean Stapeliads are *Caralluma incarnata* and *Caralluma mammillaris* plus *Stapelia variegata* were all figured in the Decades of Rare African Plants, 1938, by Johannes Burman (1707-1780), Professor of Botany at the University of Amsterdam, and he was first botanist to adopt Linnaeus' generic name, *Stapelia*. Linnaeus came from Sweden to Amsterdam in 1735, for a year he lived in Burman's home, and in all possibilities the name was decided then.

Peter Forsskal (1736–1753)

The first Stapeliads discovered after the four species known to Burman in 1738 were collected a quarter of a century later by Peter Forsskal. Linnaeus recommended this young Swedish naturalist to Fredrick V of Denmark, when the latter was planning an expedition to Egypt, Arabia and India, to be headed by Karsten Niebuhr, a German traveler. This was an ill fated expedition, for every member of the small party, except Niebuhr, died on the journey, first the philologist, then Forsskal, then the artist, and finally the surgeon. Forsskal contracted the plague in Arabia, so even without a terrorist threat it was not safe to travel in those days. Niebuhr reached Bombay alone, and got back to Copenhagen in 1767. Later he published the works of his companion Forsskal in a series of books, included Flora Aegyptiaco - Arabica, 1775, and Icones Rerum Natur., 1776. Forsskal collected five Stapeliads, the ones that have been identified are only two, *Caralluma quadrangula* and *Caralluma subulata*.

Karl Peter Thunberg (1743–1828)

Karl Peter Thunberg was a Swedish naturalist and pupil of Linnaeus. He worked his way to South Africa as assistant surgeon on a vessel of the Dutch East India

STAPELIAD CONTRIBUTORS AND THEIR DISCOVERIES

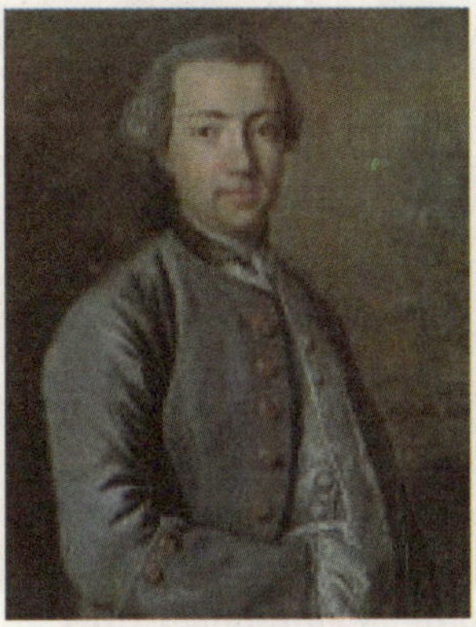
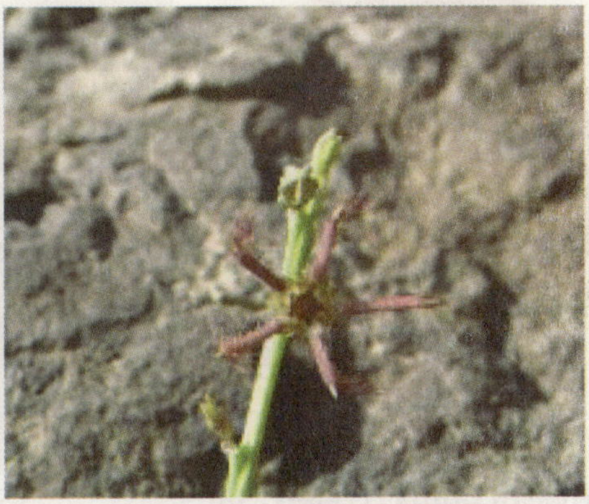

Peter Forsskal (1736–1753) ***Caralluma subulata* Forsskal**

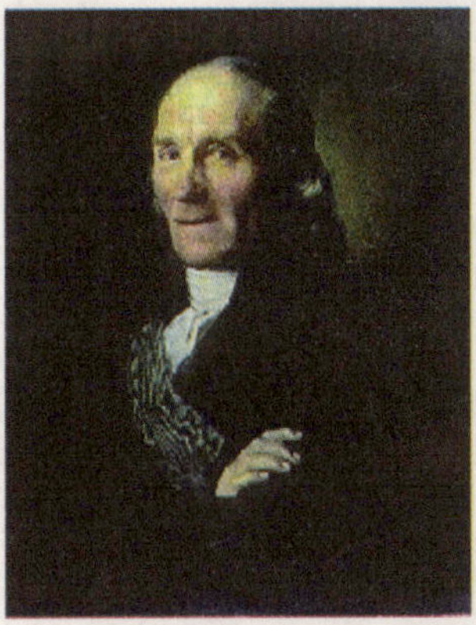
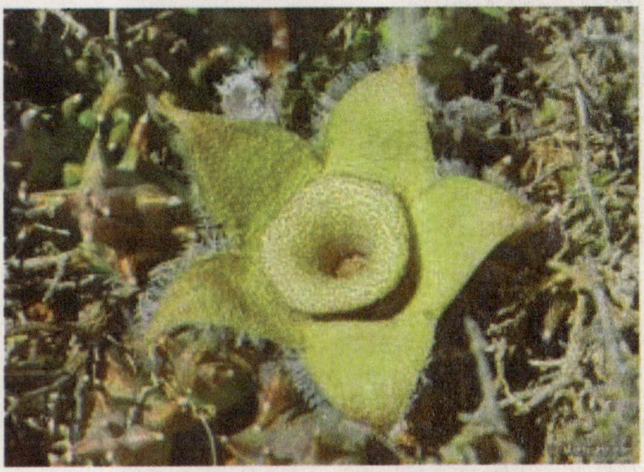

Karl Peter Thunberg (1743–1828) ***Orbea ciliata* Thunberg**

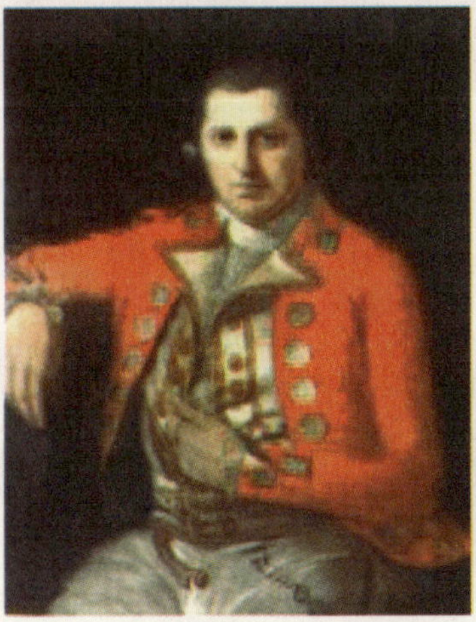
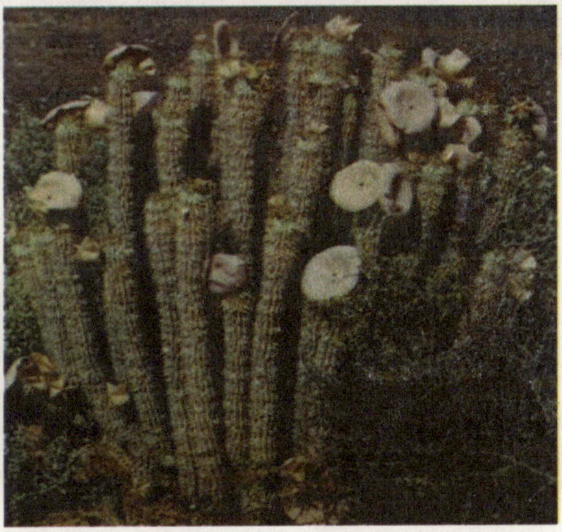

Col. Robert Jacob Gordon (1743–1795) ***Hoodia gordonii***

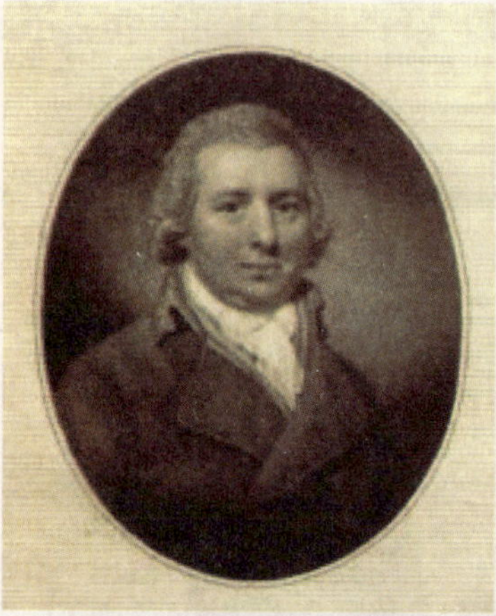

William Curtis (1746–1799)

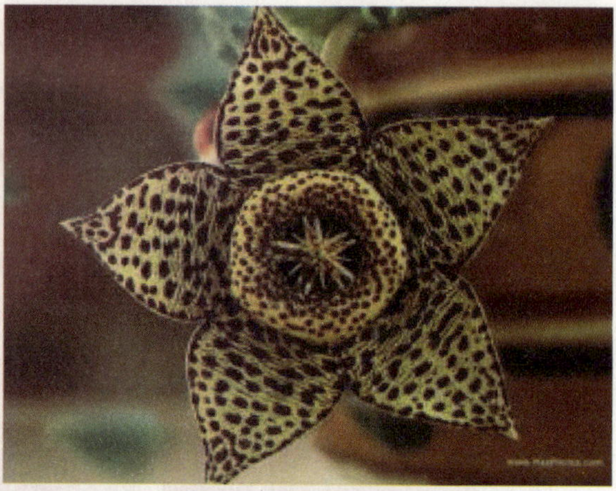

***Stapelia variegata* Curtis**

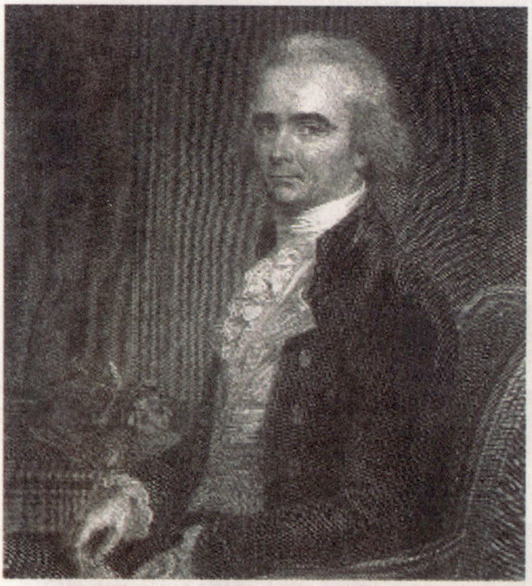

William Roxburgh (1751–1815)

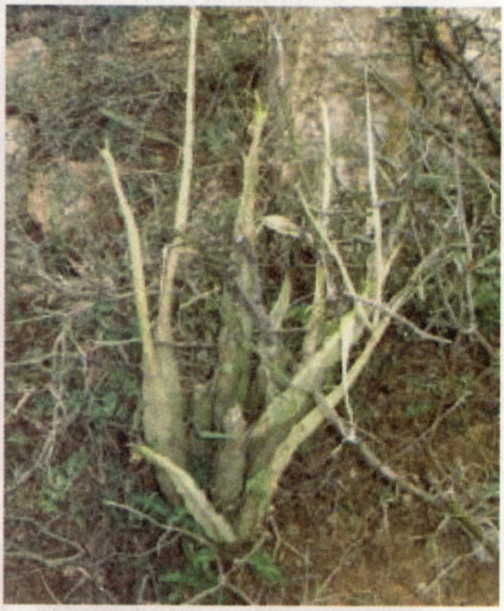

***Caralluma adscendens* Roxb.**

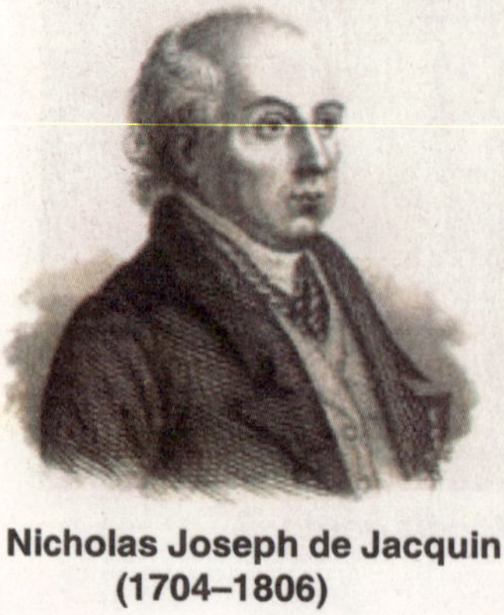

Nicholas Joseph de Jacquin (1704–1806)

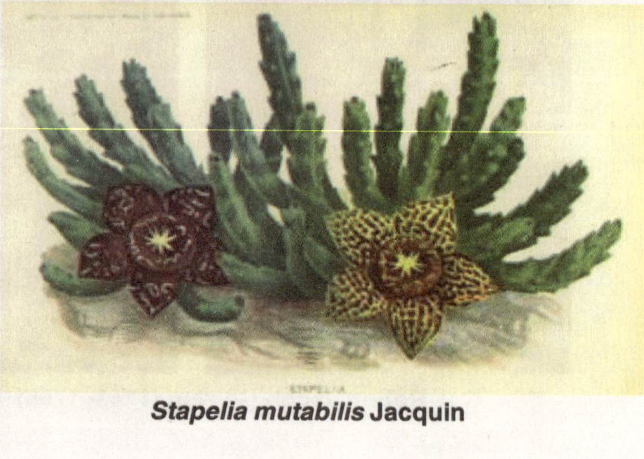

***Stapelia mutabilis* Jacquin**

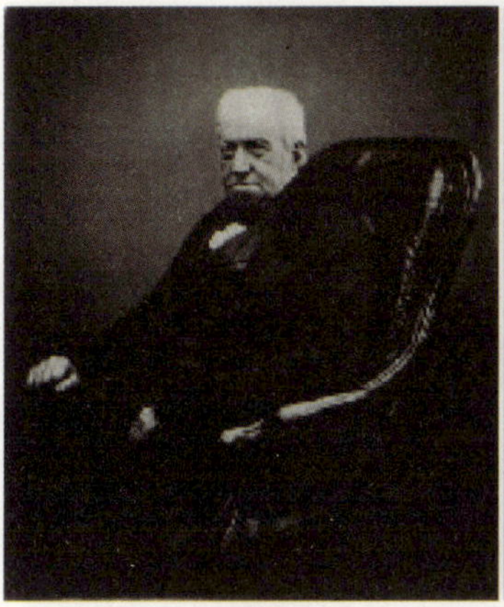

Robert Brown (1773–1858)

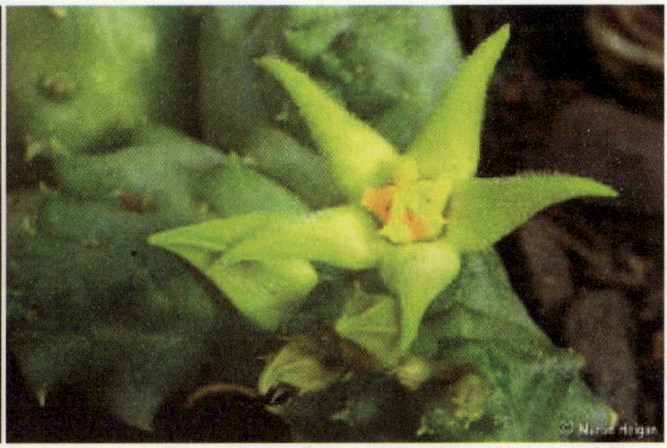

Piaranthus decorus

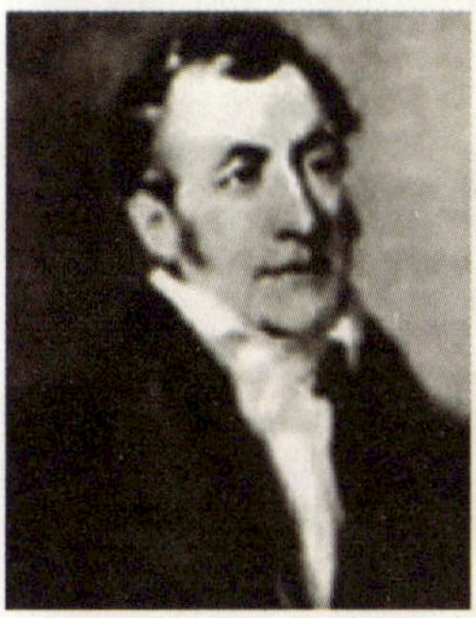

Nathaniel Wallich 1786–1854)

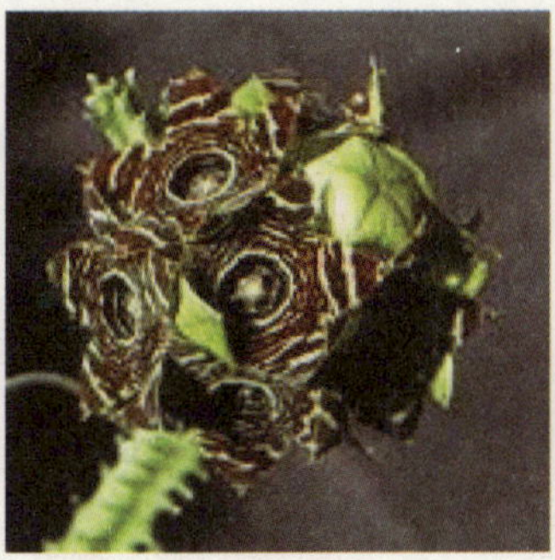

Caralluma crenulata

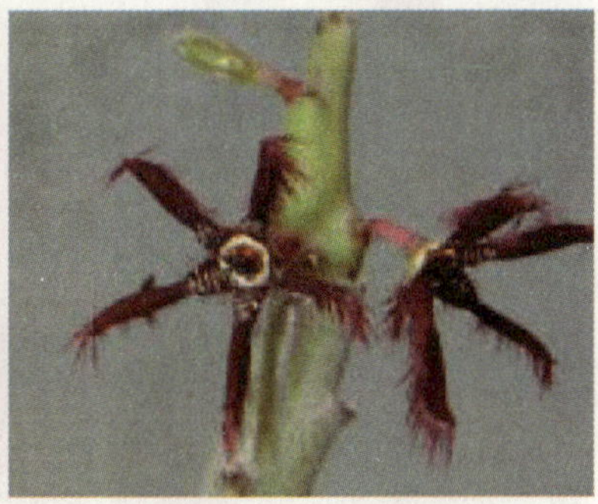

Caralluma adscendens* var. *fimbriata

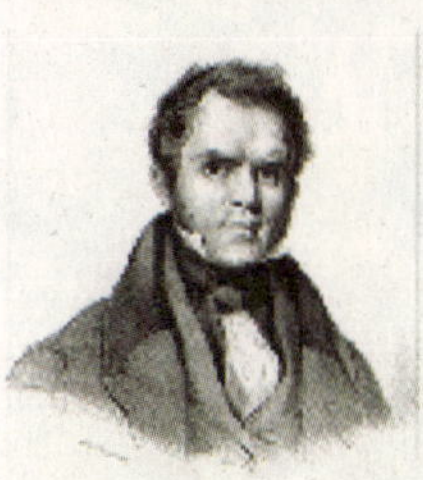

Robert Wight (1796–1872)

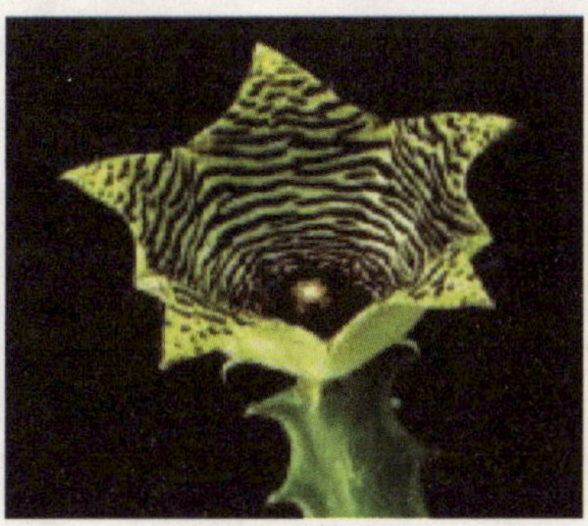

***Caralluma pauciflora* Wt.**

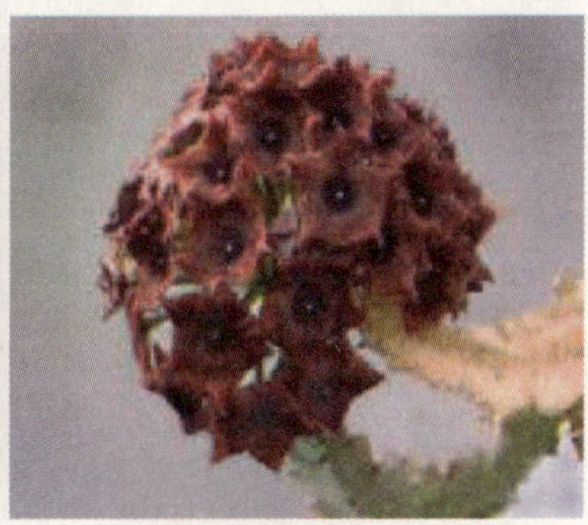

***Caralluma diffusa* Wt.**

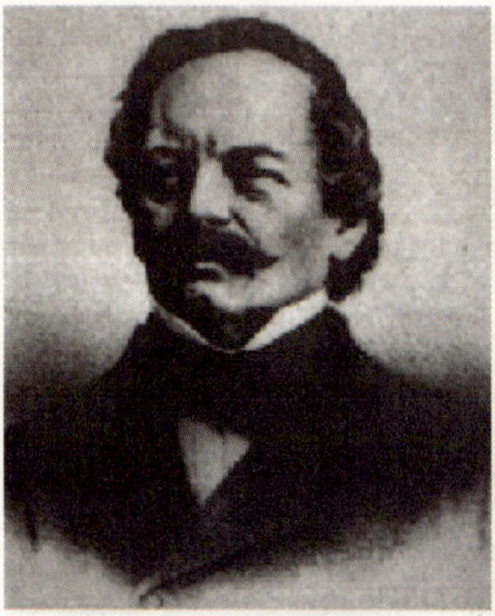

Friedrich Welwitsch (1806–1872)

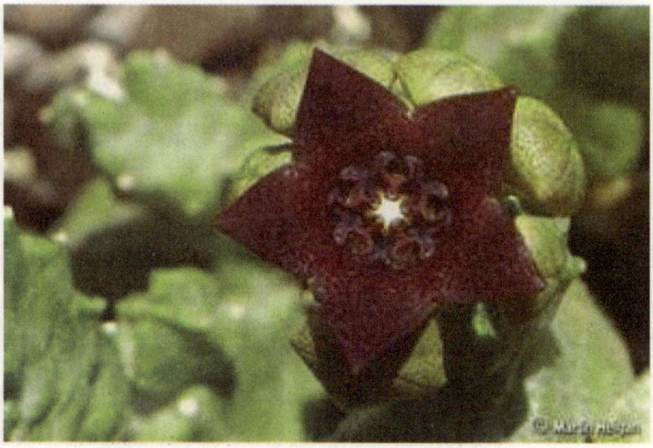

***Caralluma huillensis* Welwitsch**

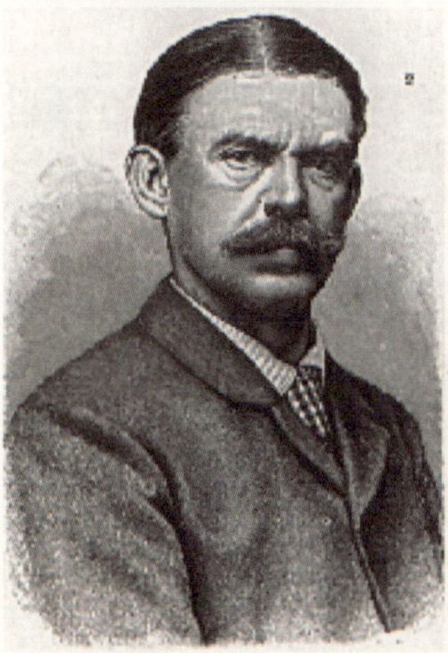

Georg August Schweinfurth (1836–1925)

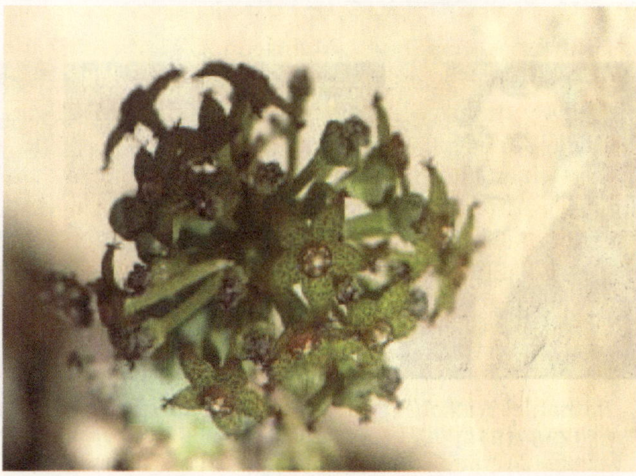

***Caralluma penicillata* Schew.**

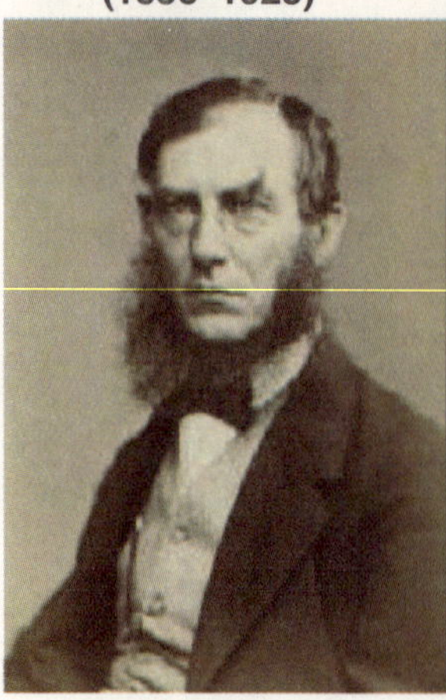

Sir Joseph Dalton Hooker (1817–1910)

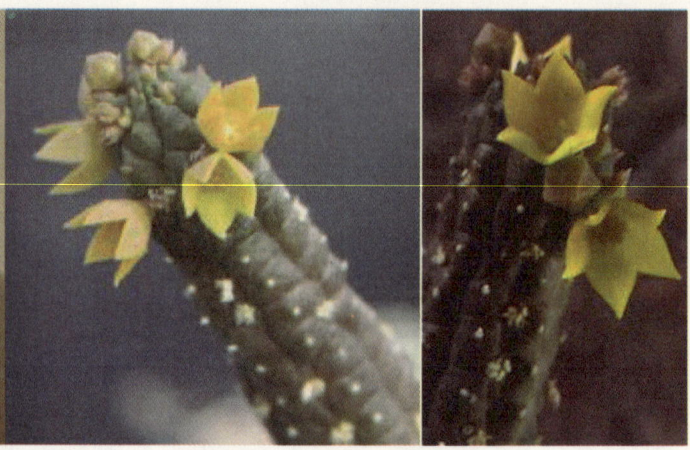

Echidnopsis cereiformis

Company and reached the Cape in April 1772. He remained in South Africa for nearly three years, almost coincided with Francis Masson's first visit. He overcame all difficulties, and the accounts of his travels were published in four volumes, in 1788-1793. He has been translated all his books into English, French and German. His Flora Capensis, his own collections, enumerates 3100 species. This was published in parts in 1807, 1823, 1818, and a complete edition by J. A. Schultes in Stuttgart in 1828. He left the Cape, visited Japan, and other eastern islands, and he returned to Sweden. In 1783 he was appointed to the chair at the University of Uppsala, which Linnaeus the father, and Linnaeus the son occupied before him. He died in 1828, crowned by honours, and honorary member of no less than 66 scientific societies in all parts of Europe. He has discovered new Burman's species *Diplocyatha ciliata* (*Orbea ciliata*), *Pectinaria articulata*, and *Trichocaulon piliferum* (*Larryleachia piliferum*). His plant *Stapelia caudata* turned out to be a *Brachystelma*, another tribe of the Asclepiads.

Francis Masson (1741–1805)

Francis Masson (born, Aberdeen, 1741; died in Montreal, Canada, 1805) stayed for two and a half years in Cape. For part he travelled with Thunberg, two excursions of about 4 months each, one began September 1773, the other the same season the following year. North they reached the Olifants river, east they reached the Zwartkops and Fish River. He spent time writing up his journeys and his stay in the cape, in this time he produced his little book, Stapeliae Novae or A Collection of several new species of that genus that he discovered in the interior parts of Africa. London. 1796. It appeared about June 1797, there was no colour printing so they were lithographs that he coloured by hand. It contained figures and descriptions of 41 plants.

Gordon and Patterson (1777–1779)

Col. Robert Jacob Gordon (1743-1795) he was a Dutch officer by Scotch extraction, he reached the river in 1777, named it the Orange River after the Dutch Stadtholder the Prince of Orange. William Patterson (1755 - 1810) reached the lower course of the river, and in 1779 Patterson and Gordon explored the river together. Gordon discovered *Hoodia gordoni*, and Patterson *Trichocaulon cactiforme*. Patterson wrote an account of his travels, narrative of Four Journeys into the Country Of The Hottentots and Caffraria, London. 1789. Patterson left South Africa in 1781, travelled to India, 1781-1785, Australia in 1791, he died at sea on the return voyage from Australia to England, 1810.

William Curtis (1746–1799)

William Curtis have edited several Botanic Magazines, includes Flora Londinensis. He spoke of the magazine and the flora as the one brings him pudding, the other one praise. He continued as editor until his death. Dr. John Simms (1749-1831) edited until 1826. Whilst they were editors the stapeliads were best represented in Curtis's Bot. Mag. In the first volume *Stapelia variegata* was featured, a note on their care was published, "If these plants be kept in a very moderate stove in winter, and in summer placed in an airy glass-case where they may enjoy much free air, but screened from wet and cold, they will thrive and flower very well". Well there goes the wife's stove for the next winter. At the turn of the 19th century stapeliads were really the flavour of the month, supplied by nurserymen, 1800 Grimwood and Wykes, 1825 Whitley, Brame and Milne, most important was Mr Loddiges, nurseryman at Hackney had a large Stapeliad collection. Conrad Loddiges, (1743-1826) was a Dutch gardener, set up his nursery in Hackney in 1771, then continued by his son, George Loddiges (1784-1846), also editor of the Botanical Cabinet, from 1817-1834. This periodical contained numerous stapeliads drawn by Loddiges.

William Roxburgh (1751–1815)

Dr. William Roxburgh was born at Underwood in the parish of Craigie, Ayrshire. He studied medicine in Edinburgh. He had been a surgeon's mate on an East India Company ship at the age of 17 and had completed two voyages to the East in that capacity until the age of 21. He also studied botany in Edinburgh under John Hope. He joined the Madras Medical Service as an assistant surgeon in 1776 and became a surgeon in 1780. At Madras he turned his attention to botany. The East India Company recognized his botanical knowledge and made him superintendent in the Samalkot garden in the Northern Circars in 1781. Here he conducted economic botany experiments. He employed native artists to illustrate plants. He had 700 illustrations by 1790. He then succeeded Patrick Russell (1727-1805) as Naturalist to the Madras Government. He made rapid progress and acquired a good reputation and was in a short time invited by the government of Bengal, to take charge of the Calcutta Botanical gardens from Colonel Robert Kyd. In 1793 he succeeded Colonel Robert Kyd as Superintendent of the Company garden at Sibpur near Calcutta. A catalog of the garden was made in 1814 - *Hortus Bengalensis*. He sent many of his illustrations to Sir Joseph Banks. He was succeeded by Francis Buchanan-Hamilton. He employed a full time painter to draw all his plants form a camera. In 1790, he became principal botanist for East India Company. Between 1791 and 1794, he sent 500 of his plates and descriptions to England, of which 300 were published by Sir Joseph Banks, "Plants of the Coast of Coromandel", London, 3 vols., 1795-1819. He discovered *Caralluma adscendens* and opened new account for Indian stapeliad groups.

Baron Nicholas Joseph de Jacquin (1704–1806)

Baron Nicholas Joseph de Jacquin was the first serious collector of Stapeliads, at Imperial Gardens of Schonbrunn near Vienna, at the Palace of the last Roman Emperors and the first Austrian Emperors. He began his interest in the Asclepiads in 1758, on his first visit to America; his main interest was in the reproductive mechanisms of plants in this family. He wrote an article in his Miscellanea Austriaca, 1778, *Stapelia variegata*, and *Stapelia hirsuta* were discussed. Then Masson's plants became available to collectors, he grew every species, he could get hold of, the flowers were studied for hours, artists did drawings. Soon seeds and new plants began to arrive from Boos and Scholl in South Africa.

His principal work was "Stapeliarum in hortis Vindobon cultarum descriptions", Vienna, 1806, of sixty-four plates, the work was only completed in 1819 after his death by his son Joseph Franz Jacquin, he edited a Synopsis Stapeliarum in 1816. At the Imperial Gardens, a few good species of Stapeliads were grown, also his infamous hybrid, *Stapelia mutabilis*.

Robert Brown (1773–1858)

Robert Brown, English botanist, was a Scottish botanist and palaeobotanist who made important contributions to botany largely through his pioneering use of the microscope. In 1810, he published the results of his collections in his famous *Prodromus Florae Novae Hollandiae et Insulae Van Diemen*, the first systematic account of the Australian flora. That year, he succeeded Jonas C. Dryander as Sir Joseph Banks' librarian, and on Banks' death in 1820 Brown inherited his library and herbarium. This was transferred to the British Museum in 1827, and Brown was appointed Keeper of the Banksian Botanical Collection. Brown's name is commemorated in the Australia herb genus *Brunonia* as well as numerous Australian species such as *Eucalyptus brownii*, *Banksia brownii* and the moss Brown's Tetrodontium Moss (*Tetrodontium brownianum*), a species which he discovered growing at Roslin near Edinburgh whilst still a student. The plant can still be found at the site of its discovery. He was first to divide genus *Stapelia*, established 3 new genera, namely *Huernia*, *Piaranthus* and *Caralluma*. He was the first botanist to advocate the natural system of plant identification.

Adrian Hardy Haworth (1768–1833)

Adrian Hardy Haworth an English botanist, was a very enthusiastic collector of succulents in England. In his "Synopsis Plantarum succulentarum", London, 1812, and Supplementarum, 1819 he carried on with the subdivision of the known Stapeliads, begun by R. Brown. He established new genera, *Duvalia*, *Pectinaria*, *Obesia* [now in *Piaranthus*], and *Gonostemon*, *Tromotriche*, *Tridentia*, *Caruncularia* and *Podanthes*. He died in 1833, and interest waned. He has discovered Indian succulent stapeliad *Boucerosia umbellata* but controversy existed whether the specimen was collected from Southern India or Sri Lanka.

Nathaniel Wallich (1786–1854)

Dr. Nathaniel Wallich, Dane by birth, went to India in 1807 as surgeon to a Danish settlement there, when it was taken over by Dutch East India Company in 1813, he was appointed in charge of the Botanic Gardens at Calcutta, he returned to London on 1847. In 1828 he was temporarily invalided in London, but took 8000 dried specimens of plants with him. In 1830 - 1832 he published 3 volumes of Plantae Asiaticae rariores (description and figures of a select number of East Indian Plants). He discovered *Caralluma crenulata*, and *Caralluma adscendens* var. *fimbriata*.

Christian Gottfried Ehrenberg (1795-1876)

Dr. Christian Gottfried Ehrenerg (1795 - 1876), was a famous German physician and a naturalist. In 1820 he went with the scientific expedition of General van Minutoli to Egypt, the Libean dessert, Ethiopia and Arabia. On this journey, on Dahlac Island in the Red Sea, he discovered the giant stapeliad taxa *Caralluma retrospiciens*.

George Samuel Perrottet (1793–1850)

Perrottet was a gardener-botanist from the Museum of Natural History Paris. He was a Swiss-born, French botanist and horticulturalist who was a native of Vully, canton Vaud. He worked as a gardener at the *Jardin des Plantes*, and in 1819-21 was as a naturalist on an expedition commanded by Naval Captain Pierre Henri Philibert. Perottet's duties on the journey involved collecting plants in Réunion, Java, and the Philippines for re-plantation and cultivation in Guyane. His collection now housed in National Museum Paris. Two type specimens, preserved in alcohol, have disappeared, *Caralluma retrospiciens* var. *acutangula* and *Caralluma decaisneana*. In 1833 he began the publication of Flora of Senegambia, with Guillemin and Richard, remained incomplete. In 1832 Perrottet was appointed correspondent of the *Museum National d'Histoire Naturelle* in Paris, and from 1834 to 1839 was assigned to the botanical garden at Pondicherry. In 1839 he returned to France, where he became involved with silkworm cultivation. From 1843 until his death in 1870, he worked as a botanist in Pondicherry.

Robert Sweet (1783–1835)

Robert Sweet in the second edition of Hortus Britannicus, London, 1830, he established the Genus *Hoodia*. He was the first to think of separating the many-angled stems from those with stems of a few angles. He was not troubled by the two *Trichocaulon* (Masson and Patterson), he just dismissed one as being a *Piaranthus*. But this strange species discovered by Col. Gordon was a real problem. In the 1827, first edition, he took it out of *Stapelia*, where it had been for 50 years, and assigned it to Haworth's genus *Gonostemon*. This was soon seen to be an unsatisfactory solution, Sweet himself realised it, he soon corrected it by the erection of his new Genus *Hoodia*. He published a number of beautifully illustrated works on plants cultivatd in British gardens and hothouses. The fine plates were mainly drawn by Edwin Dalton Smith, a botanical artist, who was attached to the Royal Botanic Gardens, Kew. His works include *Hortus Suburbanus Londinensis* (1818), *Geraniaceae* (five volumes) (1820–30), *Cistineae*, *Sweet's Hortus Britannicus* (1826–27), *Flora Australasica* (1827–28) and *British Botany* (with H. Weddell) (1831). He died at Chelsea, London in January 1835.

Aucher-Eloy (1793–1838)

Pierre Martin Remi Aucher-Eloy, a French pharmacist, then publisher, and then botanical explorer. His headquarters were in Constantinople, from where he visited, Egypt, Sinai, Palestine, Syria, and Cyprus.1832. He discovered *Caralluma aucheriana* and *Caralluma sinaica*.

Robert Wight (1796–1872)

Dr. Robert Wight, was a Scottish surgeon and botanist who spent 30 years in India. He spent the time between 1819-1853 in India and devoted most of that time to the study of plants. He has put in charge of the Madras Botanic Gardens. Invalided to England 1831 – 1834, he published his "Contributions to the Botany of India, London, 1834 in collaboration with Dr. G.A. Walker-Arnot. After his return to India, his services to the army became impossible, for on a march he needed several native carts to transport his plants, and half a dozen more for his books and kit. In 1836, he was appointed to a position in the revenue department. He then became superintendent for experimental growing of cotton and tobacco in Coimbatore, whilst in this job he completed 5 volumes of Icones Plantarum Indiae orientalis, Madras 1838 - 1853 and 2 volumes of illustrations of Indian Botany, Madras, 1841 - 1850. He had for his own expense a plant collector, and two native artists, Govindoo and Rungiah. He discovered *Caralluma adscendens* var. *attenuata, Caralluma diffusa, Caralluma indica,* and *Caralluma pauciflora*. Two others now merged into *Caralluma umbellata*.

Quartin Dillon and Petit (1839–1843)

Richard Quartin Dillon discovered *Caralluma ango* and *Huernia macrocarpa*. He was plant collector on a French mission to Ethiopia, headed by Naval Lieut. T. Lefebvre. The expedition landed at Massaua in Eritrea in 1839, and Quartin Dillon made his first shipment in 1840. He either collected alone or at times with the zoological collector, A. Petit, who incidentally discovered *Caralluma sprengeri*.

Mary Elizabeth Bowker (1819–1899)

Mary Elizabeth Bowker, came with her father from England with the 1820 Settlers. She became one of the pioneer students of nature in South Africa. She corresponded with Darwin, Hookers etc. She discovered *Stapelia glabricaulis*, and *Stapelia jucunda*. Her drawings are in the Herbarium at Kew, and at Albany Museum, Grahamstown. Her brother Col. James Henry Bowker discovered *Huernia primulina*, and *Stapelia tsomoensis*.

Joseph Decaisne (1807–1882)

In the 8th vols. of A. Pyrame de Candolle's Prodromus, Paris, 1844, the Asclepiadaceae were edited by Decaisne, he enumerated 110 species, 25 were hybrids. He also showed that 2 species known to Linnaeus in 1753, the 7 of Thunberg in 1807, and the 169 in N. E. Brown's Flora Capensis, 1909, this was a comparison made by Marloth. He showed that the great increase in the 19th century was due to the real increase that had occurred many years earlier, with Francis Masson, Jacquin and to lesser degree Haworth. Decaisne marked no increase, save a few hybrids. He was typical of Dark Ages of Stapeliads. The Parade of Systems, and Dictionaries of Botany, included Decaisne 1844, Bentham and Hooker, 1876 made a brave show of names, which they changed back and forth from one genus to another, but they had a complete lack of original material, and were simply scrambling the eggs which they found in Jacquin and Haworth's basket.

Friedrich Welwitsch (1806–1872)

Dr. Friedrich Welwitsch, Austrian physician and scientist went to Lisbon in 1839 for a short visit but stayed for 14 years, the Portuguese government sent him to a survey of Angola 1853 - 1861, he was granted a pension and permission to work on his discoveries at Kew. In 1896-1901 he published the catalogue of his African Plants, London, with William Philip Hiern (1839-1925). In a Lisbon periodical of 1854 Welwitsch established the genus *Tavaresia* for one of his new plants, *Tavaresia angolensis*. He also discovered *Caralluma huillensis, Hoodia parviflora,* and *Huernia similis*.

Michael Pakenham Edgeworth (1812–1881)

Michael Pakenham Edgeworth was an Irish naturalist, botanical writer, his half sister, Maria Edgeworth, novelist, and author of Dialogues on Botany. He entered

Bengal Civil service in 1831, in 1862 he published *Florula mallica* in the Journal of the Linnaean Society, records the discovery of *Caralluma edulis*, and was being sold for food in north western India.

Dalzell (1864)

In February 1864, N. A. Dalzell, Superintendent of Botanic Gardens in Bombay discovered *Frerea indica* in the neighbourhood of Poona. He created a new genus, dedicated to the Governor, Sir Henry Bartle Edward Frere.

Federico Delpino (1833–1905)

Federico Delpino was an Italian botanist, professor at universities of Genoa, Bologna, and Naples. 1865 - 1866 he spent on the fertilisation of the Stapelias by different flies. In 1873, he published a monograph on The Fertilisation of the Phanerogams. He also published a general classification of plants based on their floral structure in 1873. Stapeliads were placed in section called Melananti or "black flowers" with two types, Macromyiophilous attract large flies, and Sapromyiophilous flowers attracting carrion flies by their odours.

George August Schweinfurth (1836–1925)

Prof. George August Schweinfurth was a German ethnologist, botanist, scientist spent his life to study and exploration of tropical Africa. He learnt nearly all European Languages, perfected his drawing skills. At 27 yrs he bought a small boat, and had his first cruise along shores of the Red Sea explored upper Egypt and Nubia, this was so successful what he was sponsored by the Humboldt Foundation in Berlin for his later travels, Southern Arabia, Socotra, His bibliography includes 464 articles. He discovered *Caralluma adenensis, Caralluma commutata, Caralluma longidens, Caralluma penicillata, Echidnopsis nubica, Edithcolea sordida, Huernia concinna* and *Caralluma schweinfurthii*.

Sir Joseph Dalton Hooker (1817–1910)

Sir Joseph Dalton Hooker, established genus *Echidnopsis* in The Botanical Magazine, 1871, to provide a genus for *Echidnopsis cereiformis*. he was son of Sir William Jackson Hooker (1785-1865) director Royal Botanic Gardens at Kew in 1841-1865 and founder of Hooker's Icones Plantarum (in this N.E. Brown will be publishing Sir Henry Barkly's collection). Sir Joseph later succeeded his father at Kew, 1865-1885.

Johan Maria Hildebrandt (1847–1881)

Johan Maria Hildebrandt was a young German machinist. In 1872 he explored Arabia, Somaliland, East Tropical Africa and Madagascar. He had poor health and died at age 34. He discovered *Caralluma gracilipes, Echidnopsis virchowii*, and three other stapeliads.

Sir William Turner Thiselton-Dyer (1843–1928)

Sir William Turner Thiselton-Dyer has edited volumes of Flora of Tropical Africa, 1904, and Flora Capensis, 1909. They contained the revisions of The STAPELIEAE by

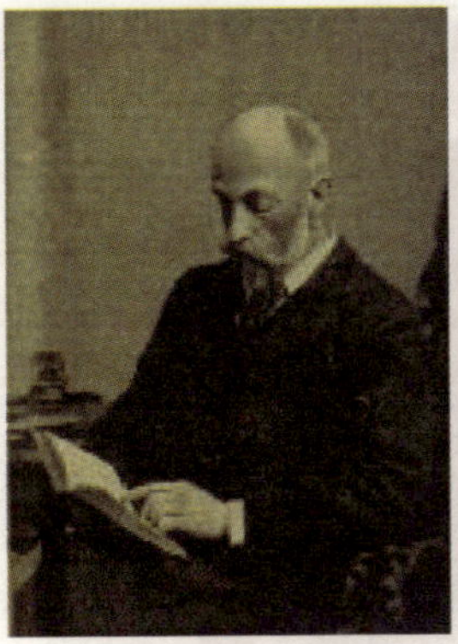

Sir William Turner Thiselton-Dyer (1843–1928)

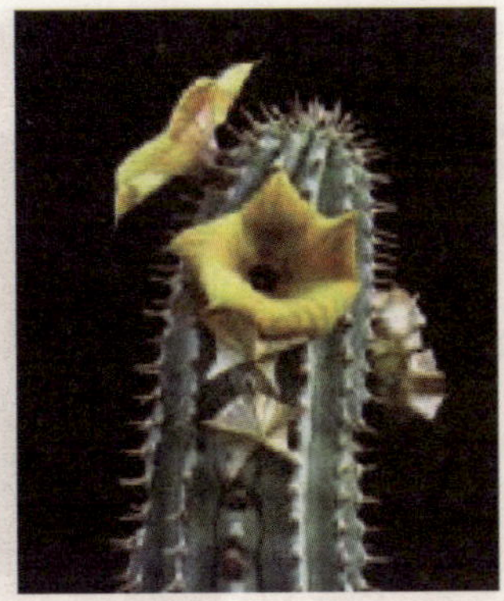

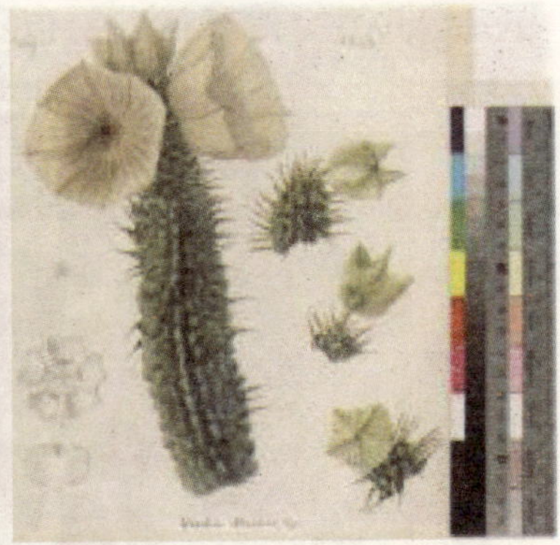

***Hoodis bainii* Dyer**

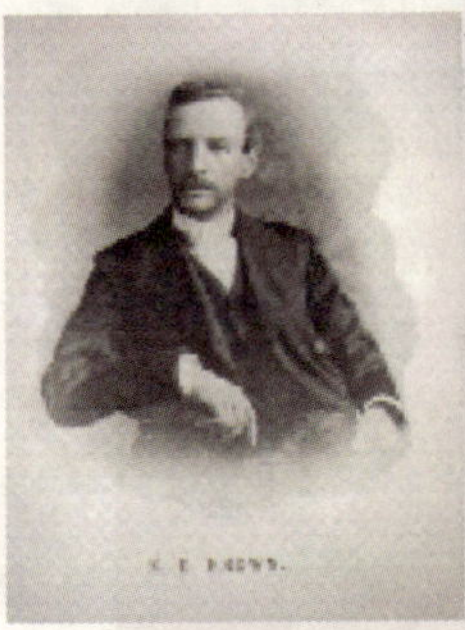

Nicholas Edward Brown (1849–1934)

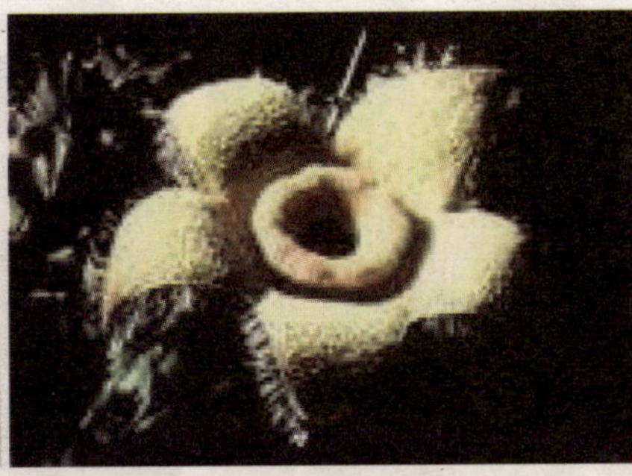

***Diplocyatha ciliata* Brown**

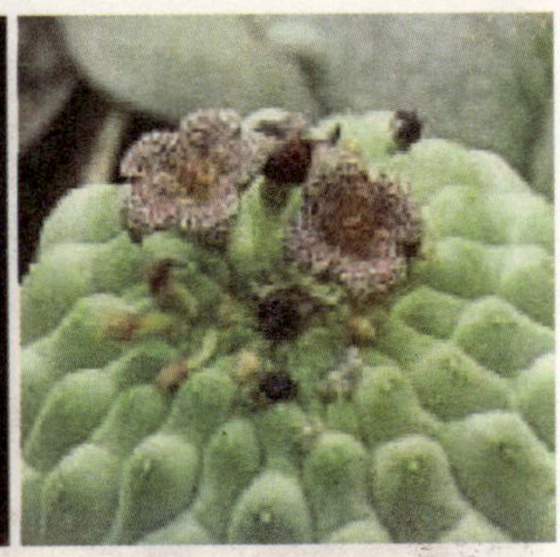

***Trichocaulon* Brown**

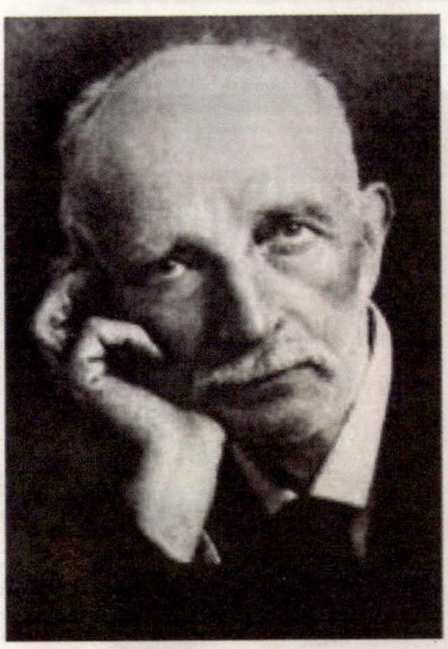

Rudolf Marloth (1855–1931)

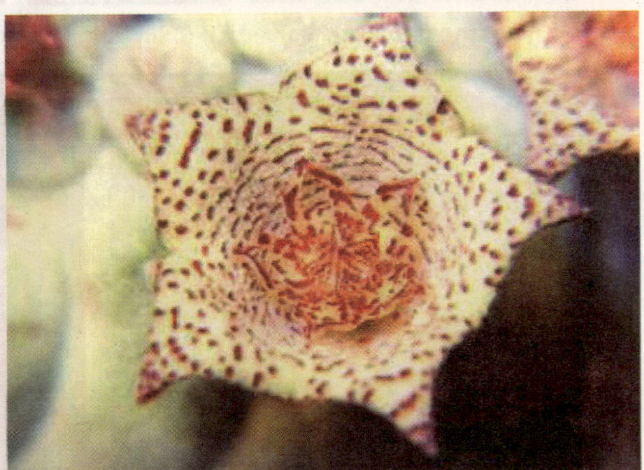

Stapelia marlothii

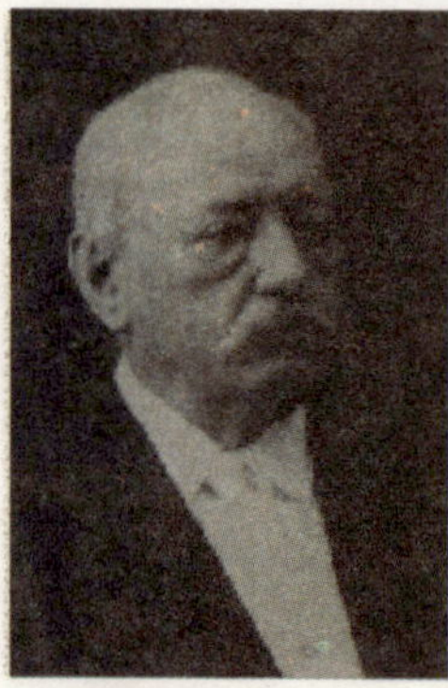

Adolph Engler (1844–1930)

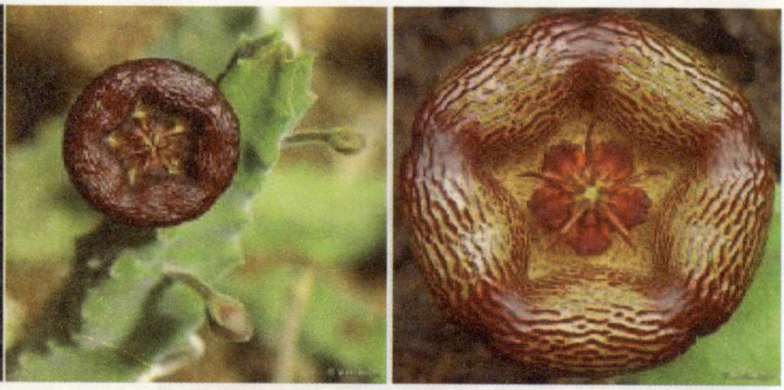

Stapelia engleriana

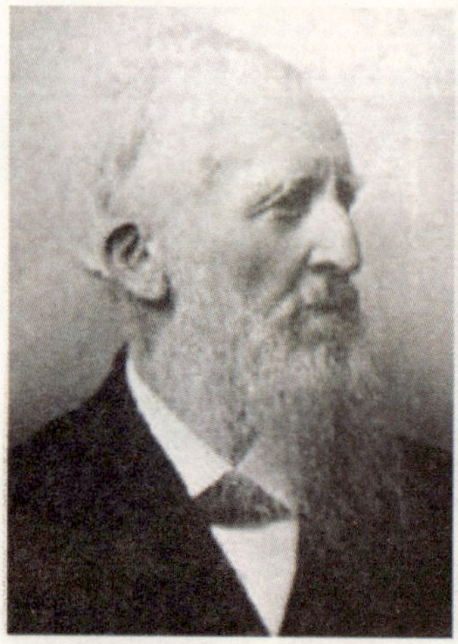

John Medley Wood (1827–1915)

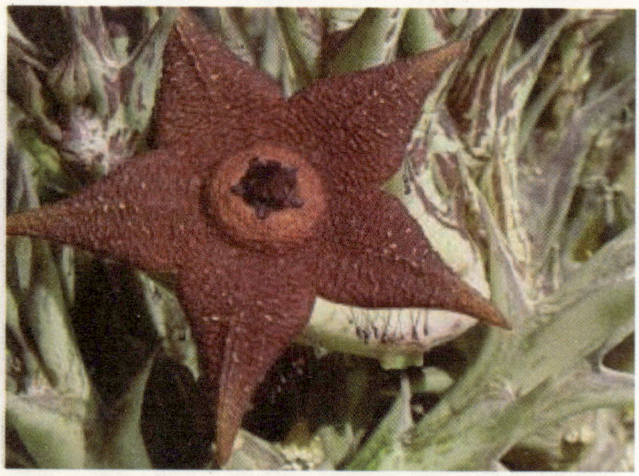

Stapelia woodii

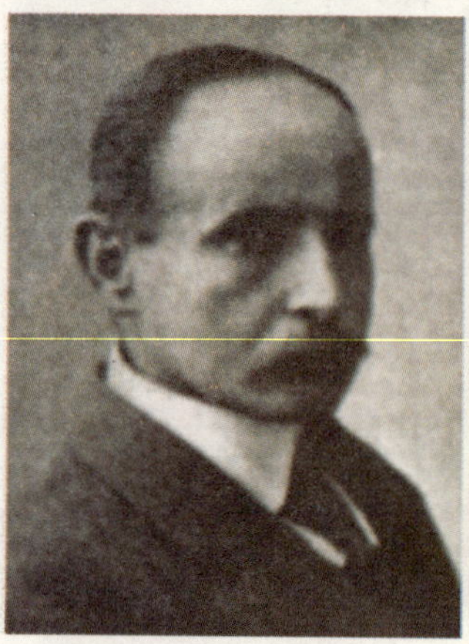

Rudolf Schlechter (1872–1925)

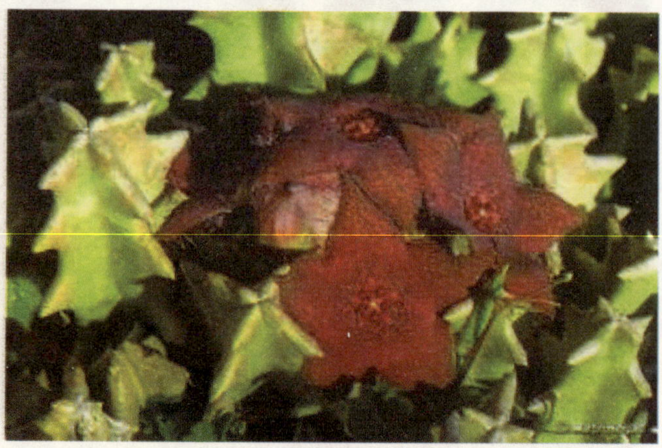

Orbea melanantha

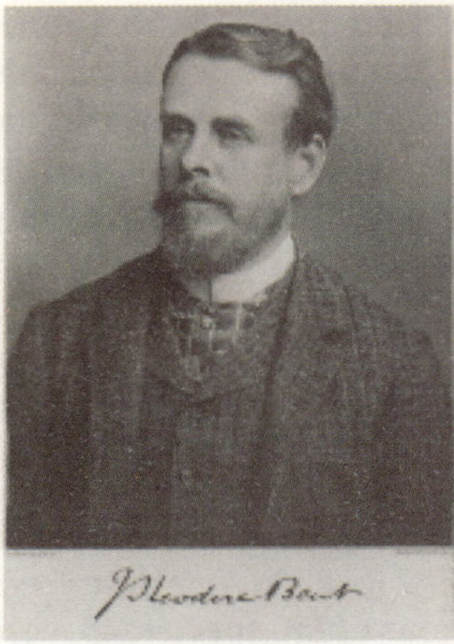

James Theodore Bent (1852–1897)

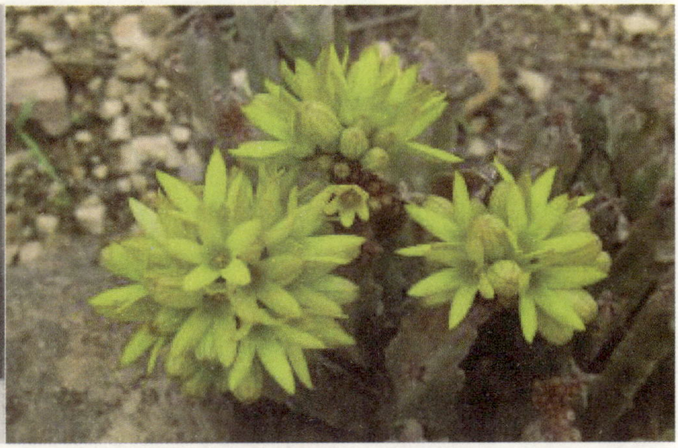

***Caralluma flava* Bent**

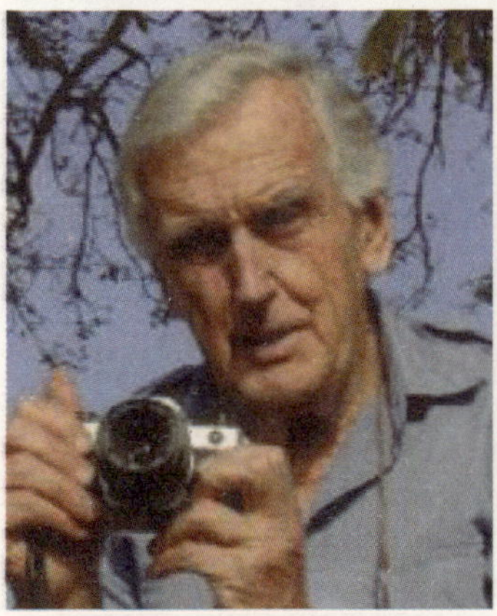

Darrel Charles Herbert Plowes (1925–)

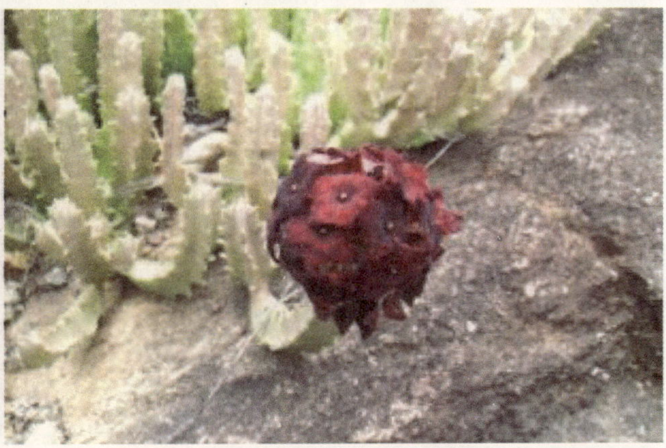

Boucerosia umbellata

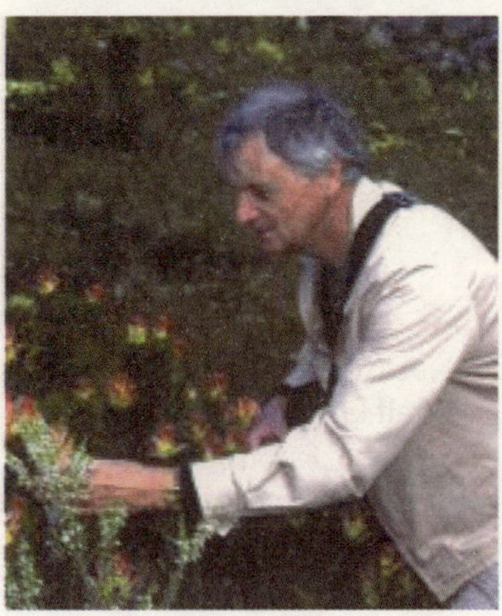

Robin Frandsen

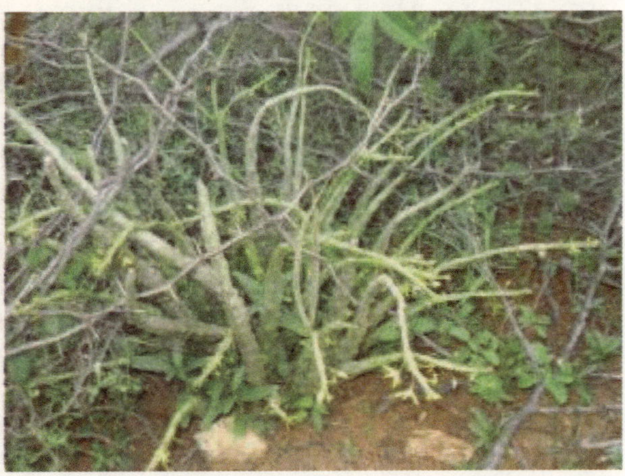

***Caralluma sarkariae* Lavranos et Frandsen**

Dr. N.E. Brown. He was himself interested in Stapeliads, and one of his occasional articles on succulents contained *Hoodia*, published in Journal of the Linnean Society in 1877. He was Director of the Royal Botanic Gardens at Kew, 1885-1905, he had the succulent house reconstructed to be more friendly to Stapelias and other succulents, these were now arriving from South Africa by the shipload, in larger numbers in any time since the death of Haworth. His most important achievement was to make Kew the botanical centre of the British Empire.

Nicholas Edward Brown (1849–1934)

The revision of the Stapelieae of Tropical and South Africa by Dr. Nicholas Edward Brown in the Flora of Tropical Africa, Vol. 4, Sect. 1, London in 1904, and in the Flora Capensis, Vol. 4 Sect. 1, London, 1909, is the starting point for the modern study of the tribe stapeliae. In the Flora of Tropical Africa 50 stapeliads were described, of which 10 were new, Flora Capensis contains descriptions of 210 species, 45 were new. The total of work done by Brown for Stapeliads can never be measured, the interest in succulents in England was at its lowest since the death of Haworth, and Brown had since a boy of 18 years been interested in Stapelias. His important contribution to the classification of Stapeliads came in 1878. He erected three new genera, *Diplocyatha*, *Huerniopsis* and *Trichocaulon* in the Journal of the Linnean Society. In 1895, he created a fourth new genus, *Edithcolea* in the Kew bulletin. He also wrote up the account of Sir Henry Barkly's plants, Stapeliae Barklyanae, in Hooker's Icones Plantarum, in 1890, and a complete enumeration of the Carallumas then known plus their synonyms in the Gardeners Chronicle 1892.

Rudolf Marloth (1855–1931)

Dr Rudolf Marloth was a German analytical chemist, came to South Africa 1883, he fell at once under the spell of the South Africa flora. He had thorough scientific training, he was interested in the living functions of plants, had an artistic skill in photography, happy literary style, friendly nature, wanted to share all his knowledge. He collected a fine herbarium, wrote many books and papers. His monumental work was "Flora of South Africa", bound in six volumes, helped to publish it through help of Sir Lionel and Lady Phillips Begun in 1913. He discovered no fewer than a dozen new species of *Stapelia*. To name but a few, *Stapelia flavopurpurea*, *Stapelia surrecta*, *Caralluma marlothii*, *Stapelia marlothii*, *Caralluma longipes*, *Caralluma simulans*, *Stapelia cincta*, *Trichocaulon meloforme*, *Trichocaulon pictum*, *Trichocaulon simile*, *Trichocaulon rusticum* and *Trichocaulon marlothii*.

Adolph Engler (1844–1930)

Geheimrath Dr. Adolph Engler director of Botanic Gardens and Museum at Dahlem, near Berlin, Germany. Principal director of Die Naturlichen Pflanzenfamilien, Leipzig, 1889. It was a monumental systematic account of all known genera of plants, and their important species. The Stapelieae was reviewed for this work by K. Schumann, in Vol. IV, 1895. New subsections of *Caralluma* and *Huernia* established. He also edited Botanische Jahrbcher, Leipzig, containing formal description of a number of Stapeliads. He made several botanic journeys into Africa, found *Caralluma priogonium* in German East Africa (Tanganyika) about 1890, *Trichocaulon engleri*

(*Larryleachia*) in South West Africa (Namibia), while on a trip with Prof. Kurt Dinter, about 1910. *Stapelia engleriana* was dedicated to him by Dr. R. Schlechter in 1905, it was first collected by Burke about 1840, and 65 years later was rediscovered growing in Dahlem Gardens.

John Medley Wood (1827–1915)

John Medley Wood was young English naval officer, retired from East Indian Merchant service in 1852, settled in Natal, appointed curator of Botanic Gardens at Durban in 1882 as well as Director of the Natal Herbarium. He established the Jubilee Palm House in 1898. He discovered *Stapelia woodii* (*Orbea woodii*). He has published Natal Plants in 6 Volumes, 1898-1912.. His name is linked also to *Encephalartos woodii*, a very rare cycad, only one plant in existence.

Rudolf Schlechter (1872–1925)

Dr. Rudolf Schlechter came to South Africa, in 1891, covered a vast territory in South Africa. He also explored Indonesia, New Guinea, South and Central America and Australia. His collection, herbarium specimens was deposited in botanical gardens at Zurich. His vast herbarium was destroyed during the bombing of Berlin in 1945. He has discovered *Caralluma chlorantha*, *Caralluma melanantha* (*Orbea melanantha*), *Huernia confusa* (*Huernia insigniflora*). *Huernia stapeliodes* was discovered on 13 February 1894 growing in the sand at Nazareth between Klipdam and Houtboschberg, about 90 km. east of Petersburg (Polokwane).

Terracino and Pappi (1862–1917)

Prof Achille Terracciano was Professor of Botany at the University of Sassari in Sardinia, from 1906 till his death. He made botanical expeditions to Eritrea 1892-93 with Augustino Pappi, discovered *Caralluma dicapuae*. Pappi was a gardener/collector for the Italian Colonial Herbarium then, he went to live at Asmara, Eritrea.

James Theodore Bent (1852–1897)

James Theodore Bent was an English traveller, made his last visit to Hadramaut, in Southern Arabia, east of the then Aden. He contracted malaria and died in London, May 5, 1897, just a few days after his return from field. Before his death he still went to Kew with a few fragments of plants he collected on his last journey. This includes 4 new species of *Stapelia*, *Echidnopsis bentii*, *Caralluma flava*, *Caralluma torta* and *Duvalia sulcata*.

Kurt Dinter (1868–1945)

Prof. Kurt Dinter's visit to South West Africa (present day Namibia) over a period of nearly 40 years, yielded a great harvest of new discoveries. He covered more than 25,000 miles, on foot, ox, cart, motor truck. He has collected upwards of 8000 plants. His publications were just as numerous, the most important for Stapeliad lovers are "Nue Pflanzen Deutch-Sudwest-Afrika", Okahandja in 1914. "Succulentenforschung in SudwestAfrik", part 1, Dahlem, 1923, and Part 2 Herrenhut published in 1928. Some of his discoveries include, *Stapelia portae-taurinae* (*Stapelia similis*), *Stapelia albocastanea* (*Orbea albocastanea*). Dinter and his wife Jutta are commemorated in the genus *Dintera* Stapf, *Dinteracanthus* C.B.Cl. ex Schinz, *Dinteranthus* Schwantes and *Juttadinteria* Schwantes, as well as a great number of specific names including *Amaranthus dinteri* Schinz, *Anacampseros dinter* Schinz, *Cissus juttae* Dinter, *Hoodia juttae* Dinter, *Stapelia dinteri* Berger, *Stapelia juttae* Dinter, *Trichocaulon dinteri* Berger and *Vigna dinteri* Harms. The botanical journal *Dinteria* was named in his honour to celebrate the centenary of his birth.

Auguste Jean-Baptiste Chevalier (1873–1956)

Auguste Jean-Baptiste Chevalier was born at Dumfront, France, June 23, 1873, Professor at the National Museum of Natural History in Paris, and director of the Revue de Botanique Appliquee. He made many botanising expeditions tropical, central and western Africa. On Jun 29, 1899 he rediscovered in the French Sudan *Caralluma decaisneana* (*Orbea decaisneana*) first collected in Senegal 70 years previously. On July 22 1899, collected *Caralluma retrospiciens* var. *tombuctuensis*, brought to his attention Yacouba-Dupuis.

Charles Eustace Pillans (1850–1919)

Charles Eustace Pillans, born at Rosebank, Cape Province in 1850. His favourite recreation was gardening, and collecting Cape succulents, grew many of the rarer plants at his home in Rosebank, includes *Stapelia jucunda, S. miscella, S.desmetiana, Huernia clavigera* var. *maritima*. Neville S Pillans (1884 – 1964) the only son of Charles Pillans, was the most eminent collector of Stapeliads, and he discovered a very large number of new species. He also rediscovered many of Masson's and other collector's plants that were not seen for years. In a visit in 1929 to Namaqualand he discovered 4 new species, one gave rise to new Genus *Stapeliopsis*. Some notable discoveries of Pillans include *Duvalia pillansii* and *Huernia pillansii*.

Alain Campbell White (1880–1951)

Alain Campbell White was an American botanist and chess champion, and Boyd Lincoln Sloane (1885 – 1955), American botanist specializing in Cacti. White was the author of several books on chess, the two were co-authors of the three volumes editions of *The Stapelieae* (1933, 1937), considered a major work in the field, and they also co-authored with R.A. Dyer, *The succulent Euphorbiae*. For their contribution a stapeliad genus named *Whitesloanea crassa* (now *Caralluma crassa*).

Frederic Henry Gravely (1885–1965)

Dr. Frederic Henry Gravely was an eminent arachnologist, entomologist, zoologist and student of archaeology, who conducted pioneering research and wrote extensively on various subjects during his tenure at the Indian Museum, Calcutta, and the Government Museum, Madras. When working as Assistant Superintendent at the Indian Museum, Calcutta, Dr. Gravely conducted pioneering classification work on the family *Passalidae*. He unified the monographs of early observers with the notes of Arrow and Zang to bring to the oriental passalids (1914), and the family itself in general (1918), the classification that is in vogue today with minor alterations. Dr. Gravely became the Superintendent of the Government Museum of Madras in 1920. Over the next two decades, he undertook the investigation of the littoral fauna of Krusadai Island, Gulf of Mannar, revived the Bulletin of the museum, and embarked on the scientific preservation, study and interpretation of the museum's collections. The most important of Dr. Gravely's many contributions to the subject was the monograph he collaborated on with T. N. Ramachandran (Curator of Archaeology 1925-1935) on the scientific basis for identifying the period of metal images. Dr. Gravely and P.V. Mayuranathan considerably enhanced the Herbarium and the botanical collections of the Madras museum and they worked out the Indian species of the genus *Caralluma*. In this monographic study, they have described one new species and four new varieties in the genus *Caralluma*.

Dr. J.S. Sarkaria (1987–1995)

Dr. Sarkaria was a succulent plant collector and gardener, he established seven and half acres of succulent garden with personal collections of about 3,500 succulent species in 1987. It has become a National Cactus and Succulent Botanical Garden and Research Institute at Panchkula, Chandigarh. He was maintained almost all native succulent asclepiads including his new discovery of *Caralluma bhupinderiana* and *Caralluma sarkariae*. He has explored extensively for Indian scculents over the subcontinent of India and has preserved all his collections both living and herbarium specimens at Chandigarh. After his death, the garden and herbarium lost its original beauty due to negligence of maintenance.

Darrel Charles Herbert Plowes (1925–)

Darrel C.H. Plowes is one among the greatest all-round naturalists of Zimbabwe. He is an authority on stapeliadas, orchids, butterflies, birds and has published numerous articles, books and even award-winning film. He has made numerous discoveries during his career with a number of newly described taxa named in his honour. He also was an outstanding photographer throughout his career and has a vast collection of excellent field photographs of nearly all the plants he has collected. He has revised several major groups of stapeliads, including descriptions of new genera and species. His taxonomic views are informed by extensive field work in 15 countries. His botanical collections included several new species: *Dissotis pulchra, Gazacloa, Dierama plowesii, Aloe plowesii, Huernia plowesii* and *Euphorbia clivicola*. His reclassification of *Caralluma* appeared in 1995, after his classification and generic delimitations of the genus *Caralluma* has much attracted many for molecular systematists. Even though he execratively segregated in the genus but also his classification made remarkable contribution for the modern classification of *Caralluma*.

M.G. Gilbert (1943–)

Gilbert is working in the herbarium, Royal botanic garden at Kew from 1985. He has botanized in Ethiopia for Flora of Ethiopia and he has described more than 50 new species to Ethiopian flora. His discoveries include in the section *Caralluma* are; *Caralluma lanellosa* and *Caralluma abayensis* from Somalia and several subspecies *Caralluma gracilipes* subsp. *edwardsiae, C. sprengeri* subsp. *foetida, C. sprengeri* subsp. *ogadensis, C. sprengeri* subsp. *laticorona*, and C. *arachnoidea* var. *breviloba*. His review of *Caralluma* and its segregates in 1990 created much attention on the taxonomy and classification of this group among modern taxonomists.

Ulrich Meve and Sigrid Liede (2002–)

Both of them are working in the Department of Plant Systematics, University of Bayreuth at Bayreuth. They are focussing on delimitation of monophyletic units on tribal, subtribal and generic level using molecular and classical tools. On this base, their study the morphological characters in an evolutionary context and try to identify causes for the surprising homologies between phylogenetically distant groups. On this ground they have found the many solutions for taxonomic problems in Asclepaids and in particularly succulent tuberous stapeliads. Based on the molecular data they have transferred *Caralluma dalzielli* to *C. subulata*. Similarly *Caralluma hexagona* transferred to *Monolluma hexagona*. One Indian *Caralluma* variety *Caralluma adscendens* var. *geniculata* was elevated to species level *Caralluma geniculata*. In 2004, they have published an illustrated handbook of succulent plants. It has elaborated almost all succulent asclepiads.

P.V. Bruyns (2002–)

Bruyns is working in Bolus herbarium in the section of Asclepiadoideae (Apocynaceae). He revised the genus *Ballyanthus, Orbea* and *Quaqua* in the Asclepiadaceae. The genus *Quaqua* incorporates all the 'hard stemmed' *Caralluma* species of the Western and Northern Cape of South Africa. The genus includes 13 species, 9 subspecies and 2 varieties. He spoke in an International succulents Congress in 2003 and 2006 at South Africa about the succulent plant diversity and conservations. He described the new species of *Orbea lutea* in South Africa. He also discovered a new genus *Baynesia* from Namibia. He has contributed the new classification of Asclepiadoideae in Apocynaceae. He has published revised phylogenetic classification assisted with molecular markers with Hedderson in 2005.

Dr. Ram Gandhi (1999–)

Dr. Ram Gandhi has published a book on Carallumas of the Indian subcontinent in 1999. In this book, he has given identification keys and elaborate descriptions for each species. Also he has given colorful photographs for all the species much easier to identify the species.

References

Abdel-Sattar, E., Ahmed, A.A., Heqazy, M.E., Faraq, M.A. and Al-Yahya, M.A. 2007. Acylated pregnane glycosides from *Caralluma russeliana*. *Phytochem.* **68(10):** 1459-1463.

Abdel-Sattar, E., Al-Yahya, M.A., Nakamura N. and Hattori, M. 2001. Penicillosides A-C, C-15 oxypregnane glycosides from *Caralluma penicillata*. *Phytochem.* **57:** 1213-1217.

Abdel-Sattar, E., Harraz, F.M., Al-Ansari, S.M., El-Mekkawy, S., Ichino, C., Kiyohara, H., Ishiyama, A., Otoquoro, K., Omura, S. And Yamada, H. 2008. Acylated pregnane glycosides from *Caralluma tuberculata* and their antiparasitic activity. *Phytochem.* **69(11):** 2180-2186.

Abdel-Sattar, E., Harraz, F.M., Gharieb, S.A., Elberry, A.A., Gabr, S. and Suliaman, M.I. 2011. Antihyperglycemic and hypolipidaemic effects of the methanolic extract of *Caralluma tuberculata* in streptozotocin-induced diabetic rats. *Nat. Prod. Res.* **25(12):** 1171-1179. Doi: 1080/14786419.2010.490782.

Abdel-Sattar, E., Meselhy, M.R. and Al-Yahya, M.A. 2002. New oxypregnane glycosides from *Caralluma penicillata*. *Planta Med.* **68:** 430-434.

Abdel-Sattar, E., Shehab, N.G., Ichino, C., Kiyohara, H., Ishiyama, A., Otoguro, K., Omura, S. And Yamada, H. 2009. Antitrypanosomal activity of some pregnane glycosides isolated from *Caralluma* species. *Phytomedicine* **16(6/7):** 659-664. doi: 10.1016/j.phymed.2009.02.009.

Abdul Aziz, Al-Yahya, M., Abdel-Sattar, E. and Guittet, E. 2000. Pregrane glycosides from *Caralluma russeliana*. *J. Nat. Prod.* **63(10):** 1451-1453.

Aditya, S. 2009. Habitat colour variance in *Caralluma sarkariae* Lavranos et Frandsen. *Asklepios*. **105:** 5-8.

Aditya, S. 2011a. *Caralluma moorei* Aditya *sp. nova.* A new species from East Coastal India. *Asklepios* **110:** 3-10; figs.

Aditya, S. 2011b. *Caralluma sarkariae* var. *longipedicellata var. nova.* A new *Caralluma* variety from Peninsular India. *Asklepios* **110:** 18-24.

Ahmad, M.M., Qureshi, S., Shah, A., Qazi, N.S., Rao R.M. and Al-Bakiri, M. 1983. Anti-inflammatory activity of *Caralluma tuberculata* alcoholic extract. *Fitoterapia.* **46:** 357-360.

Ahmad, V.U., Usmanghani, K. and Rizwani, G.H. 1988. New pregnane glycosides from *Caralluma tuberculata. J. Nat. Prod.* **51:** 1092-1097.

Ahmed, M.M., Quereshi, S., Al-Bekhari, Sha, A.M., Rao, A.K. and Qazi, R.M. 1993. Anti-inflammatory activity of *Caralluma tuberculata* alcoholic extract. *Fitoterapia* **64:** 357.

Ahmed, M.M., and Shaikh, M.U. 1989. Improvement in glucose tolerance by *Caralluma tuberculata, Acacia nilotica* and *Papaver somniferum. Pakistan J. Zool.* **21:** 325-332.

Al-Bekairi, I.S., Quereshi, S., Ahmed, M.M., Qazi, N.S., Khan, Z.A., Shah, A.H. 1992. Effect of *Caralluma tuberculata* on the cytological and biochemical changes induced by cyclophosphamide I mice. *Food Chem. Toxicol.* **30(8):** 719-722.

Albers, F. 1976. In IOPB Chromosome number reports LI. *Taxon* **25:** 155-164.

Albers, F. 1977. In IOPB Chromosome number reports LIII. *Taxon* **26:** 557-565.

Albers, F. 1981. In: Chromosome number reports. LXX. *Taxon* **30:** 76-77.

Albers, F. 1983. Cytotaxonomic studies in African Asclepiadaceae. In *Proceedings of the X AETFAT Congress.* AETFAT, Pretoria, Bothalia, pp. 795-798.

Albers, F. and Meve, U. 1991. Mixoploidy and cytotypes: a study of possible vegetative species differentiation in Stapeliads (Asclepiadaceae). *Bothalia* **21**: 67-72.

Albers, F. and Meve, U. 2001. A karyological survey of Asclepidaceae, Periplocoideae and Secamonoideae, evolutionary considerations in Apocynaceae *s.l.* In: Endress M, Stevens W.D. (eds). Procedings of the International Botanical Congress, St. Louis, 1999. *Ann. Missouri Bot. Gard.* **88 (4):** 624-656.

Albers, F. and Meve, U. 2002. *Illustrated handbook of succulent plants: Asclepiadaceae.* Vol. 5. Springer-Verlag, New York.

Al-Harbi, M.D., Qureshi, S., Raza, M., Ahmed, M.M., Afzal, M. and Shah, A.H. 1994. Evaluation of *Caralluma tuberculata* pretreatment for the protection of rat gastric mucosa against toxic damage. *Toxicol. Appl. Pharmacol.* **128:** 1-8.

Ali, S.I. 1983. *Flora of Pakistan.* Asclepiadaceae. 150. pp. 1-65.

Almeida, M.R. 2001. *Flora of Maharashtra.* Vol. 3. Blatter herbarium, Bombay.

Al-Yahya, M.A., Abdel-Sattar, E. and Guittet, E. 2000. Pregnane glycosides from *Caralluma russeliana. J. Nat. Prod.* **63:**1451-1453.

Al-Yahya, M.A., Tariq M., Khalifa, T.I. and Ashraf, I. 1983. Toxicity studies on *Caralluma penicillata* – a poisonous plant from Saudi Arabia. *Toxicon* (Suppl.) **3:** 9-12.

Ansari, N. M., Houlihan, L., Hussain, B. and Pieroni, A. 2005. Antioxidant activity of five vegetables traditionally consumed by South-Asian migrants in Bradford, Yorkshire, UK. *Phytoter. Res.* **19:** 907-911.

Aruna, V. 2006. *In vitro studies on micropropagation from mature explants of Caralluma spp (Asclepiadaceae).* Ph.D. thesis submitted to S.K. University, Anantapur, Andhra Pradesh, India.

Aruna, V., Kiranmai, C., Karuppusamy, S. and Pullaiah, T. 2009. Micropropagation of three varieties of *Caralluma adscendens.* – via nodal explants. *Indian J. Plant. Biochem. Biotech.* **18**(1): 121-123.

Babu, K.S., Rao, V.R., Radhakrishnan, S.V., Rao, J.M. and Rambabu, S.S. 2008. A new pregnane steroid from the stems of *Caralluma umbellata. J. Asian Nat. Prod. Res.* **10(11-12):** 1013-1016.

Bader, A., Braca, A. Tommasi, N.D. and Morelli, I. 2003. Further constituents from *Caralluma negevensis. Phytochem.* **62:** 1277-1281.

Baquar S. R. 2001. *Textbook of Economic Botany.* Ferozsons (Pvt) Ltd., Lahore.

Bhairavamurthy, P.V. and Krishna Mohan, R. 1991. A Contribution to the flora of Prakasam district, Andhra Pradesh. *J. Econ. Tax. Bot.* **15:** 49-63.

Bhandari, M.M. 1978. *The Flora of the Indian Desert* (ed. 1) Scientific Publishers.

Borchsenius, F. 2009. *FastGap 1.1.* Department of Biological Sciences, University of Aarhus, Denmark, Available at: http://192.38.46.42/aubot/fb/FastGap_home.htm.

Braca, A., Bader, A., Morelli, I., Scarpato, R., Turchi, G., Pizza C. and Tommasi N.D. 2002. New pregnane glycosides from *Caralluma negevensis. Tetrahedron.* **58:** 5837-5848.

Bramwell, D. 1990. The role of *In vitro* cultivation in the conservation of endangered species. In: J.E. Harnandez Bermejo, M. Demeute and Y. Hey wood (eds); *Conservation techniques in Botanic gardens,* Koeltz Scientific Books, Koenigstein, pp. 3-15.

Brown, N. E. 1878. The Stapeliae of Thunberg's Herbarium, with description of four new genera of Stapeliae. *Journ. Linn. Soc.* **17**: 162-172.

Brown, N. E. 1879. Stapeliae Barklyanae. *In Hook. Icon. Plant.* **10:** 1-13.

Brown, N. E. 1892. *Caralluma campanulata.* (With an enumeration of the other species of the genus, and description of several). *Gardener's Chronicle* (3) **12** (2): 369-370.

Brown, R. 1810. On the Asclepiadeae, a natural order of the plants separated from the Apocineae of Jussieu. *Mem. Wern. Nat. Hist. Soc.* I, 12-78.

Brummitt, R.K. 1992. *Vascular plant families and genera.* Royal Botanical Gardens, Kew.

Bruyns, P. V. 1981. A review of *Pectinaria* Haw., Stapeliopsis Pillans and a new genus, *Ophionella* (Asclepiadaceae). *Cactus and Succulent Journal of Great Britian* **43**: 61-83.

Bruyns, P. V. 1982. Notes on two little-known stapeliads from southern Africa. *Excelsa* **10**: 103-111.

Bruyns, P. V. 1983. Resurrection of the genus *Quaqua* N.E.Br. *Bradleya,* **1**: 33–78.

Bruyns, P. V. 1984. Uber *Caralluma subulata* (Forsskal) Decaisne von der arabischen Halbinsel. *Kakt.and Sukk.* **35(12):** 276-280.

Bruyns, P. V. 1986. Miscellaneous notes on Ceropegieae (Asclepiadaceae). *Bradleya* **4:** 29-38.

Bruyns, P. V. 1987. The genus *Caralluma* R. Brown in Isreal. *Israel. J. Bot.* **36:** 73-86.

Bruyns, P. V. 1988. A revision of the genus *Echidnopsis* Hook, f. (Asclepiadaceae). *Bradleya* **6:** 1-48.

Bruyns, P. V. 1989. Miscellaneous notes on Stapeliae. *Bradleya* **7:** 66-67.

Bruyns, P. V. 1990. Miscellaneous notes on Stapeliae (Asclepiadaceae). *Bradleya* **8:** 33-38.

Bruyns, P. V., 1993. A revision of *Hoodia* and *Lavrania* (Asclepiadaceae - Stapelieae). *Botanische Jahrbücher fiir Systematik* **115:** 145-270.

Bruyns, P. V. 1995. A re-assessment of the genera *Tridentea* Haw. and *Tromotriche* Haw. *South African J. Bot.* **61:** 180-208.

Bruyns, P. V. 1999a. The relationships of *Huerniopsis* and *Piaranthus* (Apocynaceae Asclepiadoideae) with a critical revision of the species. *Bot. Jahrb. Syst.* **121 (3):** 311-402.

Bruyns, P. V. 1999b. The systematic position of *Quaqua* (Apocynaceae Asclepiadoideae). *Systematic Botany* **24:** 379-397.

Bruyns, P. V. 1999c. A systematic assessment of *Ophionella* (Apocynaceae; Asclepiadoideae; Stapeliae). *Bot. J. Linn. Soc.* **131 (4):** 383-398.

Bruyns, P. V. 2000a. New combinations in the genus *Orbea*. *Aloe,* **37**: 72–76.

Bruyns, P. V. 2000b. Phylogeny and Biogeography of the Stapeliads. *Plant Syst. Evol.,* **221**, 199–226.

Bruyns, P. V. 2000c. *Baynesia,* a new genus of stapeliad from the northwestern-most corner of Namibia (Apocynaceae). *Novon,* **10:** 354–358.

Bruyns, P. V. 2002a. A Monograph of *Orbea* and *Ballyanthus* (Apocynaceae - Asclepiadoideae - Ceropegieae). *Systematic Botany Monographs* **63:** 1-190.

Bruyns, P. V. 2002a. The Southern African genera of the Stapeliads. *Aloe,* **39**: 52–63.

Bruyns, P. V. 2002b. A new species of *Stapeliopsis* from Namaqualand and a new combination in *Stapeliopsis* (Apocynaceae - Asclepiadoideae - Ceropegieae). *Aloe* **39 (3&4):** 80-82.

Bruyns, P. V. 2005. *Stapeliads of Southern Africa and Madagascar.* Umdaus Press, Hatfield, South Africa.

Bruyns, P. V. 2007. A new species of *Huernia* (Asclepiadoideae–Ceropegieae) from southern Angola. *Bothalia* **37(1):** 23-25.

Bruyns, P.V., Al Farsi, A. and Hedderson, T. 2010. Phylogenetic relationships of *Caralluma* R.Br. (Apocynaceae). *Taxon* **59:** 1031-1043.

Bruyns, P. V. and Jonkers H. A. 1993. The genus *Caralluma* R. Br. (Asclepiadaceae) in Oman. *Bradleya* **11:** 51-69.

Bruyns P. V. and Meve, U. 1995. The generic position of *Caralluma dodsoniana* (Asclepiadaceae). *Edinburgh J. Bot.* **52(2):** 195–203.

Bruyns, P. V. and Miller, A. G. 2002. *Socotrella*, a new genus of Stapeliad (Apocynaceae-Asclepiadoideae) from the Island of Socotra. *Novon.* **12(3):** 330–333.

Burkill, I.H. 1909. *A working list of the flowering plants of Baluchistan.* Govt. Press, Quetta, p.66.

Chopra, R.N., Nayar, S.L. and Chopra, I.C. 1956. *Glossary of Indian Medicinal Plants.* C.S.I.R, New Delhi.

Carmen, F., Felice, S., Giovanna, D.P., Mariarosa, S., Maurizio, B., Antonella, M., Sergio, R., Pietro, Z., Maurizio, S. 2009. Headspace volatile composition of the flowers of *Caralluma europaea* N.E.Br. (Apocynaceae). *Molecules* **14**: 4597-4613.

Castro, R.V.A., Francisco, C.G., Gonzalez, A.G., Hernandez, R. and Suarez, E. 1980. A 3,4-seco-triterpene from *Caralluma buchardii. Phytochem.* **19**: 2210-2212.

Chase, M.W. and James L, R. 2009. A phylogenetic classification of the land plants to accompany APG III. Botanical J. Lin. Soc. **161:** 122-127.

Cook, T. 1905. *Flora of Presidency of Bombay.* Botanical Survey of India, Howrah.

Courrier, K. 1992. Losses of biodiversity and their causes. In: K. Courrier (ed.) Global biodivertsity strategy- Guidelines for action to save, study and use earths biotic wealth sustainably and equitably. Pp. 7. WRI, IUCN and UNEP Publication. U.K.

Deepak, D., Khare, A. and Khare, M.P. 1989. Plant pregnanes. *Phytochem.* **28:** 3255-3263.

Deepak, D., Srivastav, S. and Khare, A. 1997. Pregnane glycosides. *Progress in the chemistry of organic natural products.* **71:** 169-325.

De Leo, M., Braca, A., De Tommasi, N., Saroga, R., Autore, G., Marzocco, S., Pizza, C., Morelli I. and Braca A. 2005. New Pregnane glycosides from *Caralluma dalzelli. Steroids* **70**: 573-585.

Doyle, J. J. and Doyle, J. L. 1987. A rapid DNA isolation procedure for small quantities of fresh leaf material. *Phytochem. Bull.* **19:** 11–15.

Edgeworth, M. P. 1862. Florula Malica. *J. Linn. Soc.* (Bot.) **6:** 179-210.

Ehrenberg, C.G. 1829. De antheris et polline Asclepiadearum. *Linnaea.* **4:** 94-97.

Endress, M. 2004. Apocynaceae: Brown and Now. *Telopea* **10:** 525-541.

Endress M. E. and Bruyns, P. V. 2000. A revised classification of the Apocynaceae *s.l. Botanical Review.* Lancaster **66:** 1-56.

Fischer, C. E. C. 1925. *Caralluma stalagmifera. R. Bot. Gard. Kew. Bull. Misc. Infor.* **1925:** 430-431.

Forster, P.I. 1991. The correct publication dates for some genera and species of Asclepiadaceae described by Robert Brown. *Asklepios* **52:** 78-79.

Gamble, J. S. 1915-35. *Flora of the Presidency of Madras.* Bishen Singh Mahendra Pal Singh, Dehra Dun.

Gautheret, R.J. 1945. Une voie nouvelle enbiologie vegetale: la culturedes tissue, Gallimard, Paris.

Gilbert, M. G. 1980. *Duvaliandra*: A new genus of stapeliad. *Cact. Succ. J. Gr. Brit.* **42:** 99-101.

Gilbert, M. G. 1990. A review of *Caralluma* R. Br. and its segregates. *Bradleya* **8:**1-32.

Gilbert, M. G. 1993. Notes on the Ceropegiae (Asclepiadaceae) of Ethiopia. *Nordic J. Bot.* **22 (2):** 209.

Girach R. D., Khan, H. and Ahmad, M. 2003. Botanical identification of Thuhar, seldom used as unani medicine. *Hamdard Medicus* **46(1):** 27-33.

Gomez-Dompa, A., Vazquez-Yanes, G. and Guevara, A. 1972. The tropical rain forest: A renewable resources. *Science.* **117:** 762-765.

Gravely, F.H. and Mayuranathan, P.V. 1931. The Indian species of the genus *Caralluma* (Fam.Asclepiadaceae). *Bull. Madr. Gov. Mus., new ser. Nat. Hist. Sect.* **4:** 1-28.

Habibuddin, M., Daghriri, H.A., Humaira, T., Qahtani, M.S.A. and Hefzi A.AH. 2008. Antidiabetic effect of alcoholic extract of *Caralluma sinaica* L. on streptozotocin-induced diabetic rabbits. *J. Ethnopharmacol.* **117**: 215-220.

Hajra, P.K. and Mudgal, V. 1997. *Plant diversity Hot spots in India- An overview.* Botanical Survey of India. Calcutta.

Halaweish, F.T., Huntimer, E. and Khalil, A.T. 2004. Polyoxypregnane glycosides from *Caralluma retrospiciens. Phytochem. Anal.* **15**.189-194.

Halim, A. and Khalil, A.T. 1996. Pregnane glycosides from *Caralluma retrospiciens. Phytochem.* **42**: 1135-1139.

Hall, T. A. 1999. BioEdit: a user-friendly biological sequence alignment editor and analysis program for Windows 95/98/NT. *Nucleic Acids Symposium Series,* **41**: 95–98.

Hansel R. 1975. Medicinal Plants and Empirical Drug Research. In. Tony Swain (ed.) *Plants in the Development of Modern Medicine* (1st Edition) Published by Harvard University Press, Cambridge. England. pp 161-174.

Haworth, A. H. 1812. *Synopsis Plantarum Succulantarum.* Taylor, London.

Hayashi, K., Iida, I., Nakao, Y. and Nakeko, K. 1998. Four pregnane glycosides, Boucerosides. AI, AII, BI and BII from *Boucerosia aucheriana. Phytochemistry.* **27:** 3919-3924.

Heneidak, R. 2001. Biosystematic studies on the species of subfamilies Asclepiadaceae and Periplocaceae (Family Apocynaceae *sensu lato*) in Egypt. Ph.D. thesis, Faculty of science, Suez Canal University.

Henry, A.N., Kumari, G.R. and Chithra, G.R.V. 1987. *Flora of Tamilnadu.* Ser. 1. Analysis Vol. 2. Botanical Survey of India. Coimbatore.

Hooker, J.D. 1885. *Flora of British India.* Vol. IV. London.

Hoope, H.A. 1975. *Drogen Kunde. Band I.* Angiospermen 8. Auflage Walterde Gruyter, Berlin. P.176.

Iwu, M.M. 1993. *Handbook of African Medicinal Plants.* CRC Press, Boca Raton.

Jadge, D.R and Naik, J.B. 2009. Anti-inflammatory activity of ethanolic and aqueous extracts of *Caralluma adscendens*. *J. Pharmacy Res.* **2**: 1228-1229.

Jagtap, A.P and Singh, N.P. 1999. *Fascicles of Flora of India.* Fascicle 24. Botanical Survey of India. Calcutta.

Jain, S.K. and Rao, R.R. 1977. *Field and Herbarium methods.* New Delhi.

Jayakar, B., Rajkapoor, B. and Suresh, B. 2004. Effect of *Caralluma attenuata* in normal and alloxan induced diabetic rats. *J. Herb. Pharmacother.* **4:** 35-40.

Jena, B.S., Jayaprakash, G.K., Singh, R.P. and Sakaria, K.K. 2002. Chemistry and biochemistry of hydroxycitric acid from *Garcinia. J Agric. Food Chem.* **50**:10-22.

Jonkers, B., and Walker, C.C. 1993. The Aslepiads of Morocco- a short commentary. *Asklepios.* **59:** 14-21.

Kamalakkannan, S., Rajendran, R., Venkatesh, R.V., Clayton, P., Akbarsha, M. 2010. Antiobesogenic and antiatherosclerotic properties of *Caralluma fimbriata* extract. *J. Nutrition and Metabolism* **10:** 1155-1561.

Kamil, M., Jayaraj, A.F., Ahmed, F., Gunasekhar, C., Samuel, S., Chan K. and Habibullah. 1999. Flavone glycosides from *Caralluma arabica. J. Pham. Pharmacol.* 225.

Kamil, M., Sheikh El, O.M., Jayaraj, A.F., Faizan, A., Gunasekhar, C., Samuel, S., Mazen, A.N. 2002. Quality control studies and standardisation of *Caralluma arabica* – A herbal Medicine. *Emirates Medical Journal* **20(2):** 131-137.

Karthikeyan, S., Sanjappa, M. and Moorthy, S. 2009. *Flowering Plants of India, Dicotyledons, volume I (Acanthaceae – Avicenniaceae).* Botanical Survey of India, Howrah.

Karuppusamy, S. 2011. Notes on the stapeliad genus *Boucerosia* (Asclepiadaceae) of South Peninsular India. *Aloe* **48(1):** 4-8.

Karuppusamy, S. and Pullaiah, T. 2007. Two new varieties of *Caralluma stalagmifera* C.E.C. Fisch. (Asclepiadaceae) from Peninsular India. *Rheedea.* **17 (1 & 2):** 41-45.

Karuppusamy, S., Ugraiah, A. and Pullaiah, T., 2012. Morphological and reproductive variations within the *Boucerosia umbellata* complex (Family: Apcyanceae; sub family: Ascleopidoideae) in South India. *Int. J. Plant Repr. Biol.,* **4:** 53-58.

Kaur, G., Rathore, T.S., Rama Rao, S. and Shekhawat, N.S. 1992. *In vitro* micropropagation of *Caralluma edulis* (Edgew.) Benth. et Hook.f. a rare edible plant species of Indian desert. *Indian J. Plant Gen. Res.* **5:** 51-56.

Khalil, A.T. 1995. Pregnane esters from *Caralluma retrospiciens. Fitoterapia.* **67**: 261-264.

Khatoon, S. And Ali, S.I. 1993. *Chromosome atlas of the Angiosperms of Pakistan.* Department of Botany, University of Karachi, Karachi.

Kiranmai, C. 2006. Tissue culture studies of *Pergularia daemia* (Forsk.) Chiov. and *Caralluma pauciflora* (Wight) N.E. Br (Asclepiadaceae). Ph.D. thesis submitted to S.K. University, Anantapur, Andhra Pradesh, India.

Kirtikar K.R and Basu, B.D. 1935. *Indian Medicinal Plants.* Vol. 2. L.M.Basu, Allahabad.

Kishore, M., Surendrababu, K., Hanumantharao, Y., Himabindu, G.N. and Janardhanan, M. 2010. Chemical examination of medicinal plant *Caralluma umbellata* (Asclepiadaceae) roots. *Int. J. Appl. Biol. Pharm. Tech.* **1(2):** 545-549.

Kumar, K.P., Khan, K.A., Anupama, K. And Prakash, K.V. 2008. Antifungal and anthelmintic activity of *Caralluma fimbriata* stem: a herb. *Int. J. Chem. Sci.* **6(3):** 1486-149.

Kumari, G.R. and Subba Rao, G.V. 1976. A new species of *Caralluma* (Asclepiadaceae) from India. *J. Bombay Nat. His. Soc.* **73:**194–196.

Kunert O., Simic, N., Ravinder, E., Adavi Rao, B. V., Ravi Kumar, B., Alex, R. M., Kuehnelt, D. and Appa Rao, A. V. N. 2009. Steroidal glycosides from *Caralluma umbellata. Phytochemistry Letters.* **2(3):** 134-138.

Kunert, O., Adavi Rao, B. V., Babu, G. S., Padmavathi, M., Ravi Kumar, B., Alex, R. M., Schfhly, W., Simic, N., Fhnelt, D. K. and Appa Rao, A. V. N. 2006. Novel Steroidal Glycosides from two Indian *Caralluma* species, *C. stalagmifera* and *C. indica. Helv. Chim. Acta.* **89:** 201-209.

Kunert, O., Gurunath Rao, V., Babu, G. S., Sujatha, P., Sivagamy, M., Anuradha, S., Adavi Rao, B. V., Ravi Kumar, B., Alex, R. M., Schühly, W., Kühnelt, D., Venkateshwara Rao,G. and Appa Rao, A. V. N. 2008. Pregnane Glycosides from *Caralluma adscendens* var. *fimbriata. Chemistry and Biodiversity.* **5:** 239-250.

Kuriyan, R., Raja, T., Srinivas, S.K., Vaza, M., Rajendran, R., Anura, V. and Kurpada, 2007. Effect of *Caralluma fimbriata* extract on appetite, food intake and anthropometry in adult Indian men and women. *Appetite* **48(3):** 338-344. doi:10.1016/j.appet.2006.09.013.

Lakshminarasimhan. P. and Sharma, B.D. 1991. *Flora of Nasik District.* Botanical Survey of India, Calcutta.

Lakshminarayana, K., Venkanna, P. and Pullaiah, T. 1997. *Flora of Krishna District,* M.D. Publications, New Delhi.

Lassmann, T. and Sonnhammer, E. L. 2005. Kalign – an accurate and fast multiple sequence alignment algorithm. *BMC Bioinformatics,* **6:** 298.

Lavrnos, J.J. and Frandsen, M.I. 1978. *Caralluma sarkariae. Cact. and Succ. J.* (U.S.A). **50:** 211.

Lawrence, R.M. and Choudary, S. 2004. *Caralluma fimbriata* in the treatment of obesity; 12th Annual world congress on antiaging medicine. December, 2-5, U.S.A.

Leach, L. C. 1975. The lectotype species of *Stapelia* L. and the reinstatement of *Orbea* Haw. (Asclepiadaceae). *Kirkia* **10:** 287 291.

Leach, L.C. 1978. A contribution towards a new classification of stapelieae (Asclepiadaceae) with a preliminary review of *Orbea* and description of three new genera. *Excelsa. Tax. Ser.* **1:** 1-75.

Leach, L. C. 1980. A revision of *Tridentea* Haw. (Asclepiadaceae). *Excelsa Tax. Ser.*, **2:** 1-68.

Leach, L. C. 1984. A revision of *Tromotriche* Haw. (Asclepiadaceae). *South African J. Bot.* **50:** 549-562.

Leach, L. C. 1985. A revision of *Stapelia* L. (Asclepiadaceae). *Excelsa Taxon. Ser.* **3:** 1-157.

Leach, L. C. 1988. A revision of *Huernia* R. Br. (Asclepiadaceae). *Excelsa Taxon. Ser.* **4:** 1-197.

Leach, L.C and Plowes, D.C.H. 1966. *Stapelieae* from South Tropical Africa, III. *J. S. Afr. Bot.* **32:** 299-303.

Leo, M.D., Tommasi, N.D., Sanogo, R., Giuseppina, A., Marzocco, S., Pizza, C., Morelli, I. and Braca, A. 2005. New pregnane glycosides from *Caralluma dalzielii*. *Steroides.* **70**: 573-585.

Liede, S. and Albers, F. 1994. Tribal disposition of Asclepiadaceae genera. *Taxon* **43:** 201-231.

Lin, L.J., Lin, L.Z., Gill, R.R., Cordell, G.A., Ramesh, M., Srilatha, B., Reddy, B. and Appa Rao, A.V.N. 1994. Pregnane glycosides from *Caralluma umbellata*. *Phytochem.* **35**: 1549-1553.

Loewenstein, A.B. and Garbari, F. 2004. Cytotaxonomic contribution to the Jordanian flora.3. The Stapelieae (Asclepiadaceae) in the Hisma basin (South Jordan). *Caryologia* **57(1):** 73-77.

Mabberley, D.J. 1993. *The plant book.* Cambridge University press, Cambridge.

Madhava chetty, K., Sivaji, K. and Tulasi Rao, K. 2008. *Flowering plants of Chittoor district, Andhra Pradesh, India.* Students offset Printers, Tirupati.

Madhuri, V., Amrutha, V.A. and Murthy, K.S.R. 2010. Evaluation of immunostimulating activities of *Caralluma* spp. *Int. J. Pharmacogn. Phytochem. Res.* **2(4):** 1-4.

Madhuri, V., Amrutha, V.A. and Murthy, K.S.R. 2011a. DNA fingerprinting profile of *Caralluma* species: An approach to molecular taxonomy. *Asian J. Biochem. Pharm. Res.* **1(2):** 500-506.

Madhuri, V., Amrutha, V.A. and Murthy, K.S.R. 2011b. Biochemical study of *Caralluma* species to understand species morphology. *Int. J. Appl. Biol. Pharm. Tech.* **2(1):** 139-144.

Mahmood, T., Muhammad, S. and Shinwari, Z.K. 2010. Molecular and morphological characterization of *Caralluma* species. *Pak. J. Bot.* **42(2):** 1163-1171.

Mali, K.K., Dias, R.J., Havaldar, V.D., Mahajan, N.S. 2009. Hypoglycemic activity of *Caralluma adscendens* in alloxan induced diabetic rats. *Ind. J. Chem.Sci.* **7**: 517-522.

Marwah, R.G., Fatope, M.O., Al Mahrooqi, R.S., Varma, G.B., Al Abadi, H. and Al-Burtamani, K.S. 2007. Antioxidant capacity of some edible and wound healing plants in Oman. *Food Chem.* **101**: 465-470.

Mary, S. 2006. Indian cactus is promising appetite suppresant and weight loss aid. Your guide to Thyroid Disease Newsletters at Thyroid info.com.

Matthew. K.M. 1983. *Flora of the Tamilnadu Carnatic.* Rapinat Herbarium, Tiruchirapalli.

Mc Corkle C. M. 1992. *Plants, Animal and People-Agropastoral Systems Research* (1st Edn). Published by Westview Press, Inc. Colorado.

Menon, A.R., Bhatti, K.M. and Menon, A.N. 1984. A new pregnane sterod from the stems of *Caralluma edulis. J. Chem. Soc. Pak.* **6(1):** 71-72.

Meve, U. 1994. The genus *Piaranthus* R. Br. (Asclepiadaceae). *Bradleya* **12:** 57-102.

Meve, U. 1995. Cytological and morphological differentiation in *Caralluma burchardi* (Asclepiadaceae). *Nordic J. Bot.* **15(5):** 459-467. Doi: 10.1111/j.1756-1051.1995.tb00178.x.

Meve, U. 1997. The genus *Duvalia* (Stapelieae): stem-succulents between the Cape and Arabia. *Pl. Syst. Evol. Suppl.*, suppl. **10**: 11-26.

Meve, U. and Heneidak, S. 2005. A morphological, karyological and chemical study of the *Apteranthes (Caralluma) europaea* complex. *Bot. J. Linn. Soc.* **149(4):** 419-432. Doi: 10.1111/j.1095-8339.2005.00448.x

Meve, U. and Liede, S. 1994. Floral biology and pollination in Stapeliads – new results and literature review. *Pl. Syst. Evol.* **192:** 99-116.

Meve, U. and Liede, S. 2002. A molecular phylogeny and generic rearrangement of the stapeloid Ceropegieae (Apocynaceae- Asclepiadoideae). *Plant Syst. Evol.* **234:** 171-209.

Meve, U. and Liede, S. 2004. Subtribal division of *Ceropegieae* (Apocynaceae-Asclepiadaceae). *Taxon.* **53:** 61-72.

Mikan, J.C. 1835. Curiosourum Exhibentie Ephemerides give observations *Apteranthes gussoneana.* Histories et Nova Acta Physico-medica Academeae Caesavece Leopodine-Carolinae Naturae. **17:** 594-623.

Muhammad, T.A. 1999. *Phytochemical studies on Caralluma tuberculata, Caralluma edulis and Pharmacological studies on Sida pakistanica.* Ph. D. Thesis, Univ. Karachi, Pakistan.

Müller, B. and Albers, F. 2002. *Caralluma.* In *Illustrated handbook of succulent plants: Asclepiadaceae.* Albers, F. and Meve, U. (eds.), Springer, pp 45–63.

Munster, R. 1990. *Angolluma,* a new genus. Part I. *Cact. Succ. J.* (*Woollhara*) **17:** 63-65.

Murashige, T. and Skoog, F. 1962. A revised medium from rapid growth and bioassays with tobacco tissue culture *Physiol Plant.* **15:** 473-497.

Munster, R. 1990. *Angolluma,* a new genus. *Cact. Succ. J. N.S.W.* vol. **17 (4):** 63-65.

Naik J.B and Jadge, D.R. 2009. Antiinflammatory activity of ethanolic and aqueous extracts of *Caralluma adscendens. J. Pharm. Res.* **2(7):** 1228-1229.

Navaneetham, N. 1980. On the chromosome numbers of some Asclepiadaceae from South India. *Proc. Indian Sci. Congr. Assoc.* (IIIC) **67**: 57.

Navaneetham, N. 1981. In: Chromosome number reports. LXXII. *Taxon* **30:** 696.

Navaneethan, N. and Sampathkumar, R. 1984. Chromosome number reports LXXXII. *Taxon* **33:** 126.

Naveen, M. 2011. *In vitro* propagation studies of *Boucerosia indica* Wt. and Arn., Determination of Nutritive Value, Mineral Elements and Protein Analysis of a few species of *Boucerosia* and *Caralluma.* Ph.D. thesis, Sri Krishnadevaraya University, Anantapur, India.

Nayar, M.P. 1996. *Hot spots of endemic plants of India, Nepal and Bhutan.* Tropical Botanic Garden and Research Institute. Trivandrum. India.

Nayar, M.P. and Sastry A.R.K. 1990. *Red Data Book of Indian plants.* Vol.3. Botanical Survey of India, Calcutta.

Neuwinger, H.D. 1994. *African Ethnobotany: Poisons and Drugs.* Chapman and Hall, New York, pp.238-239.

Neuwinger, H. D. 2000. *African Traditional medicine: a dictionary of plant use and applications with supplement search systems for diseases.* Medpharm Scientific Publishers, Stuttgart.

Nikaido, H., Shimizu, Y. and Mitsuhashi, H. 1967. Components of *Boucerosia aucheriana* Decne. *Chem. Pharm. Bull.* **15**: 725.

Ohia, S.E., Olubusayo, A., LeDay, A.M., Opere, C.A. and Bagchi, D. 2001. Effect of hydroxycitric acid on serotonin release from isolated rat brain cortex. *Res Comm Molec Pathol Pharmacol.* **109**: 210-216.

Oyama, M., Iliya, I., Tanaka, T. and Iinuma, M. 2007. Five new steroidal glycosides from *Caralluma dalzelli. Helvetica Chimia Acta* **90(1):** 63-71.

Pietro, Z., Maurizio, S., Maurizio, B., Antonella, M., Sergio, R., Carmen, F., Felice, S. 2010. Essential oil composition of stems and fruits of *Caralluma europaea* (Guss.) N.E.Br. (Apocynaceae). *Molecules* **15**: 627-638.

Plowes, D. C. H. 1990. An introduction to stapeliad genera. *Cactus and succulent journal* (U. S.), **62 (3):** 111-129.

Plowes, D. C. H. 1992. A preliminary reassessment of the genera *Hoodia* and *Trichocaulon* (Stapelieae: Asclepiadaceae). *Asklepios* **56:** 5-15.

Plowes, D. C. H. 1993. The taxonomy of *Quaqua* N. E. Brown. *Excelsa* **16:** 83-102.

Plowes, D.C.H. 1995. A reclassification of *Caralluma* R. Brown (Stapelieae: Asclepiadaceae). *Haseltonia* **3:** 49-70.

Plowes, D. C. H. 1997. *Larryleachia* and *Hoodia* (Stapelieae: Asclepiadaceae): some new nomenclatural proposals. *Excelsa* **17:** 3-28.

Plowes, D. C. H. 2003. *Huernia mccoyi* Plowes, a new asclepiad from western Yemen. *Cactus and succulent journal* (U. S.), **75 (2):** 81-83.

Plowes, D. C. H. 2007. Two new stapeliads from Yemen. *Excelsa* **21**: 9-14.

Plowes, D. C. H. 2008. *Angolluma taitica* (Bruyns) Plowes comb. nov. *Asklepios* **103:** 3-4.

Posada, D. 2008. ModelTest: phylogenetic model averaging. *Mol. Biol. Evol.,* **25**: 1253.

Preuss, H.G., Bagchi, D., Bagchi, M., Rao, C.V.S., Dey, D.K, Das, S., Satyanarayana, S. 2004. Weight management and mechanisms of action of a novel, natural extract of (-)- hydroxycitric acid (HCA-SX) and a combination of HCA-SX plus niacin-bound chromium and *Gymnema sylvestre* extract. *Diabetes, Obesity Metabolism.* **6**:171-180.

Pullaiah, T. 2008. Biodiversity and Conservation of Eastern Ghats. in Forest Biodiversity. **1:** 96-99 Muthuchelian, K., S.Kannaiyan and A. Gopalam (eds.). 2008. Forest biodiversity. Vol. 1. Associated Publishing Co., New Delhi.

Pullaiah, T. and Ali Moulali, D. 1997. *Flora of Andhra Pradesh,* Vol. II. Rubiaceae-Ceratophyllaceae. Scientific Publishers, Jodhpur.

Pullaiah, T., Prabhakar, C. and Ravi Prasad Rao, B. 1997. *Flora of Medak District (Andhra Pradesh).* Daya Publishing House, New Delhi.

Pullaiah, T., Prasanna, P.V. and Olulesu, G. 1992. *Flora of Adilabad District, Andhra Pradesh, India,* CBS Publishers and Distributor, Delhi.

Pullaiah, T., Ramakrishnaiah, V., Sandhya Rani, S. and Rao, P.N. 2000. *Flora of Guntur District, Andhra Pradesh, India.* Regency Publications, New Delhi.

Pullaiah, T. and Ravi Prasad Rao, B. 1995. *Flora of Nizamabad, Andhra Pradesh, India,* Bishen Singh Mahendra Pal Singh, Dehra Dun.

Pullaiah, T. and Silar Mohammed, M. 2000. *Flora of Ranga Reddi district.* Regency Publications, New Delhi.

Pullaih, T., and Yesoda, N. 1989. *Flora of Anatapur District, Andhra Pradesh, India.* Bishen Singh Mahendra Pal Singh, Dehra Dun.

Qiu, S.X., Cordell, G.A., Ravi Kumar, B., Nageshwara Rao, Y., Ramesh, M., Kokate C.K. and Appa Rao, A.V.N. 1999. Bisdesmosidic pregnane glycosides from *Caralluma lasiantha. Phytochem.* **50:** 485-491.

Qiu, S.X., Lin, L.Z., Cordell, G.A., Ramesh, M., Ravi Kumar, B., Radha Kishan, M., Krishna Mohan, G., Reddy, B.M., Nageshwara Rao, Y., Srinivas, B., Thomas N.S. and Appa Rao, A.V.N. 1997. Acylated C-21 steroidal Bisdesmosidic glycosides from *Caralluma umbellata. Phytochem.* **46:** 333-340.

Radhakrishnan, R., Zakaria, M., Islam, M.W., Liu, X.M., Chan, K. and Habibullah, M. 1999. Antihyperglycemic effects of *Caralluma arabica* in diabetic mice. *J. Pharm. Pharmacol.* **51:**116.

Raja Sreelatha, V. 2007. *In vitro* studies on mature explants of *Caralluma sarkariae* Lavranos et Frandsen and *Caralluma stalagmifera* Fischer (Asclepiadaceae). Ph.D. thesis, Sri Krishnadevaraya University, Anantapur, India.

Raja Sreelatha, V., Karuppusamy, S. and Pullaiah, T. 2011. Micropropagation of *Caralluma sarkariae* Lavranos et Frandsen: An important medicinal plant. *Plant Tissue Culture and Biotechnology* (in press)

Raja Sreelatha, V., S.Karuppusamy, B.Susheela, M.Sowgandhika and T.Pullaiah. 2008. *In vitro* propagation of *Caralluma sarkariae*. *J.Tropical Med. Plants* **9**: 390-393.

Raja Sreelatha, S.Sandhya Rani, P.V.Krishna Reddy, M.Naveen, A. Ugraiah and T.Pullaiah. 2009. *In vitro* propagation of *Caralluma sarkariae* Lavranos et Frandsen – An endemic and endangered medicinal plant. *Indian J. Biotech.* **8**: 236-239.

Ramachandran, V.S., Joseph, S., John, H.A. and Sofiya, C. 2011. *Caralluma bicolor sp. nov.* (Apocynaceae, Asclepidoideae) from India. *Nordic J. Bot.* **29:** 447-450.

Ramachandran, V.S., Thomas, B., Sofiya, C. and Sasi, R. 2011. Rediscovery of an endemic plant *Caralluma diffusa* (Wight) N.E.Br. (Asclepiadaceae) from Coimbatore district, Tamil Nadu, India, after 160 years. *J. Threatened Taxa* **3(3):** 1622-1623.

Ramakrishna, T.M. and Afzalunnisa, K. 1981. In: Chromosome number reports LXXIII. Taxon **30**: 851-852.

Rambaut, A. 2007. FigTree, a graphical viewer of phylogenetic trees. *See http://tree. bio. ed. ac. uk/software/figtree.*

Ram Gandhi. 1999. *Carallumas of the Indian sub-continent.* Indian Society of Cactii and Succulents, New Delhi.

Ramesh, M., Nageshwar Rao, Y., Appa rao, A.V.N., Prabhakar, M.C., Seshagiri Rao, C., Muralidhar, N. and Madhava Reddy, B. 1998. Antinociceptive and anti-inflammatory activity of a flavonoid isolated from *Caralluma attenuata. J. Ethnopharmacol.* **62(1):** 63-66. doi: 10.1016/So378-8741(98)00048-8.

Ramesh, M., Nageshwar Rao, Y., Rama Kumar, M., Appa rao, A.V.N., Prabhakar, M.C. and Madhava Reddy, B. 1999a. Antinociceptive and anti-inflammatory activity of carumbelloside-I isolated from *Caralluma umbellata. J. Ethnopharmacol.* **68:** 349-352.

Ramesh, M., Nageshwar Rao, Y., Rama Kumar, M., Krishna Mohan, G., Ravi Kumar, B., Appa Rao, A.V.N., Radhakishan, M. and Madhava Reddy, B. 1999b. Flavone glycosides from *Caralluma* species. *Biochemical Syst. Ecol.* **27:** 271-276.

Ramesh, M., Rao, Y.N., Kumar, Mohan, G.K., Kumar, B.R., Appa Rao, A.V.N., Krishna, M.R. and Reddy, B.M. 1999. Flavone glycosides from three *Caralluma* species. *Biochemical Syst. Ecol.* **27:** 85-86.

Rathore, M.S., Dagla, H.R., Singh, M. and Shekhawat, N.S. 2008. Rational development of *in vitro* methods for conservation, propagation and characterization of *Caralluma edulis*. *World J. Agric. Sci.* **4(1):** 121-124.

Rathore, M.S. and Shekhawat, N.S. 2009. Biotechological approaches for conservation of germplasm, problems of propagation and sustainable utilization of some important asclepiadaceae plants of India Thar Desert. *Global J. Environ. Res.* **3(1):** 45-61.

Rathore, M.S., Gehlot, H.S. and Shekhawat, N.S. 2010. Biotechnological approaches for propagation and prospecting of important medicinal plants from Indian Thar desert. *Int. J. Plant production.* **4(1):** 67-72.

Rebecca, K., Tony, R., Srinivas, S.K., Mario, V., Rajendran, R., Acura, V. 2007. Effect of *Caralluma fimbriata* extract on appetite, food intake and anthropometry in adult Indian men and women. *Appetite* **48**: 338-344.

Reddy, B.M., Byahatii, V., Appa Rao, A.V.N. and Ramesh, M. 1996. Anti-inflammatory activity of *Stapelia nobilis* and *Caralluma stalagmifera*. *Fitoterapia.* **67:** 545-547.

Repetto R and Gillis, M. 1990. *Public policies and the misuse of forest resources* (1st Edition). Published by Cambridge University, New York. USA.

Rizwani, G.H. 1991. *Phytochemical and biological studies on medicinal herbs Caralluma tuberculata and Caralluma edulis.* Ph.D. thesis, University of Karachi, Pakistan.

Rizwani, G.H., Usmanghani, K., Ahmed, M. and Ahmed, V.U. 1990. Flavone glycosides of *Caralluma tuberculata* N.E. Brown. *Pakistan J. Pharm. Sci.* **3:** 27-32.

Rizwani, G.H., Usmanghani, K., Ahmed, M. and Ahmed, V.U. 2006. Pregnane glycosides from *Caralluma tuberculata.* Natural product Letters **2(2):** 97-104.

Ronquist, F. and Huelsenbeck, J. P. 2003. MrBayes 3: Bayesian phylogenetic inference under mixed models. *Bioinformatics,* **19:** 1572–1574.

Rowley, G. 1980. *Name that succulent: 91.* Stanley Thornes, Cheltonham.

Roxburgh, W. 1795. *Plants of the Coast of Coramandel.* London.

Sallanon, H. and Maziere, Y. 1992. Influence of growth room and vessel humidity on the *in vitro* development of rose plant. *Plant Cell Tiss. Org. Cult.* **30:** 12-125.

Samata, A and Vastavaya Raju, S. 2004. *Caralluma adscendens* var. *fimbriata* (Asclepiadaceae): Another overlooked succulent from Andhra Pradesh. *J. Econ. Tax. Bot.*

Sang, T., Crawford, D. J. and Stuessy, T. F. 1995. Documentation of reticulate evolution in peonies (*Paeonia*) using internal transcribed spacer sequences of nuclear ribosomal DNA: implications for biogeography and concerted evolution. *Proc. Nat. Acad. Sci. USA,* **92:** 6813–6817.

Santapau, H. 1955. *Botanical collector's manual.* Calcutta.

Sarkaria, J.S. 1980. In search of *Frerea indica* Dalz. In *Asclepiadaceae* **21:** 29-34.

Saxena, H.O. and Brahmam, M. 1995. *The Flora of Orissa.* Bhubaneswar.

Schumann, K. 1895. Asclepiadaceae. Engler and Prantl's *Die Naturalichen Pflanzen familien Gattugen wichtigeren Arten inbesondre den Nutzpflanzen* IV (2) pp. 189-306. (*Caralluma*, pp. 265 and 277-278.).

Sedgwick, L. J. 1921. New Bombay species. *J. Indian Bot.* **2:** 125-126.

Shabbir G., Bahadur, S. and Choudhry, M. R. 2003. Botanical description, significance and production technology of some important medicinal herbs. *Hamdard Medicus* **46 (1):** 23-26.

Sharma, B.D., Singh, N.P., Raghavan, R.S. and Deshpande, U.R. 1984. *Flora of Karnataka*. Botanical Survey of India, Howrah.

Shetty, B.V. and Singh. V. 1991. *Flora of Rajasthan*.

Simmons, M.P. and Ochoterena, H. 2000. Gaps as characters in sequence-based phylogenetic analyses. *Syst. Biol.* **49:** 369–381.

Singh, M. P., Srivastava, J. L. and Pandey, S. N. 2003. *Indigenous Medicinal Plants, Social Forestry and Tribals* (1st Edition). Published by Daya Publishing House Delhi-110035.

Singh, N.P., Mudgal, V., Khanna, K.K., Srivastava, S.C., Sahoo, A.K., Bandopadyay, S., Aziz, N., Das, M., Bhattacharya, R.P. and Hajra, P.K. 2001. *Flora of Bihar Analysis.* BSI, Calcutta.

Singha, S. and Bhatia, S.K. 1988. Short proliferation of pear cultures on medium containing thidiazuron and benzyl amino purine. *Hort. Sci.* **23:** 227-228.

Soni, M.G., Burdock, G.A., Preuss, H.G., Stohs, S.J., Ohia, S,E,, Bagchi, D. 2004. Safety assessment of (-) –hydroxycitric acid and Super Citrimax ®, a novel calcium/ potassium salt. *Food and Chemical Toxicology.* **42(9):** 1513-1529.

Subba Rao, G.V. and Kumari, G.R. 2002. *Flora of Visakhapatnam District, Andhra Pradesh,* Volume. 1, BSI, Calcutta.

Suresh Babu. K., Subba Rao, V. R., Madhusudana Rao, S. V. R. J. and Rambabu, S. S. 2008. A new pregnane steroid from the stems of *Caralluma umbellata*. *J. Asi. Nat. Prod. Res.* **10 (11):** 1013 – 1016.

Suryanarayana, B. and Sreenivasa Rao, A. 2001. *Flora of Nellore district Andhra Pradesh.* Gurudev Prakashan, Shrirampur, Maharashtra.

Swofford, D, L. 2002. *PAUP*:Phylogenetic Analysis Using Parsimony (and other methods), Version 4 beta 10.* Sinauer Press, Sunderland, Mass,

Taberlet, P., Gielly, L., Pautou, G. and Bouvet, J. 1991. Universal primers for amplification of three non-coding regions of chloroplast DNA. *Plant Mol. Biol.*, **17**: 1105–1109.

Tambe, D.A., Chaudhari, T.B. and Chaudhuri, S.R. 2010a. Analgesic activity of *Caralluma adscendens* Roxb. (aerial parts). *Int. J. Pharm. Res. Dev. – Online.* **2(7):** 1-4.

Tambe, D.A., Chaudhari, T.B. and Chaudhuri, S.R. 2010b. Phyto-pharmacology of *Caralluma adscendens* Roxb: A review. *Phacos. J.* **2**: 33-38.

Tanaka, T., Tsukamoto, S. and Hayashi, K. 1990. Pregnane glycosides from *Boucerosia aucheriana*. *Phytochem.* **29:** 229-237.

Tatiya, A.U., Kulkarni, A.S., Surana S.J. and Bari N.D. 2010. Antioxidant and hypolipidemic effect of *Caralluma adscendens* Roxb. in alloxanized diabetic rats. *Int. J. Pharmacol.* **6:** 400-406. doi: 10.3923/ijp.2010.400.406.

Tatiya, A.U., Petal, U.K., Kulkarni, A.S. and Surana, S.J. 2007. Evaluation of antibacterial activity of *Caralluma adscendens* Roxb. *Indian Drugs* **44(8):** 622.

Tetali, P.S., Kulkarni, D.K., Kumbhhojkar, M.S. 1997. Studies on the status and conservation of *Frerea indica*. *J. Bomaby Nat. Hist. Soc.* **94**: 115-121.

Tideman, J. and Hawker, J.S. 1982. *In vitro* propagation of latex-producing Plants. *Ann Bot.* **49:** 273-279.

Tilman, D. 2000. Causes, consequences and ethics of biodiversity. *Nature.* **405:** 208–211.

Ugraiah, A. 2010. *Diversity of the genus Caralluma in India and In vitro propagation of Caralluma bhupinderiana Sarkaria and Boucerosia truncato-coronata Sedgewick (Asclepiadoideae: Apocynaceae).* Ph.D.thesis, Sri Krishnadevaraya University, Anantapur, India.

Ugraiah, A., Karuppusamy, S., Sandhya Rani, S. and Pullaiah, T. 2010. Notes on *Boucerosia indica* (Wight. and Arn.) Plowes (Family: Asclepiadaceae). *J. Econ. Tax. Bot.* **34(4):** 886-889.

Ugraiah, A., Raja Sreelatha, V., Krishna Reddy, P.V., Rajasekhar, K., Sandhya Rani, S., Karuppusamy, S. and Pullaiah, T. 2011. *In vitro* shoot multiplication and conservation of *Caralluma bhupinderiana* Sarkaria – an endangered medicinal plant from South India. *Afr. J. Biotech.* **10(46):** 9328-9336.

Usmanghani, K., Rizwani, G.M. and Ahmad, M. 1987. Chemical investigations of medicinal herb *Caralluma tuberculata* Decne. *J. Pharm. Univ. Karachi* **5(2):** 133-

Vajravelu, E. 1990. *Flora of Palghat.* Botanical Survey of India. Calcutta.

Venkata Raju, R.R. and Pullaiah, T. 1995. *Flora of Kurnool.* Bishen Singh Mahendra Singh, Dehra Dun.

Venkatesh, S., Dayanand Reddy, G., Madhava Reddy, B., Ramesh, M. and Appa Rao, A.V.N. 2003. Antihyperglycemic activity of *Caralluma attenuata*. *Fitoterapia.* **74(3)**: 274-279.

Ventateswarlu, J., Murthy, P.V.B. and Rao, P.N. 1972. *Flora of Visakhapatnam.* Andhra Pradesh Akademi of Science. Hyderabad. Andhra Pradesh.

Villalba, M.B.C. 2006. Nomenclatural changes in *Apteranthes* Mikan (Asclepiadoideae, Apocynaceae). *Flora Montiberica* 32: 15-20.

Von Eum, J. and Reichstein, T. 1948. *Helv. Chim. Acta.* **27:** 1146.

Wadood, A., Wadood, N. and Shah, S.A. 1989. Effects of *Acacia arabica* and *Caralluma edulis* on blood glucose levels of normal and alloxan diabetic rabbits. *J Pak. Med. Assoc.* **39(8):** 208-212.

Waheed, A., Barker, J., Barton, S.J., Khan, G.M., Najm-Us-Saqib, Q., Hussain, M., Ahmed, S., Owen, C. and Carew, M.A. 2011. Novel acylated steroidal glycosides from *Caralluma tuberculata* induce caspase-dependent apoptosis in cancer cells. *J. Ethnopharmacol.* (e pub ahead of print).

Wallich, N. 1830. *Plantae Asiaticae Rariores.* I. Llondon.

Wealth of India. 1950. Council of Scientific and Industrial Research, New Delhi.

Wealth of India. 1992 Council of Scientific and Industrial Research, New Delhi.

White, A. and Sloane, B.L. 1937. *The stapelieae* ed. 2, vol. I. Abbey San Encino Press, Pasadena, California.

White, T.J., Bruns, T., Lee, S., Taylor, J., *et al.* 1990, Amplification and direct sequencing of fungal ribosomal RNA genes for phylogenetics. *PCR protocols: a guide to methods and applications.* **18:** 315–322.

Wight, R. 1850. *Icones Plantarum Indiae Orientalis.* IV. Madras.

Wight, R. and Walker- Arnott, G. A. 1834. In Wight's *Contributions to the Botany of India.*

Wight. R. and Walker-Arnott, G. A. 1834. *Prodromus Florae Peninsulae Indiae Orientalis* containing abridged descriptions of the plants found in the Peninsula of British India, arranged according to the natural system. Parbury, Allen and Co., London,

Wink, M., Alfermann, A.W., Franke, R., Wetterauer, B., Distl, M., Windhovel, J., Krohn, O., Fuss, E., Garden, H., Mohagheghzaden, A., Wildi, E. and Ripplinger, P. 2005. Sustainable bioproduction of phytochemicals by plant *in vitro* cultures: anticancer agents. *Plant Genetic Resour.* **3:** 90-100.

Wyk, B.E.V. and Wink, M. 2004. *Medicinal plants of the world.* Pretoria, Briza.

Yadav, S.R and Sardesai, M.M. 2002. *Flora of Kolhapur District.* Shivaji University Kalhapur.

Zakaria, M.N.M., Islam, M.W., Radhakrishnan, R., Chen, H.B., Ismail, A., Chan, K. and Habibullah, M. 1999. Evaluation of antinociceptive and anti-inflammatory properties of *Caralluma arabica. J. Pharm. Pharmacol.* **51:** 117.

Zakaria, M.N.M., Islam, M.W., Radhakrishnan, R., Chen, H.B., Kamil, M., Al-Gifri, A.N., Chan, K. and Al-Attas, A. 2001. Antinociceptive and anti-inflammatory properties of *Caralluma arabica. J. Ethnopharmacol.* **76:** 155-158.

Zakaria, M.N.M., Islam, M.W., Radhakrishnan, R., Liu, X.M., Ismail, A., Kamil, M., Chan, K. and Al-Attas, A. 2002. Anti-gastric ulcer and cytoprotective properties of *Caralluma arabica. Pharmaceutical Biology.* **40:** 225-230.

Zwickl, D. J. 2006. *Genetic algorithm approaches for the phylogenetic analysis of large biological sequence datasets under the maximum likelihood criterion.* Ph. D. dissertation, The University of Texas at Austin.

Index to Scientific Names

(Italicized Names Indicate Synonymy)